W9-AGF-523

Herbal Therapy & Supplements

A Scientific & Traditional Approach

Merrily A. Kuhn, RN, PhD
President, Educational Services, Inc.
Hamburg, New York
Associate Professor, Daemen College
Amherst, New York

David Winston, AHG
Herbalist AHG and Ethnobotanist
Herbal Therapeutics, Inc.
Washington, New Jersey

TEXT CONSULTANT

Ara DerMarderosian, PhD
Professor of Pharmacognosy
Research Professor of Medicinal Chemistry
Roth Chair of Natural Products
University of the Sciences in Philadelphia
Philadelphia, Pennsylvania

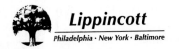
Lippincott
Philadelphia · New York · Baltimore

Acquisitions Editor: Margaret Zuccarini
Editorial Assistant: Helen Kogut
Senior Project Editor: Sandra Cherrey Scheinin
Senior Production Manager: Helen Ewan
Senior Production Coordinator: Michael Carcel

Art Director: Carolyn O'Brien
Manufacturing Manager: William Alberti
Indexer: Ellen Brennan
Printer: R. R. Donnelly & Sons

Copyright © 2000 by Lippincott Williams & Wilkins. All rights reserved. This book is protected by copyright. No part of it may be reproduced, stored in a retrieval system, or transmitted, in any form or by any means—electronic, mechanical, photocopy, recording, or otherwise—without the prior written permission of the publisher, except for brief quotations embodied in critical articles and reviews and testing and evaluation materials provided by publisher to instructors whose schools have adopted its accompanying textbook. Printed in the United States of America. For information write Lippincott Williams & Wilkins, 530 Walnut Street, Philadelphia, PA 19106.

Materials appearing in this book prepared by individuals as part of their official duties as U.S. Government employees are not covered by the above-mentioned copyright.

9 8 7 6 5 4 3 2 1

Library of Congress Cataloging-in-Publication Data
Kuhn, Merrily A., 1945-
   Herbal therapy and supplements : a scientific and traditional approach / Merrily A. Kuhn, David Winston ; text consultant, Ara DerMarderosian.
      p. ; cm.
   Includes bibliographical references and index.
   ISBN 0-7817-2643-3 (alk. paper)
   1. Herbs—Therapeutic use—Handbooks, manuals, etc. 2. Dietary supplements—Handbooks, manuals etc. I. Winston, David (David E.) II. Der Marderosian, Ara Harold, 1935-III. Title.
      [DNLM: 1. Medicine, Herbal—Handbooks. 2. Alternative Medicine—Handbooks. WB 39 K96h 2000]
RM666.H33 K84 2000
615'.321—dc21
                                                                    00-065514

Care has been taken to confirm the accuracy of the information presented and to describe generally accepted practices. However, the authors, editors, and publisher are not responsible for errors or omissions or for any consequences from application of the information in this book and make no warranty, express or implied, with respect to the contents of the publication.

The authors, editors, and publisher have exerted every effort to ensure that drug selection and dosage set forth in this text are in accordance with current recommendations and practice at the time of publication. However, in view of ongoing research, changes in government regulations, and the constant flow of information relating to drug therapy and drug reactions, the reader is urged to check the package insert for each drug for any change in indications and dosage and for added warnings and precautions. This is particularly important when the recommended agent is a new or infrequently employed drug.

Some drugs and medical devices presented in this publication have Food and Drug Administration (FDA) clearance for limited use in restricted research settings. It is the responsibility of the health care provider to ascertain the FDA status of each drug or device planned for use in his or her clinical practice.

To my parents, Audrey and Norbert Kuhn, who taught me perseverance;

To my husband, James, the love of my life, for his devotion, care, and daily concern;

To Martha Kulwicki, a loving and beautiful person, who taught me to laugh and appreciate life day to day;

To Susan Doherty, my administrative assistant, for her organization and typing of this manuscript; and

To all readers who are willing to take a step beyond their comfort zone into complementary medicine!

Merrily A. Kuhn, RN, PhD

I would like to dedicate this book to the generations of herbalists who, by practicing their craft, have left us the legacy of traditional herbal medicine. Specifically, I sincerely thank my teachers, colleagues, patients, and students for all they have taught me.

David Winston, Herbalist, AHG

Reviewers

Susan M. Cohen, DSN, C-FNP
Associate Professor
Yale University
New Haven, Connecticut

M. Katherine Crabtree, DNSc, ANP, RNCS
Associate Professor
Oregon Health Sciences University School of Nursing
Portland, Oregon

Carol DeCicco, RN, CS, CNSN, MSN
Nutrition Support Consultant
West Jersey Hospital
Voorhees, New Jersey

Margaret De Jong, RN, MS, FNP
Nurse Practitioner and Interchurch Medical Assistant
Mennonite Central Committee
Fort Lauderdale, Florida

Margaret H. Doherty, RN, MS, CCRN
Instructor, Department of Nursing
Sonoma State University
Rohnert Park, California

Sara Douglas, RN, MS, FNP
Student
Indiana Wesleyan University
Marion, Indiana

Mary Rebecca Harry, RN, BSN, MEd
Clinical Instructor
Crowder College
Neosho, Missouri

Kimberly Thomas, RN
Wound Care and Infection Control Coordinator
Integrated Health Services at Mountian View
Greensburg, Pennsylvania

Michelle R. Wolfe, RN, MSN, ANP-C
Faculty
George Washington University Nurse Practitioner Program
Washington, District of Columbia

Foreword

As text consultant for this book I was pleased to see that it has been produced as a joint venture by a registered nurse with a PhD in physiology and a noted herbalist. This blend of the best of reductionist science and holism has resulted in a well-balanced overview of herbals and supplements. Theory and rationale are covered in the front, while the majority of specific items is covered in a monographic format. Overall, it represents a welcome addition to the number of references now appearing on the topics of natural agents with possible preventable and possibly curative properties. While we are still in the early period of rediscovery of new agents from nature, this reference offers a good stepping-stone into the ultimate acceptance of many new modalities for the management of illness and the promotion of wellness. It is well referenced and should be useful to all health professionals.

Ara DerMarderosian, PhD
Professor of Pharmacognosy and
    Medicinal Chemistry
Roth Chair of Natural Products
Scientific Director
Complementary and Alternative
    Medicines Institute
University of the Sciences in
    Philadelphia

Preface

Herbal therapy has its roots in history and folk medicine. As we enter the new millennium, herbal therapy is reaching a turning point. It is becoming a field of science with its own research and data base. Socrates once said, "There is only one good: knowledge; and one evil: ignorance." Certainly this statement should guide us as health care professionals to learn as much as we can from both worlds of herbal therapy: the traditional use passed on from eclectic physicians and folk practitioners, and now the scientific evidence that supports the traditional approach.

I have had the distinct pleasure to coauthor this book with a noted herbalist, David Winston, AHG. We have both learned much in the process! Together, we have combined the traditional and scientific worlds so that we can educate today's practitioner in the use of herbal products. Often, patients know more (or think they do) about herbal products than their health care provider. This text attempts to enlighten the orthodox health care provider about both traditional and mounting scientific evidence available on herbal products.

My roots are secure in the traditional and scientific medical background as a RN with a PhD in physiology and as an author of two pharmacology texts and a critical care handbook. Since beginning to study herbal therapies, I have come to appreciate the power of herbs to improve and heal simple conditions such as the common cold, flu, and nail fungus, to more complex problems such as hypertension and menopausal changes, and, finally, to serious health problems such as cancer. Seeing and experiencing the effects of herbal and supplemental therapy is believing!

ORGANIZATION

The handbook is organized into three parts: an introductory section, the main section, which presents herbal monographs, and the third section, which presents monographs of supplements that are commonly used singly or in combination with herbal or traditional medicinal products.

Part I. The introductory chapter reviews the concept of herbal therapy. What is an herb? How herbs have been used in traditional systems of medicine (ie, Chinese, Indian, Cherokee, and Ayurvedic). The research process to evaluate herbs. The use of herbs to treat various conditions. The types of products available. The chapter also addresses the issue of standardization—is it appropriate?

Part II. The body of the text presents the most recent and up-to-date research on both herbal therapies and supplements. The format for each herbal monograph includes common names; scientific names; plant family; description; medicinal part; constituents; nutritional ingredients; traditional use; current use; available forms, dosage and administration guidelines; pharmacokinetics; toxicity; contraindications; side effects; long-term safety; use in pregnancy/lactation/children; drug/herb interactions; special notes; and a bibliography.

The most common herbs available in the United States and Canada are reviewed. Many herbs have demonstrated scientific value; however, some herbs that have not had scientific research support are discussed because they are commonly sold.

Part III. The supplemental section includes products that are very popular, such as glucosamine, chondroitin, and co-enzyme Q10. The format for presenting each supplement includes its name; common name; biologic activity; nutritional sources; current use; available forms, dosage and administration guidelines; pharmacokinetics; toxicity; contraindications; side effects; long-term safety; use in pregnancy/lactation/children; drug/herb interactions; and bibliography.

Some supplements, like herbs, have a scientific base, but some do not. We have chosen to include some supplements, even though scientific studies on them are not yet available.

APPENDICES

Several appendices present important reference material and resources as well as a glossary of commonly used terms.

Appendix A reviews herbs contraindicated during pregnancy.

Appendix B is a listing of medical disorders and their appropriate herbal or supplemental therapy. People should be encouraged not to self-diagnose and treat, but to consult with a clinical herbalist, naturopathic physician, or medical doctor versed in herbal practice. As Chapter 1 points out, two people with the same diagnosis will be treated with different herbal protocols when seen by an herbalist/naturopath.

Appendix C is an annotated guide to recommended references for further study.

Appendix D is a list of common abbreviations.

In addition to the appendices, there is a glossary of herbal/medical terms that may not be in current medical dictionaries.

Let us all enhance our own healing and health and share our knowledge with our patients. The ultimate goal of this book is to place health and healing within the grasp of all people!

Enjoy maximal health and longevity!

Merrily A. Kuhn, RN, PhD
David Winston, AHG

Acknowledgments

This book would never have come to be without the foresight of Margaret Zuccarini, Editor, at Lippincott Williams & Wilkins. Our thanks to Helen Kogut, Editorial Assistant, for organizing this text and readying it for production. Also, our thanks to all the production staff at Lippincott Williams & Wilkins, particularly Sandra Cherrey Scheinin, Senior Project Editor.

Our thanks also go out to the reviewers of this book for their knowledge and encouraging comments. All of the reviewers with whom we worked were willing to share their knowledge and expertise with us and the medical community.

Contents

An Introduction to Herbal Medicine

David Winston

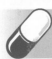

Herbs: Panaceas or Poisons?

Certain herbs have become popular during the past 20 years, but herbal medicine is still poorly understood by the public, medical practitioners, and the media. After a brief honeymoon where herbs were portrayed as "wonder drugs," we are now seeing article after article on the dangers of herbs. As in most situations, the truth lies hidden under the media hype, bad or poorly understood science, exaggerated claims, and our natural resistance to new ideas.

Seeing herbal medicines as either panaceas or as poisons blinds us to the reality that in most cases they are neither. Lack of experience, education, and good information about herbs makes consumers easy victims of marketing exploitation and herbal myths. The same lack of experience, education, and information makes many physicians and other orthodox health care providers suspicious and uncomfortable, especially with the exaggerated claims, miracle cures, and unproven remedies their patients are taking.

We as a culture are coming out of what I call the "Herbal Dark Ages," a period of time when the use of herbs virtually ceased to exist in the United States. A few ethnic communities continued to use herbs, but from the 1920s into the 1970s the only herbs that mainstream Americans used were spices in cooking. Out of this almost total lack of exposure we have seen an amazing resurgence of interest in "natural" remedies.

Along with this new interest is a profound ignorance, with many people equating "natural" with "harmless." Anyone who uses herbal products needs to understand a few basic safety rules.

The fact that something is natural does not necessarily make it safe or effective. In Cherokee medicine, we distinguish between three categories of herbs (Winston, 1992). The _food herbs_ are gentle in action, have very low toxicity, and are unlikely to cause an adverse response. Examples of food herbs include lemon balm, peppermint, marshmallow, ginger, garlic, chamomile, hawthorn, rose hips, nettles, dandelion root and leaf, and fresh oat extract. These herbs can be used in substantial quantities over long periods of time without any acute or chronic toxicity. Allergic responses are possible, as are unique idiosyncratic reactions, and even common foods such as grapefruit juice, broccoli, and okra can interact with medications.

The second category is *medicine herbs.* These herbs are stronger and need to be used with greater knowledge (dosage and rationale for use), for specific conditions (with a medical diagnosis), and usually for a limited period. These herbs are not daily tonics and should not be taken just because they are "good for you." These herbs have a greater potential for adverse reactions and in some cases drug interactions. Examples of medicine herbs include andrographis, blue cohosh, cascara sagrada, celandine, ephedra, goldenseal, Jamaica dogwood, Oregon grape root, senna, and uva-ursi.

The last category is *poison herbs.* These herbs have a strong potential for either acute or chronic toxicity and should be used only by clinicians who are trained to use them and clearly understand their toxicology and appropriate use. Even though the herb industry is often portrayed as unregulated* and irresponsible, most of the herbs in this category are not available to the public and are not sold in health food or herb stores. Examples of poison herbs include aconite, arnica, belladonna, bryonia, datura, gelsemium, henbane, male fern, phytolacca, podophyllum, and veratrum.

Another example of a traditional system of medicine that categorizes herbs according to their safety or potential toxicity is traditional Chinese medicine. The Chinese materia medica is also divided into three categories. The upper-class (superior) drugs are nontoxic and are tonic remedies. The middle-class (ministerial) drugs may have some mild toxicity, and they support the superior medicines. The last category is the lower-class (inferior) remedies, which are toxic and used only for specific ailments for limited periods.

The practitioner must have a clear understanding of an herb's benefits and possible risks and a clearly defined patient diagnosis so that he or she can counsel patients about safe and effective

*The herb industry is regulated by the FDA and laws such as the Dietary Supplement, Health and Education Act, passed by Congress in 1994.

choices in herb use. A second problem commonly experienced with the public is the belief that if a little of an herb (or medicine) is good, then more must be better. A well-publicized example is the herb ma huang (ephedra), which is being used for weight loss or as a stimulant. Serious adverse reactions, including death, have occurred; in most cases, the people were foolishly taking two to four times the recommended dose. Many herbs are useful and safe in small, appropriate doses, but, as with any medication, overdoses can cause unwanted side effects, possible injury, and, if the statistics are correct, rare fatalities.

DANGERS AND TOXICITY OF HERBAL MEDICINES

This book is divided into two sections, one on herbal products and the other on nutritional supplements. They are not the same. A recent hysterical report claimed that herbal products could cause bovine spongiform encephalitis, also known as mad cow disease. The author failed to notice that herbs are from the vegetable kingdom and do not contain animal tissue. The author of this report was correct in noting that some supplements do contain animal glandular tissue such as liver, thymus, bone marrow, and thyroid and that the possibility of contamination by infectious proteins from these products may exist. If we are going to critique herbs and supplement products, let us do it with clear knowledge and understanding of the topic.

It is not uncommon for studies to be done on animals and the results extrapolated to humans, even though we may metabolize or digest various phytochemicals quite differently. Researchers have done studies on an herb without authenticating its identity, making results meaningless (Leung, 2000).

Sometimes information on isolated constituents is confused with the whole herb, or studies on intravenous forms of herbs are confused with oral administration. This type of misinterpretation and misunderstanding gives rise to incorrect information, which often continues to be repeated even decades after the original research has been disproven. Other studies have taken hamster oocytes and human sperm, put them into extracts of herbs (St. John's wort, saw palmetto, ginkgo, and echinacea) and found that in high concentrations, some of the herbs denatured the sperm or inhibited the sperm from penetrating the hamster oocyte (Ondrizek et al., 1999). This study was widely reported in medical journals and the popular press. One medical editor said it was an important study showing a possible correlation between infertility and the use of herbs. The author of the study, Dr. Richard Ondrizek, was "flabbergasted" that his in vitro laboratory research is being reported as evidence that these herbs can cause infertility in humans. Dr. Ondrizek stated, "there is absolutely no parallel between this study and humans."

Another recent error is due to lack of knowledge about phytochemistry. Several reports have surfaced suggesting that echinacea may be hepatotoxic. There is no evidence of this whatsoever. The error comes from the fact that echinacea contains very small amounts of pyrrolizidine alkaloids, some forms of which are known hepatotoxins. Unfortunately, the authors of this misinformation failed to differentiate between unsaturated (hepatotoxic) alkaloids and the nontoxic saturated alkaloids found in echinacea. This is an easy error for the uninformed to make, but one that creates unnecessary fear and confusion.

According to the information gathered by acclaimed researcher and scientist James Duke, PhD, the statistics on deaths caused by herbs compared with other causes are quite revealing:

Herbs: 1 in 1 million
Supplements: 1 in 1 million
Poisonous mushrooms: 1 in 100,000
Nonsteroidal anti-inflammatories: 1 in 10,000
Murder: 1 in 10,000
Hospital surgery: 1 in 10,000
Car accident: 1 in 5,000
Improper use of medication: 1 in 2,000
Angiogram: 1 in 1,000
Alcohol: 1 in 500
Cigarettes: 1 in 500
Properly prescribed medications: 1 in 333
Medical mishap: 1 in 250
Iatrogenic hospital infection: 1 in 80
Bypass surgery: 1 in 20

If put into perspective, herbs (food herbs and medicine herbs) can cause problems, but they are substantially safer than over-the-counter and prescription medications. Will we find that some herbs can have side effects? Definitely. Will we find that some herbs interact with medications? Absolutely. We only have to look at a recent report that St. John's wort reduced the blood levels of cyclosporine in heart transplant patients to be aware of possible risks. At the same time, reports that followed stating that St. John's wort can interfere with birth control and would cause an epidemic of unwanted pregnancies were unfounded. Not only is there no proof of this, but millions of German women who take contraceptive pills and St. John's wort have failed, in the past 20 years, to provide any substantiation to the concerned researchers.

Recently the FDA removed two medications from the marketplace (troglitazone [Rezulin] and cisapride [Propulsid]), even though they had been through extensive testing and FDA drug approval. Any drug researcher will tell you that for many pharmaceuticals, the real test is when they are being used by the general population. Both of these medications were deemed "safe" but caused serious adverse effects and, ultimately, 60 to 70 deaths each. One benefit of the long history of human use of most herbs is that they have hundreds or thousands of years of use in the general population and a substantial record of safety or danger and effectiveness or lack thereof.

Frequently we hear complaints that herbs are poorly studied and, as such, are dangerous. It is true that the research on most herbs cannot compare to the 10 years of FDA clinical trials required for new drugs. Because herbs are rarely patentable, it is highly unlikely that any company is going to invest the time (approximately 10 years) and money (approximately $350 million to $500 million) to have an herbal product approved as a new drug. Herbs and supplements are sold in the United States as dietary supplements, with no research necessary before being sold. There are significant numbers of studies being performed on herbal medicines, but most are done in Germany, France, Japan, China, and India, and many are hard to access or never translated into English. It would be of tremendous benefit to consumers and clinicians if American companies would increase funding for well-designed and relevant herbal research.

The quality of this research would also benefit if clinical herbalists who understand appropriate forms of the medication, dosage, and traditional and clinical uses were part of the research team. In 1997, a study was done on the effects of the Chinese herb dong quai on menopausal symptoms (Hirata et al., 1997). This herb is frequently used in traditional Chinese medicine formulas for female reproductive problems. Although the study clearly showed that dong quai had no estrogenic effects and did not affect menopausal symptoms, it failed to take into account why and how this herb is used in Chinese medicine. First, dong quai is never used as a simple herb. It is not used for its estrogenic effects, but for its ability to improve cardiac function, increase uterine circulation, reduce anxiety, and mildly stimulate bowel function. Someone who understood this could have helped to design a much more useful and beneficial study.

The gold standard for proof of efficacy for a medication is the controlled double-blind trial. Many herbs, probably most, have not undergone this type of study. Although these studies are very valuable and may offer proof of activity and effectiveness, we also need to understand the usefulness of other types of herbal data. In addition to controlled double-blind trials and meta-analysis, less definitive but still valuable are well-designed unblinded trials, small uncontrolled clinical trials, population (epidemiologic) studies, and some animal and phytochemical studies. The herbalist should use all of these resources while also incorporating additional information often ignored by academics. Traditional herb use, ethnobotanical use, and practical clinical experience are extremely valuable tools that stand as the basic foundation of good herbal practice. When you find three disparate groups of people using the same herb or closely related species for the exact same use, you can be fairly certain that it does indeed have the stated effect. A good example is coptis, used as an effective antibacterial and antifungal agent by Native Americans, Northern Europeans, and the Chinese.

During the 1940s and 1950s, drug companies spent millions of dollars doing random drug screenings on plants, fungi, and soil microorganisms in search of the starting materials for new drugs. There were a few notable successes, such as the Madagascar periwinkle (*Vinca rosea*), the source of vinblastine and vincristine. However, overall the programs were failures. Rarely did any new drug develop from random screenings. In the past 10 years, pharmaceutical companies have once again begun to search the plant kingdom for new bioactive phytochemicals, but now they use ethnobotanists and even old herbals to do the preliminary searching (Holland, 1996). They have realized that for hundreds or thousands of years, indigenous people depended on these herbs to treat illness. Keen observers of their world, native people used what worked. In addition to the knowledge of preliterate peoples, the accumulated folk wisdom of Europe has been printed in books since the 1500s. Some of the information is exaggerated, some fantastical, and some totally wrong, but much of this herbal wisdom is the basis for modern European phytotherapy, and we are using many of the same herbs for the same conditions as did our distant ancestors.

Traditional systems of medicine such as Ayurveda (India), traditional Chinese medicine, Tibetan medicine, unani-tibb (Greco-Arabic), and Kampo (Japan) have a long and impressive history of effectiveness. Modern research has confirmed the usefulness and safety of what has been used as primary medical care by much of the world's population.

In the United States, eclectic medicine was practiced widely from the 1830s until 1940. This sectarian medical system was founded by a physician, Wooster Beach, MD, who rejected the mainstream medical practice of bleeding, leeching, purging, and using toxic medicines such as arsenic and mercury (Winston & Dattner, 1999). As an alternative, Beach and his followers embraced and studied the American vegetable materia medica. Eclectic physicians during the 1890s represented 10% of the doctors in the United States. Their clinical experience of treating millions of patients over 100 years was carefully chronicled in their voluminous literature. Today this is an extremely valuable body of experiential knowledge about the successful clinical use of herbal medicines in a time without antibiotics or the advances of technological medicine.

Modern clinical herbalists in the United States and even more so in Great Britain and Australia (where herbalists are recognized practitioners) have also begun to chronicle their clinical experience carefully and even to conduct small-scale clinical studies of herbal treatments. All of this information is valuable and, along with personal clinical experience, it gives the clinician a strong understanding of the appropriate, safe, and effective use of an herb or herbal protocol. In my clinical experience, working from this accumulated knowledge is a highly accurate way of matching effective protocols to each patient. Where this type of proof doesn't work well is when physicians call and want to know which herbs may be useful for a liver transplant patient, a patient undergoing dialysis, or someone who has just had a bone marrow transplant. In these instances, where there is no tradition, our only guides are careful observation and research studies.

DIFFERENCES BETWEEN ALLOPATHIC USE OF HERBS AND TRADITIONAL HERBAL MEDICINE

As I mentioned earlier, during the past 10 years certain herbs (black cohosh, echinacea, garlic, kava, milk thistle, saw palmetto, and St. John's wort) have become very popular, but herbal medicine has not. There is a very real difference between the allopathic use of an herb and the practice of good herbal medicine. Different systems of herbal medicine have their own views and distinctive practices, but they all have three things in common.

First, they have an underlying philosophy that creates a foundation and structure for the practice of medicine. Frequently, the underlying belief focuses on what naturopathic medicine calls *Vis Medicatrix Naturae*, or the healing power of nature (Kirchfield & Boyle, 1994). This idea was a central tenet of medicine as taught by Hippocrates, Maimonides, the German physician C.W. Hufeland, MD, and the early American physician Jacob Bigalow, MD. In many systems of medicine, not only is the body inherently self-healing, but there is an important relationship and connection between the physical, emotional, and spiritual aspects of each patient. In Chinese, Tibetan, and Cherokee medicine (Nvwoti), attention may also be given to what we perceive as external relationships and the effects of the family, community, and the environment on each patient.

The second and third aspects of traditional systems of medicine are interrelated: a system of energetics, and differential diagnosis. Energetics is a way of describing the activity and qualities of a given herb. Does it increase (stimulate) or decrease (sedate) function? Does it increase nutrition, tonify an organ, or moisten or dry tissue? Energetics is an effective way of understanding an herb, not by its constituents, which can be very problematic,* but by its activity and effects on the human body. This traditional form of pharmacology is used along with various types of differential diagnosis, so there is an understanding of the underlying imbalances or disease and the treatment is specific to the patient.

Good herbal medicine treats people, not diseases. Physicians and nurses are always surprised that the protocols are so patient-specific. Two different patients, both with rheumatoid arthritis, can have almost entirely different treatments, because clinical herbalists do not view these patients as "two cases of rheumatoid arthritis." They might see John Smith, age 68, with achlorhydria, chronic constipation, impaired circulation, and rheumatoid arthritis, and Alice Jones, age 38, with premenstrual syndrome, depression, biliary dyskinesia, and rheumatoid arthritis. The focus in good herbal, naturopathic, Chinese, or ayurvedic medicine is affecting the terrain: strengthen the organism, improve overall function (circulation, digestion, elimination, endocrine and immune function), reduce stress, and improve sleep and nutrition.

Many diseases, especially chronic degenerative ones, respond very well to this type of treatment. Benign prostatic hyperplasia is a good example. The orthodox treatment is terazosin (Hytrin). Saw palmetto as an allopathic herbal substitute works about as well as the pharmaceuticals, costs less, and has fewer adverse effects. As an herbalist I will probably use saw palmetto as a part of my protocol, but in addition I might add nettle root, white sage, bidens, or collinsonia to improve the activity, effectiveness, and specificity of the formula. This combination of herbs, in my clinical experience, is far superior to the pharmaceutical agents or saw palmetto as an individual remedy.

Herbal medicine, like orthodox medical practice, is an art as well as a science. Knowing how to combine herbs to create a synergistic effect is more than random polypharmacy. Another example of an herbal formula that has benefits over individual

---

*Individual constituents can have widely divergent effects as isolates. Chinese ginseng (*Panax ginseng*) is a good example: ginsenoside Rb1 is sedating, whereas ginsenoside Rg1 is a central nervous system stimulant. Despite these opposing effects, the whole herb has an overall stimulating effect.

herbs would be my protocol for seasonal affective disorder. St. John's wort is touted as an effective herbal antidepressant, and in some cases it is, but for seasonal affective disorder St. John's wort alone is inadequate. In this situation, combining lemon balm and lavender with St. John's wort increases its benefits while also improving digestion and sleep quality. Other dietary and lifestyle changes would be considered as well as additional herbs specific to the patient.

It is important to recognize that serious acute illnesses such as myocardial infarction, bacterial meningitis, stroke, acute asthma attacks, head trauma, and liver and kidney failure cannot be treated in this manner. For many years, both patients and practitioners have tended to view this difference in treatment paradigms as a choice: one or the other. Nothing could be farther from the truth. Where Western medicine is most effective, herbal medicine is often ineffective, but where herbal medicine is most effective, orthodox medicine often has little to offer patients. Not only can botanicals be very useful in many chronic degenerative conditions or mild to moderate functional ailments, but they also can play an important role in recovery from serious illness. Once head trauma victims have been stabilized, the use of ginkgo, rosemary, St. John's wort, and bacopa has dramatically reduced recovery time and improved memory as well as cognitive and motor functions. Western medicine and herbal medicine working in concert offers the best of both worlds, and the patient is the beneficiary in this new relationship.

ADMINISTRATION OF HERBS

Herbs as medicines can be administered in many forms. Some can be taken as foods or consumed regularly in the diet, such as basil, blueberries, garlic, or ginger. Teas (infusions or decoctions) are a reliable way of administering some herbs. Drinking a hot cup of a pleasant-tasting tea can be a wonderfully relaxing and healing experience in itself. Liquids are also absorbed more quickly, especially in patients with impaired digestion. For certain herbs (green tea, slippery elm), tea is the most effective way to take them. The drawbacks to teas are that many herbs have constituents that are poorly water-soluble (boswellia, ginkgo, gum guggul, milk thistle) and are not effective as teas. Other herbs have an unpleasant taste (saw palmetto, feverfew, valerian), and having to drink cupfuls of a noxious-tasting brew will limit patient compliance. Some patients also find having to make teas too much of a bother.

Tinctures are hydroalcoholic extracts of herbs. Although tinctures are not very concentrated (1:5 wt/vol), the menstruum (alcohol and water) extracts a wide range of constituents, the alcohol increases absorption of the herb by approximately 30% (Anonymous, 1998), the doses are much smaller than with teas (so the taste factor is less of a problem), and tinctures are convenient. A patient can carry a small 1-oz dropper bottle and the tincture can be placed in water, tea, or juice when needed. An additional benefit to tinctures is that fresh herbs that lose potency when dried (echinacea, eyebright, skullcap) can be made into fresh tinctures (1:2 wt/vol), which preserves their activity very effectively. The biggest limitation for tinctures is that they contain alcohol, and people with alcohol abuse issues or serious liver disease should avoid its consumption.

Fluid extracts, more concentrated alcohol-and-water extracts (1:1 wt/vol), offer many of the same benefits as tinctures, with greater potency and a smaller dose. True fluid extracts are not common in the American marketplace, and there is great confusion because different manufacturers use different terminology, technology, and menstruums (extracting liquids) to produce their products. The pharmaceutical definition of a fluid extract includes the use of heat in the manufacturing process, which can be useful for heat-soluble constituents or damaging for heat-sensitive constituents.

Spray-dried extracts are liquid extracts that are spray-dried onto a powdered carrier (cellulose, powdered herbs). These extracts are fairly concentrated (4:1, 5:1 wt/vol), maintain the activity of the whole herb, and are easily encapsulated, so taste is not an issue. The drawbacks of capsules in general, whether they contain ground herbs or a spray-dried extract, are that they are more difficult to digest than liquids, and patients, especially young children, who cannot swallow capsules, cannot use this type of product.

Capsules containing ground, dried herbs tend to have very limited activity and digestibility. Herbs that should be taken in this form are ones containing minerals as primary constituents (alfalfa, horsetail, nettles, oat straw). As long as the patient has reasonable digestive function, capsules are a superior way to ingest mineral-rich herbs.

Gelcaps are a useful method of ingesting oily nutrients such as vitamin E or oil-based supplements such as borage seed oil, flaxseed oil, or evening primrose seed oil. Gelcaps are easier to swallow than capsules or tablets, but the ingredients are subjected to considerable heat during processing, and rancidity of the oils is a substantial problem.

Tablets are often difficult to digest, but greater amounts of herbs and herb extracts can be squeezed into this format. Uncoated tablets are harder to swallow but are more absorbable. Most tablets contain proprietary herb/supplement formulas, and their effectiveness depends on the quality of the ingredients and the validity of the formula as a therapeutic regimen.

Standardized herbal products are frequently recommended in the popular literature, especially by authors who are not herbalists. The idea that each dose of an herb has exactly the same levels of active constituents is an attractive concept and a comfortable one for practitioners used to dealing with pharmaceutical products. They need to know that 0.25 mg digoxin is exactly that. Too much can cause arrhythmias and death; too little, and the patient may die of congestive heart failure. However, most herbs are not used for life-threatening conditions, nor do they have the toxicity of digoxin, so doses do not need to be as precise. The belief that each herb has an active constituent is false: most herbs have dozens or even hundreds of constituents that may contribute to their activity. Some of the constituents may have direct activity, whereas other "inert" ingredients may increase bioavailability, reduce toxicity, or stimulate function by means of a synergistic activity. To most herbalists, the active constituent is the herb itself.

Many manufacturers and academic "herbal authorities" would have you believe that only standardized herbal products work, and that all herbs should be standardized. This is disingenuous and is more a matter of marketing and belief system than fact. The reality is that fewer than 10% of the standardized products in the marketplace are standardized to known active constituents.

There are actually two types of standardization. The first is true standardization, where a definite phytochemical or group of constituents is known to have activity. Ginkgo, with its 26% ginkgo flavones and 6% terpenes, is a good example of real standardization. Other products that meet these parameters are milk thistle, curcumin from turmeric, *Coleus forskollii*, and saw palmetto (85%–95% fatty sterols). These products are highly concentrated; they no longer represent the whole herb and are now phytopharmaceuticals. In many cases they are vastly more effective than the whole herb (*Coleus forskollii*, ginkgo, milk thistle), but some effects of the herb may be lost and the potential for adverse effects and herb/drug interactions may increase. Curcumin may have stronger anti-inflammatory activity than whole turmeric, but in large doses it acts as a gastric mucosa irritant, whereas the whole root extract has a gastroprotective effect.* The standardized saw palmetto (serenoa) is believed to be much more effective than crude extracts of the berry, but again no comparative studies have been done. The dried berries and tincture, in addition to reducing symptoms of benign prostatic hypertrophy, have beneficial effects on the immune system, lungs, and gastrointestinal tract that are lost in the standardized saw palmetto.

The other type of standardization is based on a manufacturer's guarantee of the presence of a certain percentage of a marker compound. Rarely are these known active constituents, and although they may help to identify the herb, they are not indicators of therapeutic activity. An echinacea product standardized to caffeic acid or a St. John's wort product standardized to 0.3% hypericin is virtually meaningless because neither of these compounds represents the therapeutic activity or quality of the herb.

This is not to say that no quality standards are needed; they most certainly are. First, every herb product needs to be botanically identified to ensure the correct herb is in the product. Adulteration of scullcap with germander has resulted in liver

---

*There are no studies comparing the activity of one with the other, and many additional anti-inflammatory constituents of turmeric rhizome have been discovered since the curcuminoids were deemed "the active ingredients."

damage in several people. Recent substitution of aristolochia species for the Chinese herb stephania has caused kidney failure and renal cancers. In addition to accurate botanical identification, it is very important that the right part of the plant is used, that it is harvested at the right time and prepared properly, and that the appropriate pharmaceutical techniques are used to make the best medicines.

Herbalists have always standardized their herbal products. St. John's wort was gathered in bud or flower, and only the tops of the plants were picked. The tincture or oil of hypericum should turn a deep burgundy red and have a strong and distinctive aroma. How much hypericin is present per dose, I don't know; how much hyperforin per dose, I don't know. What I do know is that this preparation will be active and will work because the markers herbalists have always looked for are present. Herbalists have standardized their medicines to quality, not numbers.

As the herbal marketplace continues to grow, simply using the old organoleptic quality standards probably is not practical. I would suggest that simply applying random levels of an easy-to-test-for phytochemical isn't the answer either. A synthesis of traditional herbal knowledge and modern research will benefit the herbal manufacturer, the consumer, and the practitioner. The bridge between traditional herbalism and modern phytotherapy and the interface between academia and industry must be a person who has spent his or her lifetime gaining a hands-on practical knowledge of botanical medicine: the herbalist. The combined skills of the physician, the pharmacist, the herbalist, nurses, and other clinical staff, provide patients with the best of both worlds—safe, effective, and appropriate herbal medicine, as part of our health care system.

BIBLIOGRAPHY

Anonymous. (March 1998). Alcohol improves bioavailability. *Mediherb Monitor*. 25.

Eldin S, Dunford A. (1999). *Herbal Medicine in Primary Care*. Oxford: Butterworth-Heinemann.

Hirata JD, et al. (1997). Does dong quai have estrogenic effects in postmenopausal women? A double-blind placebo-controlled trial. *Fertility and Sterility*. 68(6):981–986.

Holland BK (Ed.). (1996). *Prospecting for Drugs in Ancient and Medieval European Texts*. Amsterdam: Harwood Academic Publishers.

Kirchfield F, Boyle W. (1994). *Nature Doctors*. Portland, OR: Medicina Biologica.

Leung A. (2000). Scientific studies and reports in the herbal literature: What are we studying and reporting? *HerbalGram*. 48:63–64.

McCaleb R. (1999). Research reviews: Possible shortcomings of fertility study on herbs. *HerbalGram*. 46:22.

Ondrizek PR, et al. (1999). An alternative medicine study of herbal effects on the penetration of zona-free hamster oocytes and the integrity of sperm deoxyribonucleic acid. *Fertility and Sterility*. 71(3):517–522.

Winston D. (1992). Nvwoti, Cherokee medicine and ethnobotany. In Tierra M. (Ed.). *American Herbalism*. Freedom, CA: The Crossing Press.

Winston D, Dattner A. (1999). The American system of medicine. *Clinics in Dermatology*. 17(1):53–56.

PART II

Herb Monographs

NAME: Aloe (*Aloe vera*)

Common Names: Cape, Zanzibar, Curacao, Barbados aloes; aloe vera; burn plant (*Aloe barbadenisis* is a synonym for *Aloe vera*)

Family: *Liliaceae*

Description of Plant

- More than 360 species in the Aloe genus
- Name means "bitter and shiny substance"
- Perennial succulents native to Africa, now grown throughout the world
- Short plant has 15 to 30 tapering leaves about 20" long and 5" wide.
- Leaf has three layers: outer (tough), middle (corrugate lining), and inner (a colorless mucilaginous pulp, the aloe gel). The plant contains 99% water.
- Mature plant can be 1.5′ to 4′ high and 3′ or more in diameter at the base.
- Yields both aloe gel and aloe latex. Although they share certain chemical components, the gel and latex are distinct, with different properties and uses.
  - The gel is naturally occurring. Undiluted gel is obtained by stripping away the outer layer of the leaf. It is for topical use and is famous for its wound-healing properties. It provides moisture and soothes the skin and thus is widely used in cosmetics, moisturizing creams, and lotions.
  - Aloe vera concentrate is gel from which the water has been removed. For topical use.
  - Aloe vera juice is an ingestible product containing a minimum of 50% aloe vera gel, usually mixed with fruit juice. For internal use.
  - Aloe vera latex is the bitter yellow liquid derived from the pericyclic tubules of the rind of aloe vera. The primary constituent is aloin. It is rarely used internally because of its powerful cathartic activity.

Medicinal Part
- Aloe gel: inside each leaf
- Latex: solid residue obtained by evaporating the latex beneath the skin

Constituents and Action (if known)
Latex Constituents
- Anthraquinones have antiviral, antibacterial, antitumor activity (Boik, 1996).
- Anthraquinone barbaloin: when concentrated, produces aloin, local irritants to GI tract, and soothes the skin
- Aloinosides A and B have a strong purgative effect (Muller, 1996).

Aloe Gel Constituents
- Polysaccharide glucomannan (similar to guar gum) is found in aloe gel. It has an emollient effect and hinders the formation of thromboxane, a chemical that delays wound healing (Hunter & Frunkin, 1991).
- Bradykininase, a protease inhibitor, relieves pain and reduces swelling (Vazquez, 1996; Visuthiokosol, 1995).
- Magnesium lactate blocks histamine and may contribute to antipruritic effect (Schmidt & Greenspoon, 1991).
- Tannins

Nutritional Ingredients: None known

Traditional Use
- Ancient Egypt (1500 BC) and Middle East: used to heal the skin and treat wounds, hemorrhoids, and hair loss
- In US, the latex has been used as a purgative since colonists brought it from Europe in their medicine chests.

Current Use
Topical (Gel)
- Helps to heal burns and reduce burn pain. Useful for first- and second-degree burns (sunburn, radiation burns, scalds). First report of clinical use for radiation burns was in 1935 in the *American Journal of Roentgenology*.
- May help heal venous ulcers
- Anti-inflammatory activity by inhibiting arachidonic acid
- Soothes skin and may enhance skin healing

Oral
- Soothes gastric ulcers (gel)
- Mild laxative (gel)
- Cathartic (concrete resin)

Available Forms, Dosage, and Administration Guidelines
Preparations
- *Gel:* Sunscreens, skin creams, lotions, cosmetics
- *Juice:* Available in various concentrations and as powdered dry juice. Highly concentrated products degrade quickly; check for inclusion of gums, sugars, starches, and other additives.

Typical Dosage
- *Fresh gel (topical):* Cut a leaf lengthwise, scrape out the gel, and apply externally as needed. Discontinue if burning or irritation occurs.
- *Juice (internal):* Take 1 tsp after meals, or follow manufacturer's or practitioner's recommendations.

Pharmacokinetics—If Available (form or route when known)

Toxicity: Internal use of latex can cause severe GI cramping.

Contraindications
- *Topical:* Deep, vertical wounds; hypersensitivity to aloe products
- *Internal:* Bowel obstruction, inflammatory bowel disease, kidney and liver disease

Side Effects
- *Topical:* Contact dermatitis is possible but uncommon.
- *Internal (latex):* May cause fluid and electrolyte imbalances, cramplike GI symptoms

Long-Term Safety
- *Gel:* Safe
- *Latex:* Not safe for daily long-term dosing because it is irritating to the bowel. When used for more than 1 to 2 weeks, it may cause intestinal sluggishness and laxative dependence.

Use in Pregnancy/Lactation/Children

- *Oral:* Latex contraindicated in all because of severe GI symptoms
- *Topical:* Safe in all

Drug/Herb Interactions and Rationale (if known)

- Gel, taken internally, can reduce absorption of many medications. Separate by at least 2 hours from all drugs.
- Latex, because of its cathartic effect, causes loss of K^+ and therefore may increase the likelihood of toxicity with cardiac glycosides, antiarrhythmics, steroids, loop diuretics, and other K^+-wasting drugs. Avoid concurrent use of internal latex and these drugs.

Special Notes

- Juice is nontoxic but has been found to be ineffective for arthritis.
- Unapproved use of parenteral aloe vera for cancer has been associated with death.
- An extracted polysaccharide, acemannan, has shown immune-stimulating activity and has been approved by the USDA as an adjunctive treatment for canine and feline fibrosarcoma. This product has been used clinically and for self-treatment of cancer and HIV. As far as the authors know, no human trials have confirmed the effectiveness of this product for these conditions.

BIBLIOGRAPHY

Boik J. (1996). *Cancer & Natural Medicine.* Portland: Oregon Medical Press.

Davis RH, et al. (1989). Anti-inflammatory activity of aloe vera against a spectrum of irritants. *Journal of the American Podiatric Medicine Association.* 79(6):263–76.

Dykman KD, Tone C, Ford C, Dykman RA. (1998). The effects of nutritional supplements on the symptoms of fibromyalgia and chronic fatigue syndrome. *Integrative Physiological Behavioral Science.* 33(1):61–71.

Hunter D, Frunkin A. (1991). Adverse reactions to vitamin E and aloe vera preparations after dermabrasion and chemical peel. *Cutis.* 47(3):193.

Muller SO, et al. (1996). Genotoxicity of the laxative drug components emodin, aloe-emodin, and danthron in mammalian cells: Topoisomerase II-mediated. *Mutation Research.* 371:165–73.

Phillips T, et al. (1995). A randomized study of an aloe vera derivative gel dressing versus conventional treatment after shave biopsy excision. *Wounds* 7(5):200–2.

Review of Natural Products (1997–98). St. Louis, MO: Facts and Comparisons, Wolters/Kluwer.

Sato Y, et al. (1990). Studies on chemical protectors against radiation. XXXI. Protection effects of aloe arborescens on skin injury induced by X-irradiation. *Yakugaku Zasshi.* 110(11):876–84.

Schmidt JM, Greenspoon JS. (1991). Aloe vera dermal wound gel is associated with a delay in wound healing. *Obstetrics & Gynecology.* 78(1):115.

Syed TA, et al. (1996). Management of psoriasis with aloe vera extract in a hydrophilic cream: A placebo-controlled, double-blind study. *Tropical Medicine & International Health.* 1(4):505–9.

Vazquez B, et al. (1996). Antiinflammatory activity of extracts from aloe vera gel. *Journal of Ethnopharmacology.* 55(1):69–75.

Visuthikosol V, et al. (1995). Effect of aloe vera gel to healing of burn wound: A clinical and histologic study. *Journal of the Medical Association of Thailand.* 78(8):403–9.

NAME: American ginseng (*Panax quinquefolius*)

Common Names: Sang, man root

Family: *Araliaceae*

Description of Plant: American ginseng grows from Canada to Georgia. It is considered an endangered species, so much of the ginseng crop is cultivated. It is a slow-growing perennial and takes 5 to 7 years to produce a marketable root. The herb is a small perennial with a single stem, which has three to six long petioled compound leaves at the top.

Medicinal Part: The mature root is used and is gathered in the autumn (September), when the red berries are ripe. The berries should be replanted.

Constituents and Action (if known)

- Saponins (4.3%–4.9%) protect LDL cholesterol from oxidation (Li, 1999).
  - Ginsenoside Rb1 has a stimulant action on protein and RNA synthesis in animal serum and liver. It has

hypotensive, anticonvulsant, analgesic, antiulcer (induced by stress), and nerve regeneration-inducing activity.
  ○ Ginsenoside Re: American ginseng (3 g/day) reduced blood sugar in diabetic and nondiabetic patients (Vuksan, 2000).
- Triterpene oligoglycosides: quinquenosides 1, II, III, IV, V; quinqueginsin has anti-HIV, antifungal activity (Wang & Ng, 2000).
- American ginseng extract has antioxidant activity (Kitts, 2000).

Nutritional Ingredients: Used as a flavoring and tonic in beverages

Traditional Use
- Adaptogen, mild stimulant, bitter tonic
- Native Americans have used ginseng as a bitter tonic and for nervous afflictions (Cherokee), for short-windedness (Creek), as a general tonic and panacea (Delaware, Mohegan), for upset stomach and vomiting (Iroquois), and for strengthening the mind (Menominee).
- Among early Americans, a debate raged over this plant's effects. Some authorities claimed that it had great powers; others believed it had no activity.
- Eclectic physicians used *Panax* for neurasthenia, digestive torpor, fatigue, loss of appetite, and nervous dyspepsia.
- American ginseng has been exported to China since 1716, after its "discovery" by a Jesuit priest in Canada. In traditional Chinese medicine, American ginseng (xi yang shen) is considered much milder and less stimulating than Asian ginseng and is used to nourish the *yin* and fluids. It is used for dry coughs, hemoptysis, exhaustion after fevers, chronic thirst, and irritability.

Current Use
- Mildly stimulating adaptogen appropriate for regular use by overworked, overstressed Americans
- A useful adjunctive therapy or tonic remedy for mild depression, postperformance immune depletion in athletes, chronic fatigue syndrome, fibromyalgia, stress-induced asthma, chronic stress, age-related memory loss (Cui & Chen, 1991), and menopausal cloudy thinking

- Concurrent with antineoplastic agents, ginseng synergistically inhibits MCF-7 breast cancer cell growth (Duda, 1999).

Available Forms, Dosage, and Administration Guidelines

- *Tea:* 1 tsp root to 12 oz water. Slowly decoct 15 to 20 minutes until liquid is reduced to 8 oz. Take 4 oz three times daily.
- *Tincture:* (1:2 or 1:5, 35% alcohol), 40 to 60 gtt (2 to 3 mL) three times daily
- *Capsules:* two capsules three times daily

Pharmacokinetics—If Available (form or route when known): Not known

Toxicity: None

Contraindications: None known

Side Effects: Large amounts may cause overstimulation. If insomnia, nervousness, or mild elevation of blood pressure occurs, discontinue use.

Long-Term Safety: Safe

Use in Pregnancy/Lactation/Children: No known contraindication. Use cautiously and in small amounts.

Drug/Herb Interactions and Rationale (if known): Some studies have suggested a possible interaction with blood-thinning medications, but others show that American ginseng does not alter warfarin pharmacokinetics.

Special Notes: Avoid using wild harvested plants. The best American ginseng products are made from 5- to 10-year-old, organically woods-grown roots.

BIBLIOGRAPHY

Bensky D, Gamble A. (1993). *Chinese Herbal Medicine: Materia Medica.* Seattle: Eastland Press.

Chen SE, Sawchuk RJ, Staba EJ. (1980). American ginseng III. Pharmacokinetics of ginsenosides in the rabbit. *European Journal of Drug Metabolism & Pharmacokinetics.* 5(3):161–8.

Chen SE, Staba EJ. (1980). American ginseng II. Analysis of ginsenosides and their sapogenins in biological fluids. *Journal of Natural Products.* 43(4):463–6.

Cui J, Chen KJ. (1991). American ginseng compound liquor on retarding-aging process. *Chung Hsi I Chieh Ho Tsa Chih.* 11(8):457–60.

Duda RB, Zhong Y, Navas V, et al. (1999). American ginseng and breast cancer therapeutic agents synergistically inhibit MCF-7 breast cancer cell growth. *Journal of Surgical Oncology.* 72(4):230–9.

Foster S. (1991). American ginseng (*Panax quinquefolius*). Austin, TX: American Botanical Council.

Hobbs C. (1997). *Ginseng, the Energy Herb.* Loveland, CO: Botanica Press.

Kitts DD, Wijewickreme AN, Hu C. (2000). Antioxidant properties of a North American ginseng extract. *Molecular and Cellular Biochemistry.* 203(1–2):1–10.

Li J, Huang M, Teoh H, Man RY. (1999). *Panax quinquefolius* saponins protect low-density lipoproteins from oxidation. *Life Science.* 64(1):43–62.

Moerman D. (1998). *Native American Ethnobotany.* Seattle: Timber Press.

Sloley BD, Pang PK, Huang BH, et al. (1999). American ginseng extract reduces scopolamine-induced amnesia in a spatial learning task. *Journal of Psychiatry & Neuroscience.* 24(5):442–52.

Vuksan V, Sievenpiper JL, Koo VYY, et al. (2000). American ginseng (*Panax quinquefolius* L.) reduces postprandial glycemia in nondiabetic subjects and subjects with type 2 diabetes mellitus. *Archives of Internal Medicine.* 160(7):1009–13.

Wang HX, Ng TB. (2000). Quinqueginsin, a novel protein with anti-human immunodeficiency virus, antifungal, ribonuclease and cell-free translation-inhibitory activities from American ginseng roots. *Biochemical & Biophysical Research Communications.* 269(1):203–8.

Yoshikawa M, Murakami T, Yashiro K, et al. (1998). Bioactive saponins and glycosides. XI. Structures of new dammarane-type triterpene oligoglycosides, quinquenosides I, II, III, IV, and V, from American ginseng, the roots of *Panax quinquefolius* L. *Chemical Pharmaceutical Bulletin (Tokyo).* 46(4):647–54.

Yuan CS, Attele AS, Wu JA, Liu D. (1998). Modulation of American ginseng on brain stem GABA-ergic effects in rats. *Journal of Ethnopharmacology.* 62(3):215–22.

NAME: Andrographis (*Andrographis paniculata*)

Common Names: Chiretta, kalmegh (Hindi), chuan xin lian (Chinese)

Family: *Acanthaceae*

Description of Plant: Common annual plant native to India and cultivated in China

Medicinal Part: Herb

Constituents and Action (if known)

- Diterpenoid lactones (andrographolides): greater hepatoprotective activity than silymarin (Bone, 1996); andrographolide (antipyretic, anodyne); neoandrographolide, and dehydroandrographolide. The whole herb extract was shown to have greater activity than andrographolide alone (You-ping Zhu, 1998) and to inhibit PAF-induced platelet aggregation (Amroyan, 1999).
- Flavones (oroxylin, wogonin)
- Andrographis extract mildly inhibits *Staphylococcus aureus*, *Pseudomonas aeruginosa*, *Proteus vulgaris*, *Shigella dysenteriae*, *Escherichia coli*.

Nutritional Ingredients: None

Traditional Use

- Anti-inflammatory, antipyretic, antifertility activity, anthelmintic, immune stimulant, bitter tonic, cholagogue, antihepatotoxin, antimalarial
- Used in ayurvedic medicine and traditional complementary medicine to treat diarrhea, dysentery, dyspepsia, impaired bile secretion, hepatitis, malaria, pyelonephritis, pneumonia, and tonsillitis

Current Use

- Prophylaxis and treatment of colds, sinusitis, and pharyngotonsillitis, with reduction of many symptoms, including headache, fatigue, earache, sore throat, nasal and bronchial catarrh, and cough (Caceres, 1999)
- As prophylaxis, patients treated with andrographis for 3 months caught colds 2.1 times less than the placebo group (Melchior, 1997; Mills & Bone, 1999).

- Numerous Chinese studies have shown andrographis is useful for acute bacterial dysentery and enteritis.
- Recent clinical trials show this herb is useful for leptospirosis.

Available Forms, Dosage, and Administration Guidelines

- *Dried herb:* 1.5 to 5 g/day
- *Tea:* $^1/_2$ to 1 tsp dried herb in 8 oz hot water, steep 30 minutes, take 4 oz three times daily
- *Tincture:* (1:5, 30% alcohol), 20 to 60 gtt (1–3 mL) three times daily
- *Standardized tablets:* 100-mg tablets containing 5 mg andrographolide and deoxyandrographolide, four tablets three times daily

Pharmacokinetics—If Available (form or route when known): Rapidly absorbed and distributed to the gallbladder, kidney, ovary, and lung. Ninety percent is excreted in the urine and feces in 24 hours and 94% after 48 hours (Tang & Eisenbrand, 1992).

Toxicity: Low potential for toxicity

Contraindications: Pregnancy

Side Effects: Nausea, vomiting; rarely urticaria

Long-Term Safety: No serious adverse effects expected; long-term human use and animal studies have found no safety issues.

Use in Pregnancy/Lactation/Children: Possible antifertility effect; contraindicated in all

Drug/Herb Interactions and Rationale (if known): None known

Special Notes: Capsule or pill form will achieve the highest patient compliance because the herb is intensely bitter.

BIBLIOGRAPHY

Amroyan E, et al. (1999). Inhibitory effect of andrographolide from *Andrographis paniculata* on PAF-induced platelet aggregation. *Phytomedicine.* 6(1):27–32.

Bone K. (1996). *Clinical Applications of Ayurvedic and Chinese Herbs*. Queensland, Australia: Phytotherapy Press.

Caceres DD, et al. (1999). Use of visual analogue scale measurements (VAS) to assess the effectiveness of standardized Andrographis paniculata extract SHA-10 in reducing the symptoms of common cold. A randomized double-blind placebo study. *Phytomedicine*. 6(4):217–23.

Kapoor LD. (1990). *CRC Handbook of Ayurvedic Medicinal Plants*. Boca Raton, FL: CRC Press.

Madau SS, et al. (1996). Anti-inflammatory activity of andrographolide. *Fitoterapia*. 67(5):452–8.

Melchior J, et al. (1997). Controlled clinical study of standardized *Andrographis paniculata* extract in common cold: A pilot trial. *Phytomedicine*. 3(4):315–8.

Mills S, Bone K. (1999). *Principles and Practice of Phytotherapy*. Edinburgh: Churchill-Livingstone.

Puri A, et al. (1993). Immunostimulant agents from *Andrographis paniculata*. *Journal of Natural Products*. 56:995–9.

Tang W, Eisenbrand G. (1992). *Chinese Drugs of Plant Origin*. Berlin: Springer-Verlag.

You-ping Zhu. (1998). *Chinese Materia Medica - Chemistry, Pharmacology, and Applications*. Amsterdam: Harwood Academic Publishers.

🌿 NAME: Angelica (*Angelica archangelica*)

Common Names: Wild angelica, garden angelica

Family: *Apiaceae*

Description of Plant: Commonly cultivated, aromatic biennial plant in the parsley family; numerous species in Europe, North America, Asia

Medicinal Part: Root, rhizome

Constituents and Action (if known)

- Angelica root oil (alpha angelica lactone) augments Ca^{++} binding in cardiac microsomes (in canines), which may increase contractility; antibacterial activity against *Mycobacterium avium*; antifungal activity against 14 types of fungi (Blumenthal, 2000)

- Coumarin
  - Osthol: anti-inflammatory and analgesic properties (Chen, 1995)
  - Umbelliferone
- Furanocoumarins (angelicin, bergapten)
- Volatile oil
  - Monoterpenes: beta-phellandrene (13%–28%), alpha-pinene (14%–31%), alpha-phellandrene (2%–14%)
  - Sesquiterpenes: beta-bisabolene, bisabolol, beta-caryophyllene
- Resins (6%)

Nutritional Ingredients: Young leaves used as a vegetable; stems candied

Traditional Use
- Antibacterial, carminative, bitter and digestive tonic, diaphoretic, diuretic, antispasmodic, emmenagogue, cholagogue, sedative
- According to legend, angelica was revealed to humans by an angel as a cure for the plague, hence its name.
- A popular European herbal medicine. It has been used for dyspepsia, nausea, borborygmus, flatulence, menstrual cramps, colds, fevers, headaches, and nervous stomach.

Current Use
- GI complaints: feeling of fullness, mild intestinal spasms, flatulence, achlorhydria, nausea
- Stimulates gastric secretions and pancreatic juices (Karnick, 1994)
- In India, used to treat anorexia nervosa and dyspepsia

Available Forms, Dosage, and Administration Guidelines
- *Dried root and rhizome:* 1 to 2 g, three times daily
- *Infusion:* steep 1 tsp of the fine-cut root in 8 oz boiled water for approximately 10 to 20 minutes. Take 4 oz a half-hour before meals.
- *Tincture:* (1:5, 45% alcohol), 20 to 40 gtt (2–4 mL), three times daily

- *Essential oil (Oleum angelicae):* 5 to 10 drops in a carrier oil for topical application in neuralgic and rheumatic complaints (see Side Effects)

Pharmacokinetics—If Available (form or route when known): None known

Toxicity: Generally recognized as safe

Contraindications: None known

Side Effects: Possible photosensitivity with topical application. Avoid excess sun or ultraviolet radiation exposure.

Long-Term Safety: Probably safe; long history as a medicine, tea, and in liqueurs

Use in Pregnancy/Lactation/Children: Not recommended in pregnancy. Small doses have been and are regularly used in Europe by children and breast-feeding women.

Drug/Herb Interactions and Rationale (if known): None known

Special Notes: The cut, sifted root, if properly stored in a cool, dry environment in an airtight container, has a shelf life of 1 year to 18 months. The powdered root has a shelf life of 24 hours.

BIBLIOGRAPHY
Bisset NG, Wichtl M. (1994). *Herbal Drugs and Phytopharmaceuticals.* Boca Raton, FL: CRC Press.
Blumenthal M, Goldberg A, Brinckmann J. (2000). *Herbal Medicine: Expanded Commission E Monographs.* Austin, TX: American Botanical Council.
Chen YF, et al. (1995). Anti-inflammatory and analgesic activities from roots of *Angelica pubescens. Planta Medica.* 61(1):2.
Karnick CR. (1994). *Pharmacopeial Standards of Herbal Plants.* Dehli: Sri Satguru Publishers.
Olin B. (Ed.). (1995). *Lawrence Review of Natural Products.* St. Louis: Facts and Comparisons, Wolters/Kluwer Co.

NAME: Arnica (*Arnica montana*)

Common Names: Leopard's bane, wolf's bane, mountain tobacco, Mexican arnica, mountain snuff, mountain arnica

Family: *Asteraceae*

Description of Plant: Perennial; grows 1' to 2' and has bright yellow, daisy-like, aromatic flowers. Native to mountain regions of Europe to southern Russia; Alaska to Mexico in western North America (*Arnica cordifola*)

Medicinal Part: Dried flower heads, rhizome

Constituents and Action (if known)

- Flavonoid glycosides (betuletol, eupafolin, flavonol glucuronides, hispidulin, luteolin, quercetin, others; Duke, 1989; Leung & Foster, 1996): improves circulation, reduces cholesterol, stimulates CNS (Bisset, 1994; Chevallier, 1996; Newall, 1996)
- Terpenoids (arnifolin, arnicolides; Chevallier, 1996)
- Sesquiterpene lactones (helenalin, dihydrohelenalin)
  - Anti-inflammatory and mild analgesic (Newall, 1996)
  - Antibacterial effect (Schaffner, 1997)
  - Antifungal activity (Bisset, 1994)
  - May inhibit platelet activity (Baillargeon, 1993)
  - Oxytocic activity (Bisset, 1994)
  - Displays cytotoxic activity (Willuhn, 1994)
- Amines (betaine, choline, trimethylamine)
- Coumarins (scopoletin, umbelliferone)
- Carbohydrates (mucilage and polysaccharides) (Chevallier, 1996)
  - Marked phagocytosis in vivo
  - Immunostimulating activity
- Volatile oils (thymol, free fatty acids) obtained from rhizomes and roots; used in perfumery (Duke, 1989)
- Arnicin, a bitter compound
- Phytosterols, resins, tannins, carotenoids (Chevallier, 1996; DerMarderosian, 1998; Newall, 1996)

Nutritional Ingredients: None known

Traditional Use
- *External* (creams, ointments, tinctures): for sprains, bruises and wound healing; anti-inflammatory; mild pain reliever; insect bites
- *Internal:* for bruises and trauma injuries, dilute tea for senile heart (Weiss, 1985), arteriosclerosis, angina

Current Use
- *External:* first aid cream (Europe), anti-inflammatory, mild pain reliever, arthralgia, arthritis, swelling related to fractures, improves circulation, hair tonics, antidandruff preparations
- *Internal:* homeopathic remedy for trauma, bruises, contusions, sprains and strains. No supportive evidence has been found (Ernst, 1998), but clinical and empirical use suggest benefit.

Available Forms, Dosage, and Administration Guidelines
Preparations: Dried flowers, whole or cut and sifted; creams (typically contain 15% arnica oil; salves should contain 20% to 25% arnica oil); gels, ointments; tinctures; homeopathic products

Typical Dosage
- *Topical:* Apply externally, following manufacturer's instructions. Use commercial preparations rather than homemade ones because of arnica's potential toxicity.
- *Tincture:* Use internally only under the guidance of a trained practitioner. 1:10, 70% alcohol, 1 to 3 gtt twice daily.

Pharmacokinetics—If Available (form or route when known): None known

Toxicity: Internal use irritates mucous membranes and can cause stomach pain, diarrhea, vomiting, dyspnea, and hepatic failure. One-gram doses can damage heart and in rare cases may lead to cardiac arrest.

Contraindications: Do not use on damaged, abraded, or cracked skin.

Side Effects

- *Topical:* contact dermatitis can occur in sensitive patients. A small skin test before general use may be helpful.
- *Internal:* GI irritation and kidney pain can occur at the normal therapeutic dosage of the tea or tincture in sensitive patients.

Long-Term Safety: Unknown

Use in Pregnancy/Lactation/Children

- Avoid during pregnancy; there is a risk of oxytocic activity and a lack of knowledge about teratogenic potential.
- Avoid during lactation or in children. No research available.
- Homeopathic preparations are safe during pregnancy and lactation and for children.

Drug/Herb Interactions and Rationale (if known):

Possible reduced effectiveness of antihypertensive medications. Do not take concurrently.

Special Notes

- Best to use on a short-term basis for acute conditions
- Research findings are mixed (positive and negative; Hart, 1997; Kaziro, 1984). More studies are needed to determine effectiveness.
- Avoid prolonged external use, because this increases the likelihood of contact dermatitis.
- FDA has classed arnica as an unsafe herb for internal use.

BIBLIOGRAPHY

Baillargeon L, et al. (1993). The effects of *Arnica montana* on blood coagulation: A randomized, controlled trial. *Canadian Family Physician.* 39:236–67.

Bisset N. (1994). *Herbal Drugs and Phytopharmaceuticals.* Stuttgart: CRC Press.

Chevallier A. (1996). *Encyclopedia of Medicinal Plants.* New York: DK Publishing.

DerMarderosian A. [Ed.]. (1998). *Review of Natural Products.* St. Louis, MO: Facts and Comparisons.

Duke J. (1989). *CRC Handbook of Medicinal Herbs.* Boca Raton, FL: CRC Press.

Ernst E. (1998). Efficacy of homeopathic arnica: A systematic review of placebo-controlled clinical trials. *Archives of Surgery.* 133(11):1187–90.

Hart O, et al. (1997). Double-blind, placebo-controlled, randomized clinical trial of homeopathic arnica C30 for pain and infection after total abdominal hysterectomy. *Journal of the Royal Society of Medicine.* 90:73–8.

Kaziro GS. (1984). Metronidazole and *Arnica montana* in the prevention of post-surgical complications: A comparative placebo-controlled trial. *British Journal of Oral & Maxillofacial Surgery.* 22:42

Leung A, Foster S. (1996). *Encyclopedia of Common Natural Ingredients* (2nd ed.). New York: John Wiley & Sons.

McGuffin M, et al. (1997). *American Herbal Product Association's Botanical Safety Handbook.* Boca Raton, FL: CRC Press.

Newall C, et al. (1996). *Herbal Medicines.* London: Pharmaceutical Press.

Schaffner W. (1997). Granny's remedy explained at the molecular level: Helenalin inhibits NF-kappa B. *Biological Chemistry.* 378:935.

Weiss R. (1985). *Herbal Medicine.* Gothenburg, Sweden: Ab Arcanum.

Willuhn G, et al. (1994). Cytotoxicity of flavonoids and sesquiterpenelactones from *Arnica* species against GLC4 and the COLO 320 cell lines. *Planta Medica.* 60:434–37.

🌿 NAME: Artichoke (*Cynara scolymus*)

Common Names: Globe artichoke

Family: *Asteraceae*

Description of Plant

- Warm-climate perennial native to Mediterranean; 80% of the yearly crop grown in Italy, Spain, and France
- Grows about 150 cm tall
- Large leaves; thistle-like
- Large edible flower heads made up of leaflike scales that enclose the bud

Medicinal Part: Fresh or dried leaf

Constituents and Action (if known)

- Caffeic acid derivatives (polyphenols)

- ○ Cynaroside, cynarin, cynarine are the bitter principles responsible for liver protective properties (Chevallier, 1996; Kraft, 1997; Newall et al., 1996). They increase bile flow (Kirchhoff et al., 1994) and assist with liver regeneration (rat livers) (Marcos et al., 1968; Mills & Bone, 1999).
  - ○ 3,5 dicaffeoylquinic acid and 4,5 dicaffeoylquinic acid have demonstrated anti-inflammatory activity in vivo (Mills & Bone, 1999).
- Flavonoids (luteolin, apigenin, cosmoside, quercetin, rutin, hesperitin, hesperidoside) may reduce cholesterol by inhibiting cholesterol synthesis (Leiss, 1998; Renewed proof, 1999; Wegener & Fintelmann, 1999).
- Sesquiterpene lactones (cynaropicrin)
- Volatile oils (beta selinene, eugenol, deconal)

Traditional Use

- Antiemetic, bitter tonic, choleretic, antihepatotoxin, diuretic
- Commonly used in Europe as a medicine since the 16th century. Primarily used as a digestion, liver, and urinary tract remedy, for treating dyspepsia, constipation, skin conditions, jaundice, hepatic insufficiency, urinary calculi, and nephrosclerosis.

Current Use

- Choleretic action useful to treat dyspepsia, loss of appetite, poor fat digestion, constipation, flatulence, nausea, GRD, and hyperlipidemia
- Reduces LDL cholesterol levels
- Cytoprotective actions in the liver: acts as an antioxidant and promotes regeneration of damaged liver tissue. May be used along with milk thistle, turmeric, or schisandra for hepatitis B and C and for drug- or chemical-induced liver damage.

Available Forms, Dosage, and Administration Guidelines

- *Leaf:* 2 g, three times daily
- *Dry extract* (12:1): 0.5 g in a single daily dose
- *Fluid extract* (1:1): 2 mL, three times daily
- *Tincture* (1:5, 30% alcohol): 60–100 gtt (3–5 mL), three times daily

Pharmacokinetics—If Available (form or route when known): Not known

Toxicity: None

Contraindications: Obstructions in biliary tract; use cautiously with gallstones

Side Effects: Handling the plant may cause allergic dermatitis in sensitive people.

Long-Term Safety: Long-term use as a food; no adverse effects expected

Use in Pregnancy/Lactation/Children: No restrictions known

Drug/Herb Interactions and Rationale (if known): None known

BIBLIOGRAPHY

Burnham T (ed.). (1999). *Review of Natural Products*. St. Louis: Facts & Comparisons.

Chevallier A. (1996). *Encyclopedia of Medicinal Plants* (pp. 196–197). New York: DK Publishing.

Ensiminger A, et al. (1994). *Foods and Nutrition Encyclopedia* (2d ed.). Boca Raton, FL: CRC Press.

Kirchhoff R, et al. (1994). Increase in choleresis by means of artichoke extract. *Phytomedicine.* 1:107–115.

Kraft K. (1997). Artichoke leaf extract: recent findings reflecting effects on lipid metabolism, liver, and gastrointestinal tracts. *Phytomedicine.* 1:369–378.

Leiss O. (1998). Hypercholesterolemia during medication with artichoke extracts. *Deutsche Medizinische Wochenschrift.* 123(25–26):818–819.

Maros T, et al. (1968). Effects of *Cynar scolymus* extracts on the regenerations of rat liver. *Arzneimittelforschung.* 18(7):884–886.

Mills S, Bone K. (1999). *Principles and Practice of Phytotherapy.* Edinburgh: Churchill Livingstone.

Newall C, et al. (1996). *Herbal Medicine* (pp. 36–37). London: Pharmaceutical Press.

Renewed proof: inhibition of cholesterol biosynthesis by dried extract of artichoke leaves. (1999). *Fortschritte der Komplementarmedizin.* 6(3):168–169.

Wegener T, Fintelmann V. (1999). Pharmacological properties and therapeutic profile of artichoke. *Wien Medizinische Wochenschrift.* 149(8–10):241–247.

NAME: Ashwagandha (*Withania somnifera*)

Common Names: Winter cherry

Family: *Solanaceae*

Description of Plant: A native of India, this member of the nightshade family is a semihardy evergreen shrub. The small green-yellow flowers are followed by bright orange-red berries.

Medicinal Part: Root

Constituents and Action (if known)

- Alkaloids (0.4%): isopelietierine, withasamine, somniferin, anaferine; sedative, withasomnine. *Withania* alkaloids have antispasmodic activity in intestinal, bronchial, uterine, and arterial smooth muscle. The activity is similar in action to that of papaverine (Mills & Bone, 1999).
- Steroidal lactones (2.8245%): withanolides. Anti-inflammatory and inhibit synthesis of 2-macroglobin, which stimulates inflammatory cascade (Standeven, 1999). Glucocorticoid-like effect (Mills & Bone, 1999), withaferin A-antihepatotoxin, immunosuppressive, sitoindosides–adaptogenic anabolic antidepressant, immunostimulant, memory aid, gastroprotective (Standeven, 1999), protected against stress-induced gastric ulcers (Bone, 1996).
- Ashwagandha has cardioprotective effects (Dhuley, 2000).
- Alcoholic root extract interacts with the GABA-A receptor, and it enhances benzodiazepine binding and has anticonvulsant activity.
- Root extracts have an immunomodulatory activity (Bone, 1996). Root extracts have shown the ability to work synergistically with radiation in the treatment of mouse tumors.

- A comparison of *Withania* and *Panax ginseng* showed that ashwagandha had similar potency to ginseng in its adaptogenic, tonic, and anabolic effects (Bone, 1996).

Nutritional Ingredients: Iron

Traditional Use

- Anti-inflammatory, adaptogen, astringent, nervine, hypotensive, diuretic, antispasmodic, sedative
- Root is used in Ayurvedic and Unani medicine as an aphrodisiac, a calming tonic for exhaustion, neurasthenia, anxiety, depression, impaired memory, poor muscle tone, and as an aid in recovery from debilitating diseases. It is given in milk to children and the elderly for emaciation, debility, and anemia.
- A male reproductive tonic mixed with ghee or honey for impotence

Current Use

- Calming adaptogen, for chronic fatigue syndrome (CFS), anxiety with hypertension, insomnia, stress-induced ulcers, and impotence associated with anxiety or exhaustion
- Used for fibromyalgia along with black cohosh (*Cimicifuga*) and kava (*Piper methysticum*)
- For osteoarthritis and rheumatoid arthritis, as well as other inflammatory chronic diseases (ankylosing spondylitis, multiple sclerosis, asthma, systemic lupus erythematosus)
- Supportive treatment for cancer and associated cachexia. Animal studies have demonstrated that ashwagandha can inhibit cyclophosphamide-induced damage to the bone marrow, preventing leukopenia in mice (Davis & Kuttan, 1998).
- For depleted, exhausted, underweight patients, especially the elderly with impaired memory. In a double-blind clinical trial, the effects of withania (3 g/day for 1 year) on the aging process were assessed in 101 healthy men (50–59 years old). Significant improvements in hemoglobin, red blood cell count, hair melanin, and seated stature was observed. Serum cholesterol levels decreased and nail calcium was preserved. Erythrocyte sedimentation rate decreased significantly, and 71.4% of those treated with the herb reported improved sexual performance (Kuppurajan et al., 1980).

Available Forms, Dosage, and Administration Guidelines

- *Dried root:* 2 to 6 g/day
- *Capsules:* Two 500-mg capsules three or four times per day
- *Tea:* 1 tsp dried root in 8 oz hot water; decoct 10 minutes and steep 20 minutes. Take 4 oz two or three times per day.
- *Tincture* (1:5, 45% alcohol): 40 to 80 gtt (2–4 mL) three times a day

Pharmacokinetics—If Available (form or route when known): Not known

Toxicity: Low potential for toxicity

Contraindications: None known

Side Effects: Rarely, nausea, dermatitis, abdominal pain, diarrhea

Long-Term Safety: Safe; long-term history of regular use and animal and human trials show no cumulative toxicity

Use in Pregnancy/Lactation/Children: Commonly used in India as a pregnancy tonic, as a stimulant for milk production, and for children. Use only in small amounts; large amounts (more than 3 g/day) are contraindicated during pregnancy.

Drug/Herb Interactions and Rationale (if known): May potentiate action of barbiturates and benzodiazepines

Special Notes: Considered one of the great tonic remedies in ayurvedic medicine. Research has confirmed most, if not all, traditional uses and its very low potential for toxicity.

BIBLIOGRAPHY

Agarwal R, et al. (1999). Studies on immunomodulatory activity of *Withania somnifera* (ashwagandha) extracts in experimental immune inflammation. *Journal of Ethnopharmacology.* 67(1):27–35.

Archana R, Namasivayam A. (1999). Antistressor effect of *Withania somnifera. Journal of Ethnopharmacology.* 64(1):91–93.

Bone K. (1996). *Clinical Applications of Ayurvedic and Chinese Herbs.* Queensland, Australia: Phytotherapy Press.

Davis L, Kuttan G. (1998). Suppressive effect of cyclophosphamide-induced toxicity by *Withania somnifera* extract in mice. *Journal of Ethnopharmacology.* 62(3):209–214.

Dhuley JN. (2000). Adaptogenic and cardioprotective action of ashwagandha in rats and frogs. *Journal of Ethnopharmacology*. 70(1):57–64.

Kapoor LD. (1990). *CRC Handbook of Ayurvedic Medicinal Plants*. Boca Raton, FL: CRC Press.

Kuppurajan K, et al. (1980). *Journal of Research in Ayurvedic Science*. 1:247.

Mills S, Bone K. (1999). *Principles and Practice of Phytotherapy*. London: Churchill Livingstone.

Standeven R. (1998). *Withania somnifera. European Journal of Herbal Medicine*. 4(2):17–22.

NAME: Asian Ginseng (*Panax ginseng*)

Common Names: Asian, Chinese, Korean ginseng, ren shen (Chinese)

Family: *Araliaceae*

Description of Plant

- Small herbaceous plant with divided palmate leaves and clusters of red berries in the autumn. It grows in Asia above the 38th latitude (Chinese or Korean ginseng).
- Asian ginseng is considered the strongest of the *Panax* species. It nourishes the *yin* and *qi* and energetically is hot (stimulating). American ginseng is milder and less stimulating and is believed to be cooler energetically. (See the monograph on American ginseng.)
- Wild harvested root is believed to be the most effective, even though the constituents are generally similar. Wild Asian *Panax* is virtually extinct and should not be used.

Medicinal Part: The root is most widely used. It is gathered in the fall just before defoliation.

Constituents and Action (if known)

- Ginsenosides (13 have been identified)
  - Support the adrenals by supporting the hypothalamus–pituitary–adrenal axis (Kim et al., 1999)
  - May reduce side effects (elevated lipid levels) in patients receiving corticosteroids

- ○ Improve CFS
- ○ Improve cognitive function, attention span, psychomotor performance, concentration
- ○ May reduce cancer development by increasing CD4 and NK cells, increasing apoptosis (Scaglione et al., 1990, 1996; Yun, 1993)
- ○ Block acetylcholine and gamma-aminobutyric receptors and is an antagonist of muscarinic and histamine receptors (Tachikawa et al., 1999)
- Panaxosides A through F exert a hypoglycemic effect by increasing insulin release from the pancreas and a higher number of insulin receptors and lower glycosylated hemoglobin levels (Loi, 1996; Sotaniemi et al., 1995).
- Polysaccharides support immune function (Scaglione et al., 1996), act as antioxidants and free radical scavengers, and may reduce the development of cancer.
- Many other constituents: volatile oils, sterols, flavonoids, peptides, vitamins (B_1, B_2, nicotinic acid, biotin)

Nutritional Ingredients: Vitamins B_1, B_2, niacin, biotin

Traditional Use
- The Chinese have used ginseng for 4,000 years, and it has a reputation among the lay public as a panacea, aphrodisiac, longevity herb, and energy tonic.
- Ginseng is a corruption of the Chinese name "ren shen," which means "man root" because of the root's supposed resemblance to the human form.
- Russians have used ginseng since 1855.
- In TCM, Asian ginseng is used to tonify the original *qi* and is given for shock, syncope, shortness of breath, and weak pulse.
- Ginseng is also used to tonify the lungs, Chinese spleen, stomach, and heart. It is given in complex formulas for asthma, lack of appetite, organ prolapse, diabetes, insomnia, poor memory, and palpitations.

Current Use
- Mixed research is available on uses and efficacy.
- Balances bodily functions

- Adaptogen: rather than being used to treat specific diseases, it is used to help the organism adapt to physical and mental stress:
  ○ Improves stamina (not verified by research)
  ○ Increases concentration and cognitive function (Wesnes et al., 1997)
  ○ Combats mental and physical fatigue
  ○ May help to support body during and after radiation and chemotherapy
  ○ Aids in disease resistance (cancer, diabetes, infection) (Tachikawa et al., 1999)
  ○ May decrease vaginal atrophy and increase vaginal moisture during menopause
  ○ May protect from flu and common cold
  ○ Improves symptoms of CFS
  ○ May assist with alcohol withdrawal

Available Forms, Dosage, and Administration Guidelines
Preparations: Dried root ("white"), steamed root ("red"), capsules, extracts, tablets, tinctures, teas. Fresh harvested root typically contains 2% to 3% ginsenosides, and the extracts range from 5% to 17%.

Typical Dosage
- *Capsules:* Up to four 500- to 600-mg capsules a day. For standardized products (4%–7% ginsenosides), 100 mg one or two times a day is generally recommended, or follow manufacturer's or practitioner's recommendations.
- *Dried roots:* 2 to 4 g/day
- *Tincture* (1:5, 35% alcohol): 60–100 gtt (3 to 5 mL) three times a day
- *Fluid extract* (1:1): 2 to 4 mL/day (34%–45% alcohol)

Pharmacokinetics—If Available (form or route when known): None known

Toxicity: Nontoxic

Contraindications
- Avoid during acute illness and menses and in patients with hypertension, schizophrenia, mania, brittle diabetes (may reduce blood sugar levels), cardiovascular disease (may

elevate blood pressure), estrogen-positive cancers (may stimulate tumor growth; this is theoretical, however, and no data support this).
- Most often used in elderly, deficient, and depleted patients; less appropriate in younger, healthier persons.

Side Effects: In type A people, may cause or exacerbate insomnia, anxiety, tachycardia, palpitations, high blood pressure, headache, chest pain, and hypertension. Infrequent side effects include diarrhea, skin rash, breast tenderness in men.

Long-Term Safety: Safe when taken as directed

Use in Pregnancy/Lactation/Children: Do not use. Not appropriate except rare cases of older children with chronic disease.

Drug/Herb Interactions and Rationale (if known)
- Concurrent use with caffeinated beverages increases the likelihood of side effects. Do not use concurrently.
- May potentiate the actions of centrally acting drugs. Do not use concurrently.
- Ginseng has a mild effect on platelets and may increase bleeding if taken concurrently with warfarin. Use cautiously.
- May potentiate the action of steroids. Use cautiously.
- Use caution with antidiabetic medications as a result of hypoglycemic activity.
- Increases side effects of monoamine oxidase inhibitors, such as headache, tremor, mania. Avoid concurrent use.

Special Notes
- Quality root is extremely expensive: the best grades of Korean red may sell for $50/oz. Studies have been done on many ginseng products, and as many as 25% had no ginseng and 60% did not have enough to produce activity (Cui et al., 1994).
- Asian ginseng, also referred to as Chinese, Korean, or *Panax ginseng*, primarily grows in the Orient. American ginseng is of the same family but grows in the United States. Siberian ginseng is a distant relative of a different genus (*Eleutherococcus senticosus*). All ginsengs have known adaptogenic activity. Adaptogens show a nonspecific effect

and raise the powers of resistance to toxins of a physical, chemical, or biologic nature. They bring about a normalizing or balancing action independent of the type of pathologic condition. They are harmless and do not influence normal body functions. They work through the HPA axis.

- Ginseng is often recommended to increase exercise performance, but several well-done studies suggest this is not true (Allen et al., 1998; Engels et al., 1996; Hermann et al., 1997).

BIBLIOGRAPHY

Allen JD, et al. (1998). Ginseng supplementation does not enhance healthy young adults' peak aerobic exercise performance. *Journal of the American College of Nutritionists.* 17(5):462–466.

Bensky D, Gamble A. (1993). *Chinese Herbal Medicine—Materia Medica* (pp. 450–454). Seattle: Eastland Press.

Cui J, et al. (1994). What do commercial ginseng preparations contain? *Lancet.* 344:134.

Engels HJ, et al. (1996). Failure of chronic ginseng supplementation to affect work performance and energy metabolism in healthy adult females. *Nutrition Research.* 16:1295–1305.

Hermann J, et al. (1997). No ergogenic effects of ginseng (*Panax ginseng*) during graded maximal aerobic exercise. *Journal of the American Dietetic Association.* 97(10):1110–1115.

Janetsky, K, Morreale, AP. (1997). Probable interaction between warfarin and ginseng. *American Journal of Health-System Pharmacy.* 54(6):692–693.

Kim HS, et al. (1990). Antinarcotic effects of the standardized ginseng extract G115 on morphine. *Planta Medica.* 56:158–63.

Kim YR, et al. (1999). *Panax ginseng* blocks morphine-induced thymic apoptosis by lowering plasma corticosterone level. *General Pharmacology.* 32(6):647–52.

Kwan CY. (1995). Vascular effects of selective antihypertensive drugs derived from traditional medicinal herbs. *Clinical and Experimental Pharmacology and Physiology.*(Suppl. 1):297–299.

Loi S. (1996). Ginseng. *Australian Journal of Emergency Care.* 3(3):28–29.

Scaglione F, et al. (1996). Efficacy and safety of the standardized ginseng extract G 115 for potentiating vaccination against common cold and/or influenza syndrome. *Drugs Under Experimental and Clinical Research.* 22(2):65–72.

Scaglione F, et al. (1990). Immunomodulatory effects of two extracts of *Panax ginseng. Drugs Under Experimental and Clinical Research.* 16:537–42.

Sotaniemi EA, et al. (1995). Ginseng therapy in non-insulin-dependent diabetic patients. *Diabetes Care.* 18(10):1373–75.

Tachikawa E, et al. (1999). Effects of ginseng saponins on responses induced by various receptor stimuli. *European Journal of Pharmacology.* 369(1):23–32.

Wesnes, KA, et al. (1997). The cognitive, subjective and physical effects of a gingko biloba/*panax ginseng* combination in healthy volunteers with neurasthenic complaints. *Psychopharmacology Bulletin.* 33(4):677–83.

Yan, Shu-Su, et al. (1998). Modulation of American ginseng on brainstem GABAergic effects on rats. *Journal of Ethnopharmacology.* 62:215–222.

Yun YS, et al. (1993). Inhibition of autochthonous tumor by ethanol insoluble fraction from *Panax ginseng* as an immunomodulator. *Planta Medica.* 59:521–4.

Zhang T, et al. (1990). Ginseng root: Evidence for numerous regulatory peptides and insulinotropic activity. *Biomedical Research.* 1:49–54.

NAME: Astragalus (*Astragalus membranaceus, Astragalus membranaceus var. mongholicus*)

Common Names: Milk vetch, huang chi, huang qi

Family: *Fabaceae*

Description of Plant

- Grows along forest margins in most of China, Korea, and Japan; mostly cultivated in China
- There are more than 1,750 astragalus species. Some are ornamental, some are medicinal, and others are poisonous, especially to grazing animals.
- Member of the pea family

Medicinal Part: Plants are 4 to 5 years old before the root is harvested. In most cases, astragalus is repeatedly moistened in honey water and flattened to create the typical "tongue depressor"-shaped root that is available commercially. This process is believed to make the root more active.

Constituents and Action (if known)

- Polysaccharides (astragaloglucans)
  - Enhance immunologic response, stimulate white blood cell activity, increase production of antibodies and interferon (particularly effective in patients undergoing chemotherapy and radiation) (Liu et al., 1994; Yao et al., 1992)
  - Increase phagocytic activity (Shimizu et al., 1991; Tomoda et al., 1991)
- Saponins (cycloartanes)
  - Diuretic activity, probably from local irritation of the kidney (Hostettmann et al., 1995); anti-inflammatory (Tang et al., 1992); hypotensive effects (Tang et al., 1992)
  - Stimulate growth of isolated lymphocytes (Calis et al., 1997; Lau et al., 1989)
- Triterpene glycosides (astragalosides I–IV)
- Biphenyl: antihepatoxic activity (He et al., 1991)
- Isoflovan glycosides: antioxidant activity (similar to vitamin E), mucronulatol, formononetin, demethoxyisoflavin (Shirataki et al., 1997; Toda et al., 1998)
- Flavonoids (afromosin, ordoratin, calycosin, quercetin)
- Triterpenoid saponins (astragalosides I–VII)

Nutritional Ingredients: None known

Traditional Use: The Chinese name for this herb is huang qi. *Huang* means yellow, referring to the interior of the root, and *qi* means leader, vital force, the venerable one, the superior tonic in Chinese medicine. Astragalus is thought to add years of health to the aged and to increase overall vitality and health. It is used in TCM to tonify the Chinese spleen, for organ prolapse, as a diuretic, to strengthen the lungs, and to protect against colds.

Current Use

- To treat stomach ulcers, diabetes, shortness of breath, general weakness
- To improve immune function in persons undergoing chemotherapy and radiation
- To enhance immune function in persons with HIV infection. Several Chinese reports suggest that astragalus can

induce seronegative conversion, but these reports need to be verified (Burack et al., 1996; Lu, 1995; Lu et al., 1995; Ono et al., 1989).

- In China, it is a part of *fu-zheng* therapy, where the goal is to restore immune system function in patients with cancer and to protect them from the side effects of chemotherapy (Bensky & Gamble, 1993).
- To treat recurrent colds and upper respiratory tract infections (Upton et al., 1999)
- Chinese studies have shown increased cardiac output in 20 patients with angina after 2 weeks of treatment. The herb strengthened the function of the left ventricle and reduced oxygen free radical activity. Astragalus also increased survival rates in in vivo studies with acute Coxsackie B-3 viral myocarditis infections (Upton et al., 1999).

Available Forms, Dosage, and Administration Guidelines

Preparations: Dried root, sliced (looks like a tongue depressor) or powdered; capsules, extracts, tablets, tinctures, combination products

Typical Dosage

- *Capsules:* Six to eight 400- to 500-mg capsules daily
- *Tincture* (1:5, 30% alcohol): 60 to 90 gtt (3–5 mL) four times a day
- *Tea:* 9 to 15 g dried sliced root, simmered for several hours in 1 qt water (the decoction is ready when the water is reduced to 1 pint)
- Or follow manufacturer's or practitioner's recommendation

Pharmacokinetics—If Available (form or route when known): None known

Toxicity: None known

Contraindications: Not recommended in acute infections

Side Effects: None known

Long-Term Safety: Used in China as a medicinal food, cooked in soups and stews. No safety issues expected.

Use in Pregnancy/Lactation/Children: No research available, but no adverse effects expected

Drug/Herb Interactions and Rationale (if known): None known

BIBLIOGRAPHY

Bensky D, Gamble A. (1993). *Chinese Herbal Medicine—Materia Medica* (pp. 457–459). Seattle: Eastland Press.

Burack J, et al. (1996). Pilot randomized controlled trial of Chinese herbal treatment for HIV-associated symptoms. *Journal of Acquired Immune Deficiency Syndrome and Human Retrovirology.* 12:386.

Calis I, et al. (1997). Cycloartane triterpene glycosides from the roots of *Astragalus melanophrurius. Planta Medica.* 63:183.

He Z, et al. (1991). Isolation and identification of chemical constituents of Astragalus root. *Chemical Abstracts.* 114:58918u.

Hostettmann K, et al. (1995). *Saponins* (p. 267). Cambridge, England: Cambridge University Press.

Lau B, et al. (1989). Macrophage chemiluminescence modulated by Chinese medicinal herbs *Astragalus membranaceus* and *Ligustrum lucidum. Phytotherapy Research.* 3:148.

Liu X, et al. (1994). Isolation of astragalan and its immunological activities. *Tianran Chanwu Yaniju Yu Kaifa.* 6:23.

Lu W. (1995). Prospect for study on treatment of AIDS with traditional Chinese medicine. *Journal of Traditional Chinese Medicine.* 15:3.

Lu W, et al. (1995). A report on 8 seronegative converted HIV/AIDS patients with traditional Chinese medicine. *Chinese Medical Journal.* 108:634.

Mills S, Bone K. (1999). *Principles and Practice of Phytotherapy* (pp. 273–279). Edinburgh: Churchill Livingstone.

Ono K, et al. (1989). Differential inhibitory effects of various herb extracts on the activities of reverse transcriptase and various deoxyribonucleic acid (DNA) polymerases. *Chemical Pharmaceutical Bulletin.* 37:1810.

Review of Natural Products. (May 1999). St. Louis: Facts and Comparisons.

Shimizu N, et al. (1991). An acidic polysaccharide having activity on the reticuloendothelial system from the root of *Astragalus mongholicus. Chemical Pharmaceutical Bulletin.* 39:2969.

Shirataki Y, et al. (1997). Antioxidative components isolated from the roots of *Astragalus membranaceus* Bunge (*Astragali radix*). *Phytotherapy Research.* 11:603.

Tang W, et al. (1992). *Chinese Drugs of Plant Origin.* Berlin: Springer-Verlag.

Toda S, et al. (1998). Inhibitory effects of isoflavones in roots of *Astragalus membranaceus* Bunge (*Astragali radix*) on lipid peroxidation by reactive oxygen species. *Phytotherapy Research*. 12:59.

Tomoda M, et al. (1991). A reticuloendothelial system-activating glycan from the roots of *Astragalus membranaceus*. *Phytochemistry*. 31:63.

Upton R, et al. (1999). *American Herbal Pharmacopoeia and Therapeutic Compendium: Astragalus Root*. Santa Cruz, CA: American Pharmacopoeia.

Yao X, et al. (1992). Mechanism of inhibition of HIV-1 infection in vitro by purified extract of *Prunella vulgaris*. *Virology*. 187:56.

B

 NAME: Barberry (*Berberis vulgaris*)

Common Names: Berberis, jaundice berry, wood sour, sourberry, pepperidge bush, European barberry, Oregon graperoot (a related species, *Berberis aquifolium*)

Family: *Berberidaceae*

Description of Plant
- Grows wild throughout Europe and is naturalized in eastern United States
- Shrub grows up to 10 feet tall, with ovate leaves and sharp thorns.
- Flowers bloom from May to June and develop into red oblong berries.

Medicinal Part: Root bark, stem bark (less active)

Constituents and Action (if known)
- Isoquinoline alkaloids: berberine (up to 6%), palmatine, oxyacanthine, magnoflorine, jatrorrhizine, columbamine (Ivanovska & Philipov, 1996; Leung & Foster, 1996)
- Berberine (berberine chloride): antibacterial activity against *Staphylococcus epidermidis*, *Escherichia coli*, *Neisseria meningitidis*, and others (Kutchan, 1996; Leung & Foster, 1996)
  - Inhibits endotoxins
  - Improves watery diarrhea associated with cholera (Maung et al., 1985)

- ○ Cytotoxic, antimitotic, antitumor; increases activity of other antitumor agents; inhibits carcinogens (Mills & Bone, 1999)
- ○ Uterine stimulant
- ○ Antihistaminic and anticholinergic activity (in guinea pig ileum) (Shamsa et al., 1999)
- ○ Antifungal (Mills & Bone, 1999)
- ○ Cholagogue (Mills & Bone, 1999)
- ○ Choleretic, increases bilirubin excretion
- ○ Reduces oxygen free radicals (Ryzhikova et al., 1999)
- Tannins
- Resin

Nutritional Ingredients: Berries: rich in vitamin C, sugars, and pectin

Traditional Use
- Gastrointestinal ailments, including diarrhea and dysentery
- Bitter tonic and cholagogue; used to stimulate bile secretion, for poor fat digestion, biliousness, and constipation with clay-colored stools
- Used in alterative formulas as a blood purifier for cancers, arthritis, and skin conditions

Current Use
- Eye drops (saline solution) for trachoma
- Topical use in creams for psoriasis
- Oral use for UTIs, cystitis
- Oral use for amebic infections (*Giardia*, *Blastocystis hominis*, *Dientamoeba fragilis*, diarrhea)

Available Forms, Dosage, and Administration Guidelines
Preparations: Tablets, tincture, tea
Typical Dosage
- *Berberine sulfate:* 100 mg four times a day. The oral LD_{50} is 329 mg/kg.
- *Tea:* 1 to 2 tsp dried root bark to 8 oz boiling water, decoct 10 minutes, steep 45 minutes; take 4 oz three times a day
- *Tincture* (1:5, 45% alcohol): 40 to 60 gtt (2–4 mL) four times a day

Pharmacokinetics—If Available (form or route when known): None known

Toxicity: Very little

Contraindications: None known

Side Effects
- Nausea
- Vomiting
- Higher doses of berberine sulfate (more than 0.5 g) may cause dizziness, nosebleeds, dyspnea, skin and eye irritation, GI irritation, diarrhea, and nephritis.

Long-Term Safety: No adverse effects are expected from ingestion of normal therapeutic doses of this herb.

Use in Pregnancy/Lactation/Children: Pregnancy: do not use because it is a possible uterine stimulant.

Drug/Herb Interactions and Rationale (if known): None known

Special Notes: Little scientific evidence exists as to the efficacy of the whole herb, but the major alkaloid berberine is well studied and therapeutically active.

BIBLIOGRAPHY

Ivanovska N, Philipov S. (1996). Study on the anti-inflammatory action of *Berberis vulgaris* root extract, alkaloid fractions, and pure alkaloids. *International Journal of Immunopharmacology.* 10:553–561.

Kutchan TM. (Nov. 7, 1996). Heterologous expression of alkaloid biosynthetic genes: a review. *Gene.* 179(1):73–81.

Lawrence Review of Natural Products. (1991). St. Louis: Facts and Comparisons.

Leung AY, Foster S. (1996). *Encyclopedia of Common Natural Ingredients Used in Food, Drugs and Cosmetics.* (2nd ed.). New York: John Wiley and Sons.

Maung KU, et al. (1985). Clinical trial of berberine in acute watery diarrhea. *British Medical Journal.* 291:1601.

Mills S, Bone K. (1999). *Principles and Practice of Phytotherapy.* Edinburgh: Churchill Livingstone.

Ryzhikova MA, et al. (1999). The effect of aqueous extracts of hepatotropic medicinal plants on free-radial oxidation processes. *Eksperimentalnaia Klinicheskaia Farmakologia.* 62(2):36–38.

Shamsa F, Ahmadiani A, Khosrokhavar R. (1999). Antihistaminic and anticholinergic activity of barberry fruit (*Berberis vulgaris*) in the guinea-pig ileum. *Journal of Ethnopharmacology.* 64(2):161–166.

NAME: Bilberry Fruit (*Vaccinium myrtillus*)

Common Names: Bilberries, European blueberry, whortleberries

Family: *Ericaceae* (heath family)

Description of Plant
- Known as European blueberry
- Native to northern and central Europe
- Shrubby perennial, grows in meadows and woods
- Produces shiny black berries containing many small, shiny brownish-red seeds
- Berries have a sweet taste with a slightly acrid aftertaste.
- The *Vaccinium* genus contains nearly 200 species of berries, including cranberry and American blueberry (which has similar chemistry and uses).

Medicinal Part: Ripe fruit

Constituents and Action (if known)
- Anthocyanosides (or anthocyanins)
  - Decrease vascular permeability (Bissett, 1994; Colantuoni et al., 1991)
  - Protect blood vessels (Grismond, 1981), particularly varicose veins, hemorrhoids, and delicate blood vessels in the elderly (Colantuoni et al., 1991; Lietti et al., 1976; Mian et al., 1977)
  - Long-term use may improve vision in persons with myopia (Gandolfo, 1990; Sala et al., 1979).
  - Antiedema (Detre et al., 1986)
  - Act as antioxidant and free radical scavenger (Lietti et al., 1976)
  - Reduce platelet stickiness; stimulate growth and reproduction of collagen (Detre et al., 1986; Monbiosse et al., 1983; Rao et al., 1981)

- ○ Increase prostaglandin E_2 release in stomach mucosa (Mertz-Nielsen et al., 1990)
- ○ Protect liver cells (Mitcheva et al., 1993)
- ○ Slow macular degeneration and diabetic retinopathy, speed up regeneration of rhodopsin (visual purple) (Alfieri & Sole, 1964; Gandolfo, 1990)
- ○ May have anticarcinogenic activity (Bomser et al., 1996)
- ○ Potential anticancer activity, at least in vitro studies (Bomser et al., 1996)
- Polyphenols, tannins, flavonoids (hyperoside, chlorogenic acid, quercetin) (Fraisse et al., 1996)
- Oligomeric procyanidins (OPCs)
- Pectin

Nutritional Ingredients: Rich in vitamin C, flavonoids

Traditional Use
- Used as food for its nutritive value
- Used to treat scurvy and urinary infections and stones
- Fruit was used to treat diarrhea, dysentery, and GI inflammation.
- British World War II pilots were said to have improved night vision with its use.
- Oral rinse for inflammation of the mouth and pharynx

Current Use
- Powerful antioxidant: reduces oxidative stress and has shown the ability to improve cognitive function
- Nonspecific, acute diarrhea
- Vascular disorders: varicose veins and hemorrhoids (prevents and treats, particularly during pregnancy), spider veins, and peripheral vascular disease (improves paresthesia, pain, skin dystrophy, edema), nosebleeds
- Eye conditions: simple glaucoma, myopia, diabetic retinopathy, hypertensive retinopathy, macular degeneration, hemeralopia; improves night vision
- Peptic ulcer: protects gastric mucosa
- Anticancer activity
- Allergies: reduces production of proinflammatory substances such as histamine and bradykinin

Available Forms, Dosage, and Administration Guidelines

Preparations: Dried fruit, capsules, tablets, liquid tinctures, fluid extracts. Standardized products contain 25% anthocyanosides. Fresh fruit contains only 0.1% to 0.25% anthocyanide content.

Typical Dosage
- *Solid (native) extracts:* 0.25 tsp twice a day
- *Capsules and tablets:* two or three standardized capsules or tablets a day, or follow manufacturer's or practitioner's recommendations.
- *Orally:* 600 to 1,800 mg/day standardized product to treat condition. Once improvement is seen, reduce dose to 200 to 300 mg/day; 200 to 300 mg/day for prevention; 60 to 120 mg/day to improve night vision.

Pharmacokinetics—If Available (form or route when known): None known

Toxicity: None known for fruit; long-term use of leaves can cause gastric irritation and kidney damage

Contraindications: None known

Side Effects: None known

Long-Term Safety: Very safe

Use in Pregnancy/Lactation/Children: Safe (Grismond, 1981)

Drug/Herb Interactions and Rationale (if known):
Potential for increased bleeding if taken with anticoagulants and other antiplatelet drugs; use cautiously if taking medicinal quantities. Normal food quantities are safe.

Special Notes: Most studies have been performed on animals. More human research is needed.

BIBLIOGRAPHY:
Alfieri R, Sole P. (1964). Influence des anthocyanosides administres par voie parenterale sur l'adaptoelectroretinogramme du lapin. *Comptes Rendu Societe de Biologie.* 158:23–38.

Bomser J, Madhavi DL, Singletary K, Smith MA. (June 1996). In vitro anticancer activity of fruit extracts from Vaccinium species. *Planta Medica.* 62(3):212–216.

Colantuoni A, et al. (1991). Effects of *Vaccinium myrtillus* anthocyanosides on arterial vasomotion. *Arzneimittelforschung.* 41(9):905–909.

Detre Z, et al. (1986). Studies on vascular permeability in hypertension: action of anthocyanosides. *Clinical Physiology & Biochemistry.* 4(2):143.

Fraisse D, Carnat A, Lamaison JL. (1996). Polyphenolic composition of the leaf of bilberry. *Annales Pharmacie Française.* 54(6):280–283.

Gandolfo E. (1990). Perimetric follow-up of myopic patients treated with anthocyanosides and beta-carotene. *Bulletin Oculisme.* 69:57–71.

Grismond GL. (1981). Treatment of pregnancy-induced phlebopathies. *Minerva Gynecology* 33:221–230.

Lawrence Review of Natural Products. (1995). St. Louis: Facts and Comparisons.

Lietti A, et al. (1976). Studies on *Vaccinium myrtillus* Anthocyanosides. I. Vasoprotective and anti-inflammatory activity. *Arzneimittelforschung.* 26:829–832.

Mertz-Nielsen A, et al. (1990). A natural flavonoid, IdB 1027, increases gastric luminal release of prostaglandin E_2 in healthy subjects. *Italian Journal of Gastroenterology.* 22(5):288.

Mian E, et al. (1977). Anthocyanosides and the walls of microvessels: further aspects of the mechanism of action of their protective effect in syndromes due to abnormal capillary fragility. *Minerva Medicine.* 68:3565–3581.

Mills S, Bone K. (1999). *Principles & Practice of Phytotherapy.* Edinburgh: Churchill Livingstone.

Mitcheva M, et al. (1993). Biochemical and morphological studies on the effects of anthocyans and vitamin E on carbon tetrachloride induced liver injury. *Cellular Microbiology.* 39(4):443.

Monbiosse JC, et al. (1983). Nonenzymatic degradation of acid-soluble calf skin collagen by superoxide ion: Protective effect of flavonoids. *Biochemistry & Pharmacology.* 32:53–58.

Rao CN, Rao VH, Steinman B. (1981). Influence of bioflavonoids on collagen metabolism in rats with adjuvant induced arthritis. *Italian Journal of Biochemistry.* 30:54–62.

Sala D, et al. (1979). Effect of anthocyanosides on visual performance at low illumination. *Minerva Oftalmologie.* 21:283–285.

Wichtl, M, Bissett NG. (1994). *Herbal Drugs and Phytopharmaceuticals.* Stuttgart: Medpharm Scientific Publishers.

NAME: Bitter Melon (*Momordica charantia*)

Common Names: Balsam pear, cerasee, balsam apple, carilla, bitter cucumber, karela

Family: *Cucurbitaceae*

Description of Plant
- Climbing annual vine, grows up to 6 feet tall
- A tropical fruit/vegetable, orange-yellow, edible but very bitter
- Unripened fruit is cucumber-shaped, with bumps on surface.
- Cultivated in Asia, Africa, Central and South America, and India

Medicinal Part: Unripe fruit, leaves, seeds, and seed oil

Constituents and Action (if known)
- Steroidal glycosides
  - Charantin and mormordin: hypoglycemic and antihyperglycemic effect (Murray, 1995; Handa et al., 1990; Raman et al., 1996)
  - Momordicosides G, F_1, F_2, I
  - Momordicines I and II
  - Vicine: inhibits glucose absorption so blood sugar is in better control
- Insulinomimetic lectins (P-insulin): an insulin-like, hypoglycemic peptide; reduces blood sugar (Chevallier, 1996; Raman et al., 1996)
- Oils (stearic, linoleic, oleic acids)
- Alkaloid fraction: slow-acting hypoglycemic effect (Raman et al., 1996)
- Glycoproteins (alpha and beta monorcharin): may have abortifacient activity (Cunnick et al., 1993)
- Other actions: antibiotic, antimicrobial activity (Cunnick et al., 1993), antitumor activity (Bruneton, 1995), antilymphoma, antileukemic activity (Raman et al., 1996), inhibits replication of viruses (polio, herpes simplex I, and HIV) (Cunnick et al., 1993; Raman et al., 1996), has antifertility activity in animals (no human research available)

Nutritional Ingredients: Edible fruit contains vitamins (riboflavin, niacin, ascorbic acid) and fatty acids.

Traditional Use: Treats tumors, asthma, skin infections, GI problems, hypertension, diabetes, colds, fevers, and constipation

Current Use
- Reduces blood sugar, improves glucose tolerance, reduces glycosylated hemoglobin, increases glucose utilization; does not promote insulin secretion (Leatherdale et al., 1981; Platel et al., 1997; Sarkar et al., 1996)
- Antiviral for HIV (experimental studies are being conducted)

Available Forms, Dosage, and Administration Guidelines
- *Juice:* 1–2 oz daily
- *Powder:* 100 mg, up to three times a day, in capsules

Pharmacokinetics—If Available (form or route when known): None known

Toxicity: None known, but may reduce blood sugar in susceptible patients

Contraindications: Patients with diabetes should take this herb under a practitioner's guidance. Contraindicated in hypoglycemia.

Side Effects: GI effects (nausea and vomiting), hypoglycemia

Long-Term Safety: Safe for short-term use (4–8 weeks); no long-term studies available

Use in Pregnancy/Lactation/Children
- Use in pregnancy is not recommended; may increase uterine contractions. More studies are needed.
- Use in children is not recommended. Two children, ages 3 and 4, were given the tea of the leaves and vine in the morning on an empty stomach. One to two hours later, they both experienced convulsions followed by a coma. Blood glucose was 1 mM (normal range 3.8–5.5 mM). Both children recovered after emergency treatment (Raman, 1996).

Drug/Herb Interactions and Rationale (if known): Use cautiously with all antidiabetic drugs because of the increased likelihood of hypoglycemia.

BIBLIOGRAPHY

Bruneton J. (1995). *Pharmacognosy, Phytochemistry, Medicinal Plants.* Paris: Lavoisier.

Chevallier A. (1996). *Encyclopedia of Medicinal Plants.* New York: DK Publishing.

Cunnick J, et al. (1993). Bitter melon (*Momordica charantia*). *Journal of Natural Medicine.* 4(1):16–21.

Handa G, et al. (1990). Hypoglycemic principle of *Momordica charantia* seeds. *Indian Journal of Natural Products.* 6(1):16–19.

Leatherdale B, et al. (June 6, 1981). Improvement in glucose tolerance due to *Momordica charantia. British Medical Journal.* 282(6279):1823–1824.

Murray M. (1995). *The Healing Power of Herbs.* (2nd ed.). Rocklin, CA: Prima Publishing.

Platel K, et al. (1997). Plant foods in the management of diabetes mellitus: vegetables as potential hypoglycaemic agents. *Nahrung.* 41(2):68–74.

Raman A, et al. (1996). Anti-diabetic properties and phytochemistry of *Momordica charantia L.* (Cucurbitaceae). *Phytomedicine.* 2(4):349–362.

Review of Natural Products. (1999). St. Louis: Facts and Comparisons.

Sarkar S, et al. (January 1996). Demonstration of the hypogycemic action of *Momordica charantia* in a validated animal model of diabetes. *Pharmacology Research.* 33(1):1–4.

 NAME: Black Cohosh (*Cimicifuga racemosa*)

Common Names: Black snakeroot, bugbane, bugwort, rattleroot, rattle weed, squaw root

Family: *Ranunculaceae*

Description of Plant

- A striking plant, 3 to 9 feet tall, with deeply divided trilobate leaflets, it grows in hardwood forests in both the United States and Canada.
- Grows at edges of woods, from southern Ontario to Arkansas

- Member of the buttercup family
- Has long spikes of small white flowers; blooms from July to September

Medicinal Part: Rhizome (dug in the autumn)

Constituents and Action (if known)

- Triterpene glycosides decrease vascular spasm and reduce blood pressure; actein, racemoside, cimicifugoside, 27-deoxyacetin
- Salicylic acid
- Tannins
- Cimicifugin (macrotin): an amorphous resin, accounts for approximately 15% to 20% of the root's constituents
- Isoflavones (formononetin): binds to estrogen receptors, producing estrogen-like activity (Lieberman, 1998). The presence of this compound is controversial, and recent studies have failed to confirm its presence (Struck et al., 1997).
- Methanol extracts: bind to estrogen receptors (Liske & Wustenberg,1998)
- Other actions
  - Luteinizing hormone and follicle-stimulating hormone levels remain normal; possible mechanism of action may be at level of neurotransmitters in brain (Foster, 1999; Freudenstein & Bodinet, 1999).
  - Does not stimulate estrogen-positive tumor growth. Action appears to be more like that of estriol rather than estradiol (Liske & Wustenberg, 1999; Snow, 1996).

Nutritional Ingredients: None known

Traditional Use

- Antispasmodic, anti-inflammatory, emmemagogue, antirheumatic, sedative
- Native Americans used it to treat arthritic joints/inflammation, fevers, reproductive conditions, including menstrual and menopausal symptoms, as well as for stimulating childbirth. It has been used to treat menopausal women in the United States, Canada, Great Britain, and Australia since the early to mid-19th century. Since 1988, black cohosh tinctures have been found to be as

effective as estrogen replacement therapy in menopausal women in Germany.

- Used for bronchial spasms and coughs associated with bronchitis, pertussis, and pneumonia
- Eclectic physicians used it for uterine neuralgia, migraines associated with menses, muscle spasms, optic neuralgia, muscle pain associated with influenza, lumbago, and chronic, deep-seated muscle pain.

Current Use

- Helps control signs and changes of menopause and those related to surgical removal of ovaries. Lengthens cycles. Fifty percent to 60% of women have reduction in symptoms in 6 to 8 weeks (Lieberman, 1998).
  - Reduces number and severity of hot flashes
  - Increases strength of pelvic floor muscles
  - Reduces depression, irritability, fatigue
  - Decreases headache
  - Reduces water retention
  - Reduces vaginal dryness
  - Reduces formication (skin crawling)
  - Alleviates insomnia and promotes sleep; has a calming effect, may be useful for menopausal insomnia (waking during the night and having difficulty falling back asleep)
- Anti-inflammatory for arthritis, especially of the muscles (fibromyalgia, bursitis), sciatica, and trigeminal neuralgia
- May have antiseizure activity
- Helpful during labor when woman is irritated or very tired. Small doses under the tongue are used.
- Painful menses (dysmenorrhea) and ovulatory pain (mittelschmerz). Works well in women with back pain.
- Lessens symptoms of endometriosis; stops spasm of uterus, reduces uterine pain, lengthens cycles
- May inhibit bone loss resulting from hormonal changes (Hunter, 2000)
- Research has demonstrated that black cohosh can block estrogen's ability to promote tumor growth. This effect is increased with concurrent use of tamoxifen (Foster, 1999; Freudenstein & Bodinet, 1999).

Available Forms, Dosage, and Administration Guidelines

Preparations: Dried root, capsules, tablets, tinctures. Standardized products are available.

Typical Dosage

- *Dried root:* 1–2 g
- *Capsules:* Three 500- to 600-mg capsules a day of the dried root. Remifemin, a brand-name standardized extract (standardized to 27-deoxyacetin), has been used in Germany since the 1950s for menopause symptoms (20 mg twice a day).
- *Tincture* (1:2, 60% alcohol): 10 to 20 gtt (0.5–1 mL) as often as every 4 hours
- *Tea:* 1 tsp dried root to 8 oz boiling water, decoct 10 minutes, steep 45 minutes; take 4 oz three times a day
- *Powdered root or as tea:* 1 to 2 g

Pharmacokinetics—If Available (form or route when known): None

Toxicity: Safe in normal therapeutic doses

Contraindications: None known

Side Effects

- Dizziness, headaches (frontal), and visual disturbance, usually with doses of more than 8 mL/day or with higher doses of the standardized extracts
- Nausea, vomiting in overdose
- Hypotension, usually from overdose
- Can increase or start bleeding again during menopause by stimulating ovarian function. Perimenopausal bleeding should be assessed to rule out possible disease.

Long-Term Safety: Safe

Use in Pregnancy/Lactation/Children

- Do not use if pregnant: increases risk of spontaneous abortion. Used in the last 2 weeks of pregnancy as a partus preparator by many midwives, herbalists, and naturopathic physicians.
- Use in children is not advised.

Drug/Herb Interactions and Rationale (if known)
- Research mixed: probably safe if used with estrogen
- May have an additive effect with antihypertensives. Use carefully.

Special Notes: Previously, it was thought that black cohosh suppressed luteinizing hormone, had estrogenic effects, contained compounds similar to estrogen, and should not be used in women with estrogen-positive tumors. Scientific proof negates each of these concepts (Freudenstein & Bodinet, 1999).

BIBLIOGRAPHY
Duker E. et al. (1991). Effects of extracts from *Cimicifuga racemosa* on gonadotropin release in menopausal women and ovariectomized rats. *Planta Medica*. 57(5):420–424.

Foster S. (Winter 1999). Black cohosh: a literature review. *HerbalGram*. 45:35–49.

Freudenstein J, Bodinet C. (1999). Influence of an isopropanolic aqueous extract of *Cimicifuga racemosa* rhizoma on the proliferation of MCF-7 cells. Abstracts of 23rd International LOF-Symposium on Phytoestrogens, Jan. 15, 1999, University of Ghent, Belgium.

Hunter A. (2000). *Cimicifuga racemosa*; pharmacology, clinical trials and clinical use. *European Journal of Herbal Medicine*. 5(1):19–25.

Lieberman S. (June 1998). A review of the effectiveness of *Cimicifuga racemosa* (black cohosh) for the symptoms of menopause. *Journal of Women's Health*. 7(5):525–529.

Liske E. (1998). Therapeutic efficacy and safety of *Cimicifuga racemosa* for gynecologic disorders. *Advances in Therapy*. 15(1):45–53.

Liske E, Wustenberg P. (1998). Therapy of climacteric complaints with *Cimicifuga racemosa*: herbal medicine with clinically proven evidence. *Menopause*. 5(4):250.

Liske E, Wustenberg P. (1999). Efficacy and safety for phytomedicines for gynecological disorders with particular reference to *Cimicifuga racemosa* and *Hypericum perforatum*. First Asian-European Congress on the Menopause, Bangkok, 1998.

Mills S, Bone K. (1999). *Principles and Practice of Phytotherapy*. Edinburgh: Churchill Livingstone.

Snow J. (1996). Black cohosh. *Protocol Journal of Botanical Medicine*. 1(4):17–19.

Struck D, Tegtmeier M, Harnischfeger G. (1997). Flavones in extracts of *Cimicifuga racemosa*. *Planta Medica*. 63(31):289.

🌿 NAME: Black Haw Bark (*Viburnum prunifolium*)

Common Names: Nannybush

Family: *Caprifoliaceae*

Description of Plant
- A small, shrubby, deciduous tree native to eastern North America
- Blooms in the spring with a flat cluster of white flowers, followed by purplish-black fruits

Medicinal Part: Root and stem bark

Constituents and Action (if known)
- Biflavone (amentoflavone): mildly spasmolytic
- Iridoid glycosides (2^1-0-acetyl-dihydropenstemide, patrinoside, 2^1-0-p-coumaroyl-dihydropenstemide, 2^1-0-acetylpatrinoside): uterine and intestinal antispasmodics (Upton, 2000)
- Coumarins (scopoletin: spasmolytic, may effect a blockade of autonomic neurotransmitters, causing relaxation of smooth muscle [Upton, 2000]; scopolin, aesculetin: spasmolytic)

Nutritional Ingredients: Edible berries

Traditional Use
- Antispasmodic, anodyne, astringent, mild hypotensive, bitter tonic, uterine tonic, uterine sedative, nervine
- Medicinal uses were learned from Native Americans, who used the bark for gastric upsets, female reproductive problems, childbirth, and muscle spasms.
- Used by eclectic physicians as a partus preparator, to alleviate postpartum pain and bleeding, to treat dysmenorrhea, and to prevent miscarriage. They also used it for diarrhea, intestinal spasms, and cardiac palpitations.
- Herbalists used black haw for premenstrual irritability, spasms of the bladder and diaphragm, spasmodic coughing, asthma, hiccoughs, and spasmodic testicular pain.

Current Use
- A uterine antispasmodic useful for dysmenorrhea, pelvic congestion syndrome, low back pain associated with menses,

and vaginismus. Works well with Roman chamomile, Jamaica dogwood, and black cohosh.
* Commonly used by midwives, herbalists, and naturopathic physicians to prevent miscarriage during the first and second trimester
* Can be used to control postpartum bleeding and pain, combined with yarrow, cinnamon, or shepherd's purse
* Bark is effective for abdominal spasms, especially chronic hiccoughs, hiatus hernia, and gastric or intestinal cramps.
* Can be useful for venospasm and as an adjunctive treatment for mild to moderate hypertension. Use with motherwort, hawthorn, garlic, olive leaf, dandelion leaf, or linden flower.

Available Forms, Dosage, and Administration Guidelines
* *Dried bark:* 2 to 6 g
* *Tea:* 1 to 2 tsp dried bark, 8 oz water, decoct 15 to 20 minutes, steep 30 minutes; take two or three cups per day
* *Capsules:* two or three 500-mg capsules three times a day
* *Fresh tincture* (1:2, 40% alcohol): 80 to 160 gtt (4–8 mL) three times a day; smaller doses can be taken more frequently
* *Tincture* (1:5, 40% alcohol): 80 to 160 gtt (4–8 mL) three times a day; smaller doses can be taken more frequently

Pharmacokinetics—If Available (form or route when known): Not known

Toxicity: Safe

Contraindications: Because of the presence of oxalate acid, avoid using in patients who have kidney stones or a history of them (McGuffin et al., 1997).

Side Effects: Nausea and vomiting with large amounts

Long-Term Safety: Safe in normal therapeutic doses

Use in Pregnancy/Lactation/Children: Black haw has long been used to prevent miscarriage, and no adverse effects have been reported. No adverse effects are expected in lactating women or children.

Drug/Herb Interactions and Rationale (if known): None known

Special Notes: Has a long history of empirical use as an antispasmodic, and animal studies have confirmed this activity

BIBLIOGRAPHY

Bissett NG, Wichtl M. (eds.). (1994). *Herbal Drugs and Phytopharmaceuticals.* Stuttgart: Medpharm Science.

Cometa MF, et al. (1998). Preliminary studies on cardiovascular activity of *Viburnum prunifolium* L. and its iridoid glucosides. *Fitoterapia.* 69(5):23.

Leung A, Foster S. (1996). *Encyclopedia of Common Natural Products* (2nd ed.). New York: John Wiley & Sons.

McGuffin M, et al. (1997). *Botanical Safety Handbook.* Boca Raton, FL: CRC Press.

Moermann DE. (1998). *Native American Ethnobotany.* Portland, OR: Timber Press.

Tomassini L, et al. (1998). Iridoid glucosides from *Viburnum prunifolium* and preliminary pharmacological studies. Proceedings of the Societa Italiana di Fitochimica 9th National Congress, Florence, Italy.

Upton R. (ed.). (2000). *American Herbal Pharmacopoeia and Therapeutic Compendium: Black Haw Bark.* Santa Cruz, CA: AHP.

Winston D. (2000). *Herbal Therapeutics: Specific Indications for Herbs and Herbal Formulas* (7th ed.). Washington, NJ: Herbal Therapeutics Research Library.

 NAME: Blessed Thistle (*Cnicus benedictus*)

Common Names: Cardo Santo thistle, holy thistle, Chardon, St. Benedict thistle

Family: *Asteraceae*

Description of Plant
- Small, annual thistle found primarily in Europe
- Has small yellow flowers, and the leaves have weak, innocuous spines, unlike many thistles

Medicinal Part: Leaves and flowers

Constituents and Action (if known)
- Sesquiterpene lactones
  - Cnicin (bitter part of plant) may have antibiotic activity (Barrero et al., 1997; Newall et al., 1996), stimulates taste buds, increases secretion of saliva and gastric juice and appetite (Bradley, 1992)
  - Salonitenolide (Gruenwald et al., 1998)
- Tannins (8%) (Newall et al., 1996)
- High mineral content (K+, Mg++, Ca++, manganese)
- Lignan lactones (lignanalides): trachelogenin, arctigenin, nortracheloside
- Flavonoids
- Volatile oils

Nutritional Ingredients: Ca++, Mg++, K+, manganese

History: Originally cultivated in monastery gardens and was considered a panacea, thus the epithet *benedictus*

Traditional Use: Bitter tonic and cholagogue; GI and hepatic disorders

Current Use
- Cholagogue: for inadequate bile secretion
- To treat dyspepsia and biliousness with nausea, flatulence, and bloating
- Loss of appetite: stimulates secretion of saliva and gastric juices

Available Forms, Dosage, and Administration Guidelines
Preparations: Dried herb, cut and sifted; capsules, tablets, tonics, tinctures
Typical Dosage
- *Capsules:* Three 500- to 600-mg capsules a day
- *Tea:* Steep 1 to 2 tsp cut and sifted dried herb in 8 oz of hot water for 10 to 15 minutes; take 4 oz up to three times a day a half-hour before meals; or follow practitioner's recommendations.
- *Infusion:* 1 to 2 tsp dried herb in 8 oz boiling water, steep 15 to 20 minutes; take 2 to 4 oz before meals
- *Tincture* (1:5, 30% alcohol): 30–80 gtt (1.5–4 mL) three times a day

- *Fluid extract:* (1:1 g/mL): 2 mL three times a day

Pharmacokinetics—If Available (form or route when known): None known

Toxicity: None known

Contraindications: None known

Side Effects
- Nausea, vomiting with excess dosage
- Contact dermatitis
- Allergic reaction: cross-sensitivity to other members of the *Asteraceae* family (feverfew, mugwort, chamomile)

Long-Term Safety: Long history of use in European herbal medicine and in liquors. No safety issues expected at usual therapeutic doses.

Use in Pregnancy/Lactation/Children: Not recommended (Blumenthal, 2000; McGuffin, 1997)

Drug/Herb Interactions and Rationale (if known): None known

Special Notes: Little scientific research is available on this herb.

BIBLIOGRAPHY

Barrero AF, et al. (1997). Biomimetic cyclization of cnicin to malacitanolide, a bytotoxic eudesmanolide from *Centaurea malacitana*. *Journal of Natural Products*. 60:1034–1035.

Blumenthal M, et al. (2000). *Herbal Medicine: Expanded Commission E Monographs*. Austin: American Botanical Council.

Bradley PR. (ed.). (1992). *British Herbal Compendium*, Vol. 1. Bournemouth: British Herbal Medicine Association.

Gruenwald J, et al. (1998). *PDR for Herbal Medicines*. Montvale, NJ: Medical Economics Co.

McGuffin T. (1997). *Botanical Safety Handbook*. Boca Raton, FL: CRC Press.

Newall CA, Anderson LA, Phillipson JD. (1996). *Herbal Medicines: A Guide for Healthcare Professionals*. London: The Pharmaceutical Press.

Reynolds JEF, et al. (eds.). (1996). *Martindale, The Extra Pharmacopoeia*, 31st ed. London: Royal Pharmaceutical Society of Great Britain.

NAME: Blue Cohosh (*Caulophyllum thalictroides*)

Common Names: Blue ginseng, squaw root, papoose root, yellow ginseng

Family: *Berberidaceae*

Description of Plant
- Perennial herb that grows to 2 to 3 feet; has pale yellow-green flowers
- Forest plant that grows from Georgia to Canada

Medicinal Part: Rhizome

Constituents and Action (if known)
- Caulosaponin and caulophyllosaponin: glycosides, uterine stimulants; can constrict coronary blood vessels; in rats, can inhibit ovulation (Baillie & Rasmussen, 1997; Ferguson & Edwards, 1954; Gunn & Wright, 1996)
- N-methylcytisine: a quinolizidine alkaloid, pharmacologically similar to nicotine (10%–40% less active), which can raise blood pressure and stimulate small intestine and may cause hyperglycemia (Ferguson & Edwards, 1954). Teratogenic in in vitro rat embryo culture (Kennelly et al., 1999).
- Taspine: embryo toxicity in in vitro rat embryo culture (Kennelly et al., 1999)
- Thalictroidine

Nutritional Ingredients: None known

Traditional Use
- Native Americans used small amounts of a decoction for several weeks before birth to ease delivery.
- Used for amenorrhea
- Used to treat muscle spasm, small joint (fingers, toes, wrists) arthralgias, rheumatism
- Used to induce sweating
- Used as a diuretic

Current Use
- Menstrual disorders, premenstrual symptoms, mastalgia, ovarian pain, mittelschmerz, functional ovarian cysts, pain of endometriosis

- Used by skilled midwives to stimulate labor and to help pass the placenta after delivery (usually mixed with other herbs)

Available Forms, Dosage, and Administration Guidelines

Preparations: Dried root, cut and sifted; capsules, tablets, tinctures, combination products, teas

Typical Dosage
- *Dried root:* 0.3 to 1 g three times a day
- *Capsule:* 1 (00) capsule two times a day
- *Tincture* (1:5, 60% alcohol): 5 to 20 gtt (0.25–1 mL) up to three times a day.

Pharmacokinetics—If Available (form or route when known): None known

Toxicity
- May cause congestive heart failure in newborns when used prepartum or during labor
- Overdose causes symptoms similar to nicotine overdose.
- Poisoning has been reported in children after ingestion of blue seeds.
- Ingestion of the fresh plant or root can cause gastritis.

Contraindications
- Avoid in pregnancy or when trying to get pregnant; may act as an abortifacient
- Taken as a partus preparator, it has been associated with congestive heart failure in newborns (Jones & Lawson, 1998).
- Avoid in heart disease

Side Effects
- May inhibit luteinizing hormone release and ovulation (may have some benefit as a contraceptive, but more research is needed)
- GI irritation, diarrhea, cramping
- Hypertension

Long-Term Safety: Unknown. Not recommended for long-term daily use. Recent concerns about congestive heart failure in newborns create serious doubts as to the safety of this traditional use. More research is needed to confirm whether blue cohosh was causative in these events.

Use in Pregnancy/Lactation/Children

- Do not use during pregnancy; appropriate only after labor has begun.
- Contraindicated during lactation and in children.

Drug/Herb Interactions and Rationale (if known)

- May increase side effects and toxicity of nicotine products. If used concurrently, observe for possible potentiation.
- Theoretical possibility of interaction with antihypertensives and antiangina agents exists. Use cautiously.

Special Notes: When used in small, appropriate doses for healthy adults (men and nonpregnant women), blue cohosh appears to be a relatively safe and useful herb.

BIBLIOGRAPHY

Baillie N, Rasmussen P. (1997). Black and blue cohosh in labor. *New Zealand Medical Journal.* 110:20–21.

Bone K. (2000). Adverse reaction reports. *Modern Phytotherapist.* 5(3):11–16.

Elder NC, et al. (March/April 1997). Use of alternative health care by family practice patients. *Archives of Family Medicine.* 6:181–184.

Ferguson HC, Edwards LD. (1954). A pharmacological study of a crystalline glycoside of *Caulophyllum thalictroides. Journal of the American Pharmaceutical Association.* 43:16.

Gunn TR, Wright IMR. (1996). The use of blue and black cohosh in labour. *New Zealand Medical Journal.* 109:410–411.

Jones TK, Lawson BM. (1998). Profound neonatal congestive heart failure caused by maternal consumption of blue cohosh herbal medication. *Journal of Pediatrics.* 132(3 pt 1):550–552.

Kennelly EJ, et al. (1999). Detecting potential teratogenic alkaloids from blue cohosh rhizomes using an in vitro rat embryo culture. *Journal of Natural Products.* 62(10):1385–1389.

Lawrence Review of Natural Products. (1992). St. Louis: Facts and Comparisons.

Wright IM. (1999). Neonatal effects of maternal consumption of blue cohosh. *Journal of Pediatrics.* 134(3):384–385.

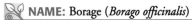 **NAME:** Borage (*Borago officinalis*)

Common Names: Common borage, beebread, starflower, ox's tongue

Family: *Boraginaceae*

Description of Plant

- Hardy annual that grows 2 feet tall and is covered with coarse hairs
- Has oval leaves and star-shaped bright-blue flowers with black anthers
- Flowers bloom from May to September.
- Grows throughout Europe and North America
- Has cucumber-like odor and taste

Medicinal Part: Borage seed oil

Constituents and Action (if known)

Herb

- Mucilage: may cause expectorant effect (Tyler et al., 1988)
- Malic acid and potassium nitrate: cause mild diuretic effect (Awang, 1990)
- Tannins: may be mildly constipating (Awang, 1990)

Seed Oil: Fatty acids are a source of gamma-linolenic acid, which may reduce prostaglandins (E_1), inhibit platelet aggregation, and have anti-inflammatory properties (Engler et al., 1992; Fan & Chapkin, 1998; Karlstad et al., 1993; Leventhal et al., 1993; Pullman-Mooar et al., 1990).

Nutritional Ingredients

- Flowers can be used to garnish salads.
- Stems and leaves can be eaten raw or cooked like spinach.
- Seeds contain gamma-linolenic acid, a dietary source of essential fatty acids (Leung & Foster, 1996).

Traditional Use

- No traditional use for the seed oil
- Leaves and flowers were seeped in wine to dispel melancholy.
- The herb is used by European herbalists as a mild amphoteric to the HPA axis. The leaf was also used to treat coughs and sore throats.

Current Use: Oil may lower blood pressure, improve psoriasis, relieve premenstrual symptoms, improve atopic eczema, improve infantile seborrhea.

Available Forms, Dosage, and Administration Guidelines: Capsules contain borage seed oil, which is 20% to 26% gamma-linolenic acid. Typical dosage is three or four 300-mg capsules a day, or follow manufacturer's or practitioner's recommendations.

Pharmacokinetics—If Available (form or route when known): None known

Toxicity: Seed oil is not associated with toxicity. Leaf contains pyrrolizidine alkaloids (supinin, lycopsamin).

Contraindications: None known

Side Effects: None

Long-Term Safety: Appears safe. Canadian government has approved this product as a dietary supplement.

Use in Pregnancy/Lactation/Children: Appears safe; approved as a dietary supplement with no restrictions

Drug/Herb Interactions and Rationale (if known): None known

BIBLIOGRAPHY

Awang DVC. (1990). Herbal medicine: borage. *Canadian Pharmacy Journal.* 123:121.

Bard JM, et al. (1997). A therapeutic dosage (3 g/day) of borage oil supplementation has no effect on platelet aggregation in healthy volunteers. *Fundamentals of Clinical Pharmacology.* 11(2):143–144.

Engler MM, et al. (1992). Dietary gamma-linolenic acid lowers blood pressure and alters aortic reactivity and cholesterol metabolism in hypertension. *Journal of Hypertension.* 10(10):1197–1204.

Fan YY, Chapkin RS. (1998). Importance of dietary gamma-linolenic acid in human health and nutrition. *Journal of Nutrition.* 128:1411–1414.

Henz BM, et al. (1999). Double-blind, multicentre analysis of the efficacy of borage oil in patients with atopic eczema. *British Journal of Dermatology.* 140(4):685–688.

Karlstad MD, et al. (1993). Effect of intravenous lipid emulsions enriched with gamma-linolenic acid on plasma n-6 fatty acids and prostaglandin biosynthesis after burn and endotoxin injury in rats. *Critical Care Medicine.* 21:1740–1749.

Leung A, Foster S. (1996). *Encyclopedia of Common Natural Ingredients.* (2nd ed.). New York: John Wiley & Sons.

Leventhal LJ, et al. (1993). Treatment of rheumatoid arthritis with gamma-linolenic acid. *Annals of Internal Medicine.* 119:867–873.

Mancuso P, et al. (1997). Dietary fish oil and fish and borage oil suppress intrapulmonary proinflammatory eicosanoid biosynthesis and attenuate pulmonary neutrophil accumulation in endotoxic rats. *Critical Care Medicine.* 25:1198–1206.

Mills DE. (1989). Dietary fatty acid supplementation alters stress reactivity and performance in man. *Journal of Human Hypertension.* 3:111–116.

Pullman-Mooar S, et al. (1990). Alteration of the cellular fatty acid profile and the production of eicosanoids in human monocytes by gamma-linolenic acid. *Arthritis & Rheumatism.* 33:1526–1533.

Tollesson A, Frithz A. (1993). Borage oil, an effective new treatment for infantile seborrhoeic dermatitis. *British Journal of Dermatology.* 129(1):95.

Tyler VE, et al. (1988). *Pharmacognosy* (9th ed.). Philadelphia: Lea and Febiger.

 NAME: Boswellia (*Boswellia serrata*)

Common Names: Shallaki (Sanskrit), sallai guggal (Hindi), Boswellin (brand name)

Family: *Burseraceae*

Description of Plant: A small to medium-size tree that grows on dry hills throughout most of India but is especially common in the northwest part.

Medicinal Part: The gum resin that oozes from the bark when the tree is cut

Constituents and Action (if known)

- Triterpene acids (alpha, beta, and gamma boswellic acids)
- Boswellic acids control the production of leukotrienes, biochemicals in the body that stimulate inflammation. Boswellic acids reduce leukotriene formation, which in turn slows progression of inflammatory conditions (Ammon et al., 1993; Gupta VN et al., 1997; Kulkarni et al., 1991; Wildfeuer et al., 1998).

- ○ Reduce morning stiffness and increase joint activity in persons with inflammatory conditions (Kulkarni et al., 1991)
- ○ Reduce symptoms in asthma (Gupta et al., 1998)
- ○ Reduce inflammation and increase remission rates in ulcerative colitis (Gupta I et al., 1997)
- Quercetin: blocks proinflammatory 5-lipoxygenase and leukotrienes (monograph from *Alternative Medicine Review*, 1998)
- Terpenoids
- Essential oils (alpha-thujene and p-cymene, alpha-pinene, alpha-phellandrine): antifungal activity (*Selected Medicinal Plants of India*, 1992)

Nutritional Ingredients: None

Traditional Use
- Anti-inflammatory, expectorant, astringent
- Used in ayurvedic medicine in India to treat liver disease, dysentery, skin diseases, ulcers, and as a general tonic and blood purifier
- Used to enhance mucous production from the respiratory system, cough, bronchitis, and asthma
- Topically, used as a gum ointment to treat boils, wounds, and sores

Current Use
- Inflammatory conditions: rheumatoid arthritis, osteoarthritis, tendinitis, bursitis, and repetitive motion injuries. Improves blood flow to joints and prevents further breakdown of all tissue (Kulkarni et al., 1991)
- Grade II or III ulcerative colitis: studies show this herb is as effective as sulfasalazine (Gupta et al., 1997).

Available Forms, Dosage, and Administration Guidelines
- Standardized ethanol extracts containing 60% to 65% boswellic acids: follow label directions.
- *Capsule* (300–400 mg standardized extract): two capsules two or three times per day

Pharmacokinetics—If Available (form or route when known): None known

Toxicity: None known

Contraindications: Extracts contain alcohol.

Side Effects: Occasional mild gastric upset

Long-Term Safety: Safe

Use in Pregnancy/Lactation/Children: Not known

Drug/Herb Interactions and Rationale (if known): None known

Special Notes
- Lacks analgesic and antipyretic activity (Singh & Atal, 1986)
- Does not affect cyclo-oxygenase activities (Ammon et al., 1993)

BIBLIOGRAPHY
Ammon HPT, et al. (1993). Mechanism of anti-inflammatory actions of curcumine and boswellic acids. *Journal of Ethnopharmacology.* 38:113–119.

(1998). Monograph: *Boswellia serrata. Alternative Medicine Review.* 3(4):306–307.

(1992). *Selected Medicinal Plants of India.* Bombay: Chemexeil.

Broadhurst CL. (January/February 1998). Herbal chemistry. *Herbs for Health.*

Etzel R. (1996). Special extract of *Boswellia serrata* (H15) in the treatment of rheumatoid arthritis. *Phytomedicine.* 3(1):91–94.

Gupta I, et al. (1997). Effects of *Boswellia serrata* gum resin in patients with ulcerative colitis. *European Journal of Medical Research.* 2(1):37–43.

Gupta I, et al. (1998). Effects of *Boswellia serrata* gum resin in patients with bronchial asthma: results of a double-blind, placebo-controlled, 6-week clinical study. *European Journal of Medical Research.* 3(11):511–514.

Gupta VN, et al. (1997). Chemistry and pharmacology of gum-resin of *Boswellia serrata. Indian Drugs.* 24:221–231.

Kulkarni RR, et al. (1991). Treatment of osteoarthritis with a herbomineral formula: a double-blind, placebo-controlled, cross-over study. *Journal of Ethnopharmacology.* 33 (1-2):91–95.

McCaleb R, Leigh E, Morien K. (2000). *Encyclopedia of Popular Herbs.* Roseville, CA: Prime Publishing.

Singh BG, Atal CK. (1986). Pharmacology of an extract of sallai guggal ex-boswellia serrata, a new non-steroidal anti-inflammatory agent. *Agents & Actions.* 18(3-4):407–412.

Wildfeuer A, et al. (1998). Effects of boswellic acids extracted from an herbal medicine on the biosynthesis of leukotrienes and the course of experimental autoimmune encephalomyelitis. *Arzneimittelforschung*. 48(6):668–674.

 NAME: Burdock (*Arcticum lappa, Arcticum minus*)

Common Names: Beggar's buttons, great burr, great burdocks

Family: *Asteraceae*

Description of Plant
- Grows throughout much of Northern Hemisphere
- Biennial; known as a pesky weed; grows 3 to 9 feet tall
- Pinkish-purple flowers that develop into a spiny burr containing the seeds

Medicinal Part: Roots (may be 5–9 feet long), leaves, seeds

Constituents and Action (if known)
- Polyacetylene compounds: antibacterial activity
- Anctropicrin (bitter component): antibacterial activity
- Bitter glycoside (arctin): reduces symptoms of common cold (Sun, 1992; Wang et al., 1993)
- Lignans: antimutagenic effect (Leung et al., 1996)
- Polyphenolic acids (caffeic, chlorogenic): may decrease urinary stones (Grases et al., 1994)
- Volatile acids (acetic, butyric, isovaleric)
- Fixed oil (from seeds)
- Inulin: a nonabsorbable polysaccharide; source of fructo-oligosaccharides

Nutritional Ingredients
- In Japan, roots are used as a vegetable called *gobo*.
- Stalk, with the outer skin removed, is a tasty raw vegetable.
- Young greens can be cooked as a bitter vegetable; thought to have antimicrobial activity (Rogers & Powers-Rogers, 1988).
- Root pulp (11% protein, 19% lipids, 34% inulin) (Tadeda et al., 1991)

Traditional Use
Internal
- Root
  - Blood purifier (alterative) to treat skin conditions (eczema, psoriasis), cancer, arthritis, and obesity. Burdock root is one of four ingredients in the "cancer formula" known as Essiac.
  - Mild diuretic and laxative
  - Used to stimulate lymphatic circulation, especially with chronically enlarged lymph nodes, mastitis, and lymphedema
- Seed tincture used by eclectic physicians to treat dry, crusty, or scaly skin conditions

Topical: Leaves were used as a poultice or wash to help heal wounds, boils, and styes.

Current Use
- Antimutagenic activity; dietary use may reduce chemically induced carcinogenesis
- Antibacterial activity, especially topically for furuncles (boils)
- Seeds, called niu bang zi in traditional Chinese medicine, are used for red, painful sore throats, coughs, mumps, and painful enlarged lymph nodes. The seeds show significant in vitro inhibitory effect against *Streptococcus pneumoniae* and many pathogenic fungi.

Available Forms, Dosage, and Administration Guidelines:
Preparations: Dried root (or leaves), whole or cut and sifted; capsules, liquid extract, tablets, tinctures
Typical Dosage
- *Capsules:* Up to six 500- to 600-mg capsules a day
- *Tea:* Steep 1 tsp dried root in a cup of hot water, decoct 15 minutes, steep 40 minutes; take up to three times a day.
- *Tincture* (1:5, 30% alcohol): 40 to 90 gtt (2–4 mL) three times a day, or follow manufacturer's recommendations
- *Seeds:* In traditional Chinese medicine, dose averages 3 to 10 g per day.

Pharmacokinetics—If Available (form or route when known): None known

Toxicity: Poisoning has been reported, but this is from contamination with other botanicals, most notably nightshades. The adverse effects are consistent with atropine toxicity.

Contraindications: None

Side Effects: Topical: contact dermatitis from plant (Rodriguez et al., 1995)

Long-Term Safety: Traditional use as a food; no toxicity expected

Use in Pregnancy/Lactation/Children: Uterine-stimulating activity has been seen in in vivo animal studies.

Drug/Herb Interactions and Rationale (if known): Do not use concurrently with insulin or oral antidiabetic agents because of possible increased hypoglycemia.

Special Notes
- Because of lack of good research, use is not recommended by the German Commission E.
- Burdock has occasionally been adulterated with belladonna (deadly nightshade plant) because the roots look vaguely similar.

BIBLIOGRAPHY

Bensky D, Gamble A. (1993). *Chinese Herbal Medicine, Materia Medica.* Seattle: Eastland Press.

Grases F, et al. (1994). Urolithiasis and phytotherapy. *International Urology & Nephrology.* 26(5):507.

Integrative Medicine Access. (2000). *Burdock Monograph. Newton, MA: Integrative Medicine Communications.*

Leung A, et al. (1996). *Encyclopedia of Common Natural Ingredients.* (2nd ed.). New York: John Wiley & Sons.

Review of Natural Products. (1996). St. Louis: Facts and Comparisons.

Rodriguez P, et al. (1995). Allergic dermatitis due to burdock (*Arcticum lappa*). *Contact Dermatitis.* 33(3):134.

Rogers B, Powers-Rogers B. (1988). *Culinary Botany.* Kent, WA: Rogers & Plants.

Sun W. (1992). Determination of arctin and arctigenin in *Fructus arctii* by reverse-phase HPLC. *Acta Pharmaceutica Sinica.* 27(7):549.

Tadeda H, et al. (1991). Effect of feeding amaranth (Food Red #2) on the jejunal sucrase and digestion-absorption capacity of the jejunum in rats. *Journal of Nutrition Science and Vitamins.* 37(6):611.

Wang H, et al. (1993). Studies on the chemical constituents of *Arcticum lappa L. Acta Pharmaceutica Sinica.* 28(12):911.

C

 NAME: Calendula (*Calendula officinalis*)

Common Names: Pot marigold

Family: *Asteraceae*

Description of Plant

- Believed to have originated in Egypt, but now has world-wide distribution
- Grows to 2 feet
- Orange or yellow ray flowers bloom from May to October.

Medicinal Part: Dried flower

Constituents and Action (if known)

- Sterols and fatty acids: calendic and oleanic acid (Szakiel & Janiszowska, 1993, 1998)
- Triterpenoids: anti-inflammatory activity (Akihisa et al., 1996; Della Loggia et al., 1994; Zitterl-Eglseer et al., 1999)
- Faradiol monoester: equals indomethacin in activity
- Essential oils
- Sesquiterpene glycosides (DeTommasi et al., 1990)
- Oleanolic acid glycosides (Kasprzky et al., 1973; Szakiel & Kasprzky, 1989)
- Flavonols (Pietta et al., 1992)
- Tocopherols
- Carotenoid pigments (coloring agents)
- Lutein and other carotenoid pigments (anti-inflammatory, antioxidant)

Nutritional Ingredients: Dried petals have a saffron-like quality and have been used in cooking and in salads.

Traditional Use

- Topically to promote wound healing and reduce inflammation, particularly for slow-to-heal wounds
- European folk use as a diaphoretic, bitter tonic, lymphatic tonic, and as treatment for jaundice
- Eclectic physicians used calendula for conjunctivitis, gastric ulcers, and topically for burns and rashes.
- Mouthwash: heals gums after tooth extraction

Current Use
Internally

- Postmastectomy lymphedema and pain (Newell et al., 1996; Zitterl-Eglseer et al., 1999)
- Chronic colitis (Chakurski et al., 1981)
- Reduces inflammation of oral and pharyngeal mucosa and skin (dermatitis, leg ulcers, bruises, pyorrhea, gingivitis)
- Promotes bile production
- Reduces HIV-1, rhinovirus, and stomatitis virus activity in vitro (DeTommasi et al., 1990; Kalvatchev et al., 1997)
- Treatment of gastric ulcers (Blumenthal et al., 2000)

Topically: Enhances epithelization of surgical wounds; reduces varicose veins; heals cracked nipples after breast feeding. Liquid preparations also show antibacterial, antiviral, and antifungal activity.

Available Forms, Dosage, and Administration Guidelines

Preparations: Dried flowers; salves, tinctures

Typical Dosage

- *Dried flowers:* 3–6 g three times a day.
- *Tincture* (1:5, 70% alcohol): 30 to 60 gtt (1.5–3 mL) three times a day
- For external use, apply tincture to affected area (dilute tincture 1:2 in water for open wounds). Or follow manufacturer's or practitioner's recommendation.

Pharmacokinetics—If Available (form or route when known): None known

Toxicity: None known

Contraindications: None known

Side Effects: Allergy possible if cross-sensitivity exists to feverfew, ragweed, chamomile, dandelion flower pollen.

Long-Term Safety: Generally recognized as safe; no adverse effects expected

Use in Pregnancy/Lactation/Children: No adverse effects known or expected

Drug/Herb Interactions and Rationale (if known): Unknown

Special Notes
- Do not confuse with the African marigold (tagetes).
- Most studies have been performed in animals; little research has been done in humans.

BIBLIOGRAPHY

Akihisa T, et al. (1996). Triterpene alcohols from the flowers of compositae and their anti-inflammatory effects. *Phytochemistry.* 43(6):1255–1260.

Blumenthal M, et al. (2000). *Herbal Medicine: Expanded Commission E Monographs.* Austin, TX: American Botanical Council.

Chakurski I, et al. (1981). Treatment of chronic colitis with an herbal combination of *Taraxacum officinale, Hypericum perforatum, Melissa officinalis, Calendula officinalis* and *Foeniculum vulgare. Vutr Boles.* 20(6):51–54.

Della Loggia R, et al. (1994). The role of triterpenoids in the topical anti-inflammatory activity of *Calendula officinalis* flowers. *Planta Medicine.* 60(6):516–520.

DeTommasi N, et al. (1990). Structure and in vitro antiviral activity of sesquiterpene glycosides from *Calendula arvensis. Journal of Natural Products.* 53(4):830.

Kalvatchev Z, et al. (1997). Anti-HIV activity of extracts from Calendula officinalis flowers. *Biomedical Pharmacotherapy.* 51(4):176–180.

Kasprzky Z, et al. (1973). Metabolism of triterpenoids in the seeds of *Calendula officinalis* germinating. *Acta Biochemistry of Poland.* 20:231.

Lawrence Review of Natural Products. (1995). St. Louis: Facts and Comparisons.

Newell C, et al. (1996). *Herbal Medicines.* London: Pharmaceutical Press.

Pietta P, et al. (1992). Separation of flavonol-2-O-glycosides from *Calendula officinalis* and *Sambucus nigra* by high-performance liquid and micellar electrokinetic capillary chromatography. *Journal of Chromatography.* 593(1-2):165.

Szakiel A, Janiszowska W. (1993). The kinetics of transport of oleanolic acid monoglycosides into vacuoles isolated from *Calendula officinalis* leaf protoplasts. *Acta Biochemistry of Poland.* 40(1):136–138.

Szakiel A, Janiszowska W. (1998). The effect of inorganic pyrophosphate on the transport of oleanolic acid monoglycosides into vacuoles isolated from *Calendula officinalis* leaves. *Acta Biochemistry of Poland.* 45(3):819–823.

Szakiel A, Kasprzky Z. (1989). Distribution of oleanolic acid glycosides in vacuoles and cell walls isolated from protoplasts and cells of *Calendula officinalis* leaves. *Steroids.* 53(3-5):501.

Zitterl-Eglseer K, et al. (1999). Anti-oedematous activities of the main triterpenoid esters of marigold (*Calendula officinalis* l.) *Ethnopharmacology.* 57(2):139–144.

 NAME: Cat's Claw (*Uncaria tomentosa, U. guianensis*)

Common Names: Samento, una de gato, saventaro

Family: *Rubiaceae*

Description of Plant

- Large woody vine (liana) found in the highlands of the Peruvian rain forest
- Vine can grow 100 feet long and climbs on trees.
- Has somewhat large, curved thorns that resemble a cat's claw
- *U. tomentosa* has two very different chemotypes with different activity.

Medicinal Part: Inner bark of plant (root is undisturbed), stem, root bark

Constituents and Action (if known)

- Pentacyclic oxinadole alkaloids (primarily found in *U. tomentosa* chemotype I): pteropodine, isopteropodine, isomitraphylline, uncarine F, speciophylline; anti-inflammatory activity (Sandoval-Chacon et al., 1998); immune enhancing activity (Hemingway & Phillipson,

1974; Rizzi et al., 1993); antileukemic activity (Stuppner et al., 1993); antimutagenic (Rizzi et al., 1993)
  ○ Mytrophylline: diuretic activity (Jones, 1994)
- Tetracyclic oxindole alkaloids (primarily found in *U. tomentosa* chemotype II): act on central nervous system and counteract the immune-enhancing activity of the pentacyclic alkaloids
  ○ Rynchophylline: inhibits platelet activity and thrombosis (Chen et al., 1992; Jones, 1994); decreases peripheral vascular resistance; has antihypertensive activity; decreases cholesterol (Hemingway & Phillipson, 1974; Jones, 1994)
  ○ Isorhynchophylline
- Six quinovic acid glycosides have antiviral activity in vitro (Aquino et al., 1989), anti-inflammatory activity (Aquino et al., 1991)
- Hirstutine: local anesthetic properties on bladder (Jones, 1994); may have an effect on Ca++ movement
- Tetracyclic and pentacyclic alkaloids: exert antagonistic effects on each other. They come from different plant chemotypes and should not be mixed together (Reinhard, 1999).
- Procyanidins: antioxidant effect, antitumor effect, immune-boosting
- Triterpinoid saponins
- Catechins (D-catechol)
- Indole alkaloid glucosides (cadambine, 3-dihydrocadambine, 3-isohydrocadambine)

Nutritional Ingredients: None known

Traditional Use: Digestive disturbances, skin problems, arthritis, contraceptive, cancer

Current Use
- Strengthens the integrity of the GI system in persons with Crohn's disease, inflammatory bowel disease, gastritis, irritable bowel disorder, and leaky gut syndrome
- Reduces side effects of chemotherapy and AZT therapy for HIV
- Used in clinical practice in Europe for cancer, HIV

Available Forms, Dosage, and Administration Guidelines

Preparations: Dried root and stem, cut and sifted or powdered; capsules, extracts, tablets, tinctures; products standardized for total alkaloid content are available.

Typical Dosage

- *Capsules:* Up to nine 500- to 600-mg capsules a day
- *Decoction:* Simmer 1 tbsp pulverized root in 1 qt water for 45 minutes; take 1 tsp in hot water before breakfast
- *Tincture:* (1:5, 60% alcohol) 20 to 40 gtt (1–2 mL) up to five times a day
- Standard cat's claw products should contain less than 0.02% tetracyclic acids.
- Or follow manufacturer's or practitioner's recommendations.

Pharmacokinetics—If Available (form or route when known): None known

Toxicity: None known

Contraindications: Use for immune problems is controversial; more research is needed. Avoid using in patients receiving immunosuppressive therapies.

Side Effects: Mild constipation, mild diarrhea; rarely, mild lymphocytosis. Monitor for signs of bleeding.

Long-Term Safety: Unknown

Use in Pregnancy/Lactation/Children: Contraindicated during pregnancy because of its traditional use as a contraceptive

Drug/Herb Interactions and Rationale (if known)

- May potentiate activity of antihypertensives; do not use together.
- Although there is no research to confirm these beliefs, European physicians recommend against using this herb with insulin, hormone therapies, or vaccines.

Special Notes

- Little concrete research exists. Well-designed human studies are needed to verify or disprove folk and current clinical use.
- Because of the two very different chemotypes that occur in this plant, only products standardized to high levels of

pentacyclic oxindole alkaloids and low levels of tetracyclic oxindole alkaloids (less than 0.02%) should be used.

BIBLIOGRAPHY

Aquino R, et al. (1989). Plant metabolites, structure and in vitro antiviral activity of quinovic acid glycosides from *Uncaria tomentosa* and *Guettarda platypoda*. *Journal of Natural Products*. 52(4):679–685.

Aquino R, et al. (1991). Plant metabolites: new compounds and antiinflammatory activity of *Uncaria tomentosa*. *Journal of Natural Products*. 54(2):453–459.

Chen, CX, et al. (1992). Inhibitory effect of rhynchophylline on platelet aggregation and thrombosis. *Acta Pharmacol Sinica*. 13:126–130.

Hemingway SR, Phillipson JD. (1974). Alkaloids from S. American species of *Uncaria* (Rubiaceae). *Journal of Pharmacy and Pharmacology*. 26(Suppl):113P.

Jones K. (1994). The herb report: una de gato, life-giving vine of Peru. *American Herb Association*. 10(3):4.

Keplinger K, et al. (1999). Ethnomedicinal use and new pharmacological, toxicological, and botanical results. *Journal of Ethnopharmacology*. 64(1):23–34.

Lawrence Review of Natural Products. (1996). St. Louis: Facts and Comparisons.

McCaleb R, et al. (2000). *Encyclopedia of Popular Herbs*. Roseville, CA: Prima Publishers.

Reinhard KH. (1999). *Uncaria tomentosa*. *Journal of Alternative & Complementary Medicine*. 5(2):143–151.

Rizzi R, et al. (1993). Mutagenic and antimutagenic activities of Uncaria tomentosa and its extracts. *Journal of Ethnopharmacology*. 38(1):63.

Sandoval-Chacon M, et al. (1998). Antiinflammatory actions of cat's claw: The role of NF-kappaB. *Alimentary Pharmacologic Therapy*. 12(12):1279–1289.

Stuppner, H, et al. (1993). A differential sensitivity of oxinadole alkaloids to normal and leukemic cell lines. *Planta Medica*. 59(Suppl. A583).

NAME: Cayenne (*Capsicum frutescens, Capsicum annuum*)

Common Names: Chili pepper, cayenne pepper, red pepper, Mexican chili, hot pepper, jalapeno

Family: *Solanaceae*

Description of Plant

- An oblong pungent fruit; a member of the *Capsicum* genus (nightshades). This same genus also includes paprika, bell, and sweet peppers.
- Originally grew in tropical America, but now is grown worldwide

Medicinal Part: Fruit (pepper)

Constituents and Action (if known)

- Capsaicinoids (up to 1.5%)
  - Oleoresin capsaicin (1.5%): powerful irritant that causes a reflex vasodilatation, probably mediated by substance P. After initial topical application, substance P is released, causing the sensation of pain. After repeated applications, substance P is depleted and a lack of pain impulses ensues. This effect usually occurs within 3 days of regular application.
  - Capsaicin is responsible for the pungency of fruit.
  - Similar to eugenol, the active principle in oil of cloves, which can induce long-lasting local analgesia
  - 6,7 dihydrocapsaicin, nordihydrocapsaicin, homodihydrocapsaicin, homocapsaicin
- Steroid glycosides: capsicosides, A to D

Nutritional Ingredients

- Carotenoids (capsanthin, capsorubin, alpha and beta carotene, lutein)
- Vitamins C, E, A, B_1, B_2, B_3
- Provitamin P (flavonoids)
- Capsaicin (the "bite" of the pepper)

Traditional Use

- To treat mouth sores (ancient Mayans)
- To restore digestive power; GI stimulant and carminative
- To restore health to blood vessels and normalize blood pressure
- A local counterirritant for sore muscles
- To stop local capillary bleeding (nose bleeds, bleeding ulcers, cuts)
- A catalyst to increase absorption in herbal formulas, commonly used in Thomsonian medicine and Southeast Asian medicine for this purpose

Current Use
- Topical application to control pain in osteoarthritis and rheumatoid arthritis; herpes zoster, shingles (Zostrix cream contains either 0.025% or 0.075% capsaicin); diabetic, postsurgical, and trigeminal neuralgias (Robbins et al., 1998); psoriasis (Ellis et al., 1993)
- Nasal spray used once weekly for 5 weeks reduces chronic, nonallergic rhinitis, runny nose, and sneezing. Nasal spray may also be helpful in decreasing the pain and number of cluster headaches.
- Used internally to stimulate digestion, reduce blood lipids, and improve circulation (this use has not been proven scientifically)

Available Forms, Dosage, and Administration Guidelines
Preparations: Fresh or dried powdered fruit; capsules, tablets, tinctures
Typical Dosage
- *Spice:* Use freely in flavoring food
- *Capsules:* Up to three 400- to 500-mg capsules a day
- *Tea:* Steep 0.25 to 0.5 tsp powdered spice in a cup of hot water for 10 to 15 minutes. If patient can tolerate the tea, he should take small sips throughout the day.
- *Tincture* (1:10, 90% alcohol): 5 to 10 gtt (0.25–0.5 mL) diluted in water
- Or follow manufacturer's or practitioner's recommendations.

Pharmacokinetics—If Available (form or route when known): None known

Toxicity
- Topically: intolerable sensation of heat and burning; milk may blunt effect
- Internal: intense GI pain and burning

Contraindications
Internal
- Peptic ulcers, acid indigestion, esophageal reflux, contact dermatitis
- Cayenne has shown inhibitory activity against *Helicobacter pylori*, and studies show that people who regularly consume

hot peppers have a lower incidence of duodenal and peptic ulcers than those who do not.

Topical

- Do not use on open, broken skin and in or near eyes or vaginal mucosa.
- Do not apply additional heat.

Side Effects

- External: contact dermatitis; does not cause blistering or redness because it does not act on capillary beds; transient stinging
- Internal: GI distress

Long-Term Safety: Safe; long-term food use

Use in Pregnancy/Lactation/Children

- Pregnancy: Safe as a food. Internally, medicinal quantities should be used cautiously because this herb may cause uterine contractions.
- Lactation: Safe as a food.
- Do not use in young children.

Drug/Herb Interactions and Rationale (if known): None known for internal use

Special Notes

- Hot peppers cause skin burning and irritation. Use rubber gloves when preparing fresh peppers. Wash hands thoroughly after preparing peppers or using the creams.
- Capsaicin is not water-soluble, so it is difficult to wash off after handling peppers.
- Avoid contact with eyes.

BIBLIOGRAPHY

Blumenthal M, et al. (2000). *Herbal Medicine: Expanded Commission E Monographs.* Austin, TX: American Botanical Council.

Ellis CN, et al. (1993). A double-blind evaluation of topical capsaicin in pruritic psoriasis. *Journal of the American Academy of Dermatology.* 29:438–442.

McCaleb R, et al. (2000). *Encyclopedia of Popular Herbs.* Roseville, CA: Prima Publishers.

Robbins WR, et al. (1998). Treatment of intractable pain with topical large-dose capsaicin: preliminary report. *Anesthesia & Analgesia.* 86:579–583.

NAME: German or Hungarian Chamomile (*Matricaria recutita*), Roman or English Chamomile (*Chamaemelum nobilis*)

Common Names: Common chamomile, true chamomile, English chamomile, wild chamomile, German chamomile, Hungarian chamomile, Roman chamomile, sweet false chamomile

Family: *Asteraceae*

Description of Plant: *Matricaria recutita* is an erect annual, growing 1 to 2.5 feet; has small daisy-like flowers in clusters.

Medicinal Part: Flower head; gather just before blooming and then dry

Constituents and Action (if known)

- Volatile oils: carminative activity, anti-inflammatory, antidiuretic, antispasmodic, sedative, muscle relaxing, antibacterial (Aggag & Yousef, 1972)
  - Alpha-bisabolol (50% of essential oil): anti-inflammatory, antipyretic (Habersang et al., 1979; Isaac, 1979) antiulcer effect (Fidler et al., 1996)
  - Alpha-bisabolol oxides A and B: papaverine-like antispasmodic activity (Achterath-Tuckerman et al., 1980)
  - Matricine: anti-inflammatory (Della Loggia et al., 1996)
  - Chamazulene: formed during steam distillation, makes up 5% of essential oil; anti-inflammatory
- Flavonoids (0.5%–3%): contain significant anti-inflammatory activity (Della Loggia et al., 1996)
  - Apigenin-7-glucoside and luteolin: bind to benzodiazepine receptors and have anxiolytic and mild relaxing effects with no sedation; anti-inflammatory activity may be greater than that of indomethacin (Hamon, 1989; Paladini et al., 1999)
  - Quercetin: equal to apigenin in strength; antispasmodic effects (Achterath-Tuckerman et al., 1980)
- Sesquiterpene lactones: matricin, matricarin

Nutritional Ingredients: None known

Traditional Use
Internal
- As a remedy for teething babies
- To quiet an upset stomach
- To relieve intestinal colic and menstrual cramps
- To reduce tension and induce sleep

Topical: For hemorrhoids, mastitis, eczema, and leg ulcers; reduces inflammation; soothes aches; heals cuts, sores, and bruises

Current Use
Internal
- Irritable bowel syndrome
- Indigestion
- Infant colic (can be given to the mother and the oils pass through the breast milk to the infant)
- Gastric reflux disease
- Mild to moderate dysmenorrhea
- Gastritis
- Stress-related insomnia
- Peptic ulcer disease
- Spastic colon
- Cramping secondary to diarrhea
- Soothes oral cavity, including irritated gingiva and aphthous ulcers

Topical
- Anogenital irritation
- Wound healing (Glowania et al., 1987)
- Eczema: ointment is as effective as hydrocortisone and superior to nonsteroidal anti-inflammatories (Aertgeerts et al., 1985)

Available Forms, Dosage, and Administration Guidelines
Preparations: Dried flowers; capsules, cream salve, tea, tincture, bath products

Typical Dosage
- *Bath:* For hemorrhoids or irritated skin, soak 1 lb dried flowers in a tub of hot water.
- *Capsules:* Up to six 300- to 400-mg capsules a day

- *Tea:* Steep 1 tbsp dried flowers in a cup of hot water 5 to 10 minutes; take three or four times a day between meals.
- *Tincture* (1:5, 40% alcohol): 60 to 120 gtt (3–6 mL) three times a day
- Or follow manufacturer's or practitioner's recommendations.
- *Topical:* For insect bites, mix 1 tsp aloe vera gel with 2 gtt chamomile essential oil and apply to bite.

Pharmacokinetics—If Available (form or route when known): None known

Toxicity: None known

Contraindications: None known

Side Effects: Topical: allergic skin reactions. Internal: bronchial constriction. Persons with severe allergies to plants in the *Asteraceae* family (ragweed, asters, chrysanthemums) should avoid chamomile. Allergic reactions are rare and need to be verified (Mann & Staba, 1986).

Long-Term Safety: Safe

Use in Pregnancy/Lactation/Children: German chamomile has a long history of use during pregnancy and breast-feeding and as a children's remedy. It is a common beverage tea throughout Europe and South America. Roman chamomile has been found to be an abortifacient in animals.

Drug/Herb Interactions and Rationale (if known): Anticoagulants may potentiate effect. Use cautiously.

Special Notes: German chamomile is better-tasting and milder in action than Roman chamomile. It is more appropriate for pregnant women and children.

BIBLIOGRAPHY

Achterath-Tuckerman U, et al. (1980). Investigations on the spasmolytic effect of compounds of chamomile and kamillosan on the isolated guinea pig ileum. *Planta Medica.* 39:38.

Aertgeerts P, et al. (1985). [Comparative testing of Kamillosan cream and steroidal (0.25% hydrocortisone, 0.75% fluocortin butyl ester) and non-steroidal (5% bufexamac) dermatologic agents in maintenance therapy of eczematous diseases] (In German). *Z Hautkr.* 60(3):270–277.

Aggag ME, Yousef RT. (1972). Study of the antimicrobial activity of chamomile oil. *Planta Medica.* 22:140–144.

Blumenthal M, et al. (2000). *Herbal Medicine, Expanded Commission E Monographs.* Austin, TX: American Botanical Council.

Della Loggia R, et al. (1996). The role of flavonoids in the anti-inflammatory activity of *Chamomilla recutita.* In: Cody V, et al. (Eds.). *Plant Flavonoids in Biology and Medicine: Biochemical, Pharmacological and Structure-Activity Relationships.* New York: Alan R. Liss.

Fidler P, et al. (1996). Prospective evaluations of a chamomile mouthwash for prevention of SFU-induced oral mucosites. *Cancer.* 77:522–524.

Glowania HJ, et al. (1987). Effect of chamomile on wound healing: a clinical double-blind study (In German). *Z Hautkr.* 62(17):1262–1271.

Habersang S, et al. (1979). Pharmacological studies with compounds of chamomile IV. *Planta Medica.* 37:115.

Hamon NW. (November 1989). Herbal medicine: the chamomiles. *Canadian Pharmaceutical Journal.*

Isaac O. (1979). Pharmacological investigations with compounds of chamomile I. *Planta Medica.* 35:118.

Lawrence Review of Natural Products. (1991). St. Louis: Facts and Comparisons.

Mann C, Staba EJ. (1986). The chemistry, pharmacology, and commercial formulations of chamomile. In: Craker LE, Simons JE. (Eds.). *Herbs, Spices, and Medicinal Plants: Recent Advances in Botany, Horticulture, and Pharmacology,* Vol. 1 (pp. 235–280). Phoenix, AZ: Oryx Press.

Mills S, Bone K. (1999). *Principles and Practice of Phytotherapy.* Edinburgh: Churchill Livingstone.

Paladini AC, et al. (1999). Flavonoids and the central nervous system: from forgotten factors to potent anxiolytic compounds. *Journal of Pharmacy & Pharmacology.* 51(5):519–526.

Rodriguez-Serna M, et al. (1998). Allergic and systemic contact dermatitis from *Matricaria chamomilla* tea. *Contact Dermatitis.* 39(4):192–193.

 NAME: Chaparral (*Larrea tridentata*)

Common Names: Creosote bush, grease wood

Family: *Zygophyllaceae*

Description of Plant: A very long-lived evergreen perennial shrub that grows in the deserts of Mexico and the American Southwest. The aromatic leaves smell like creosote.

Medicinal Part: Leaves

Constituents and Action (if known)
- Lignans: nordihydroguaiaretic acid (antioxidant), nor-isoguaiasin, dihydroguariaretic acid, larreatricin, many others
- Flavonoids: quercitin, kaempherol, rutin
- Triterpenes: larreagenin A, larreic acid

Traditional Use
- Antioxidant, expectorant, alterative, diuretic, antitumor, antifungal
- Ethnobotanical use by Native Americans and Hispanics for arthritis, bursitis, neuralgias (oral and topical), uterine fibroids, cancer, respiratory infections, and skin conditions (oral and topical)

Current Use
- Considered unsafe; not recommended for internal use
- Topical use (baths) for arthralgias, sciatica, bursitis, and psoriasis
- Research is ongoing for the use of this herb in treating lymphoma and breast cancer. Intratumoral injection has shown the greatest activity.

Available Forms, Dosage, and Administration Guidelines: No toxicity observed from tea (1 tsp dried leaf to 8 oz water). The strongly unpleasant taste may limit the amount taken and thus the possibility of side effects.

Pharmacokinetics—If Available (form or route when known)

Toxicity: Potentially hepatotoxic (Anesini et al., 1997; Katz et al., 1990; Lampe & McCann, 1985; *Morbidity and Mortality Weekly Report*, 1992)

Contraindications: Liver disease, pregnancy

Side Effects
- Idiosyncratic hepatitis (has occurred in a few people taking chaparral tablets or capsules)
- Contact dermatitis

Long-Term Safety: Not recommended for long-term use

Use in Pregnancy/Lactation/Children: Do not use.

Drug/Herb Interactions and Rationale (if known): None known

Special Notes: Nordihydroguaiaretic acid was previously used as an antioxidant in the food Industry (1940s–1970) until rat feeding studies (0.5%–1% nordihydroguaiaretic acid for 74 weeks) showed lymph node and kidney lesions.

BIBLIOGRAPHY

Anesini C, et al. (1997). In vivo antitumoural activity and acute toxicity study of *Larrea divarcata* C. extract. *Phytotherapy Research*. 11(7):521–523.

Anesini C, et al. (1998). In vivo antitumor activity of *Larrea divarcata* C. extract. *Phytomedicine*. 5(1):41–46.

Chaparral-induced toxic hepatitis, California and Texas. (1992). *Morbidity and Mortality Weekly Report*. 48:812.

Katz M, et al. (1990). Herbal hepatitis: subacute hepatic necrosis secondary to chaparral leaf. *Journal of Clinical Gastroenterology*. 12:203.

Lampe KF, McCann MA. (1985). *AMA Handbook of Poisonous and Injurious Plants*. Chicago: AMA.

Leung A, Foster S. (1996). *Encyclopedia of Common Natural Ingredients*. (2nd ed.). New York: John Wiley & Sons.

Mabry JT, et al. (1977). *Creosote Bush: Biology and Chemistry of Larrea in New Word Deserts*. Stroudsburg, PA: Dowden, Hutchinson and Ross.

Sheikh NM, et al. (1997). Chaparral: associated hepatotoxicity. *Archives of Internal Medicine*. 157:913–919.

 NAME: Chaste Tree (*Vitex agnus-castus*)

Common Names: Monk's pepper, chasteberry

Family: *Verbenaceae*

Description of Plant: A woody shrub that grows abundantly in southern Europe and the Mediterranean; likes moist riverbanks; has purple flowers in summer, gray fruit in autumn

Medicinal Part: Dried fruit

Constituents and Action (if known)

- Essential oils (0.5%–1.22%)
  - Monoterpenes: cineol (25%), alpha-pinene, beta-pinene, limonene, sabinene (Kustrak et al., 1992): sedative properties
  - Sesquiterpenes: beta-caryophyllene, beta-farnesene; may assist with regulation of luteal phase of female cycle (Milewicz et al., 1993)
- Iridoid glycosides: agnuside (0.6%), aucubin (0.3%)
- Flavonoids and flavones (glucosides): casticin, iso-orientin, isovitexin (Brown, 1994; Snow, 1996)
- Other actions: binds to dopamine receptors and inhibits release of prolactin (Jarry, et al., 1994; Snow, 1996)

Nutritional Ingredients: None known

History: Symbol of chastity in medieval European church; where it is native (Mediterranean, Greek islands), in pre-Christian times its use was sacred to Hera, protectress of women

Traditional Use

- Anaphrodisiac, diaphoretic, diuretic, carminative, galactagogue
- Has been used for more than 2,000 years to treat female problems, such as menstrual cramps, irregular cycles, breast pain, and abnormal bleeding, and to stimulate milk production in lactating women
- Believed to be an "anaphrodisiac" for men, it was called "monk's pepper." Was grown around monasteries, and monks used it regularly as a tea to lessen sexual desires.
- Used for digestive upsets, to promote sweating in fevers, to increase urination, and to relieve hysteria

Current Use

- Treats perimenopausal symptoms (hot flashes, vaginal dryness, formication); most effective if used with black cohosh, dong quai, and omega-3 fatty acids

- Relieves premenstrual anxiety and other premenstrual symptoms caused by elevated estrogen levels or deficient progesterone levels (migraines, breast tenderness, cramps, edema, constipation)
- Relieves breast pain (mastodynia) and helps to treat fibrocystic breast disease
- Relieves dysmenorrhea; use along with antispasmodics such as black haw, motherwort, or Roman chamomile
- In latent hyperprolactinemia, inhibits prolactin secretion by directly binding to the dopamine receptor in the pituitary
- Used for corpus luteum insufficiency and associated symptoms (hypermenorrhea, infertility, polymenorrhea, oligomenorrhea, anovulation, primary and secondary amenorrhea, menorrhagia)
- May be useful for women who have stopped using birth control pills and have irregular menstrual cycles
- Increases milk production during lactation. Studies on 100 nursing mothers found that vitex increased milk flow and eased milk release.
- Useful for polycystic ovarian disease, along with saw palmetto
- Can reduce the size of uterine fibroids (smooth muscle or subserous) and ovarian cysts; takes 2 to 6 months to see improvement
- Teenage acne: in a controlled study of 161 patients (male and female), after 3 months of treatment with vitex 70% reported significant improvement compared with patients using a placebo

Available Forms, Dosage, and Administration Guidelines

Preparations: Dried fruit, whole, pulverized; capsules, tinctures, tablets, and combination products. Clinical studies in Europe used a proprietary extract and capsules called Agnolyt.

Typical Dosage

- *Capsules* (nonstandardized): up to three 650-mg capsules a day
- *Standardized extracts* (standardized for 0.5% agnuside): 175 to 225 mg/day

- *Tea:* Steep 1 scant tsp dried, ground berries in 1 cup hot water for 10 to 15 minutes; take two or three cups per day.
- *Tincture* (1:5, 45% alcohol): 20 to 40 gtt (1–2 mL) once or twice per day
- Or follow manufacturer's or practitioner's recommendations

Pharmacokinetics—If Available (form or route when known): Not known

Toxicity: Nontoxic

Contraindications: May aggravate spasmodic dysmenorrhea that is not associated with premenstrual symptoms (Mills & Bone, 1999)

Side Effects: Nausea, vomiting, itching, urticaria, mild headache, increased menstrual flow

Long-Term Safety: Safe; safe in women with estrogen-positive cancers; no effect on estrogen receptors

Use in Pregnancy/Lactation/Children: Do not use until after menarche. Use cautiously in early pregnancy for insufficient corpus luteum function. Studies on lactating women show benefits and no toxicity.

Drug/Herb Interactions and Rationale (if known)
- Do not use concurrently with hormone replacement therapy or birth control pills.
- Haloperidol may weaken or block the effects of vitex.

Special Notes: This herb's ability to reduce prolactin secretions may make it useful for benign prostatic hypertrophy.

BIBLIOGRAPHY

Betz W. (1998). Commentary. *Forschende Komplementarmedizen.* 5:146–147.

Bone K. (1994). *Vitex agnus castus*: scientific studies and clinical applications. *European Journal of Herbal Medicine.* 1(2):12–15.

Brown DJ. (Summer 1994). *Vitex agnus castus* clinical monograph. *Quarterly Review of Natural Medicine.* p. 111.

Dr. Duke's Phytochemical and Ethnobotanical Databases. Agricultural Research Service. Available at: *http://www.ars-grin.gov/cgi-bin/duke/index.html.*

Halaska M, et al. (1998). Treatment of cyclical mastodynia using an extract of *Vitex agnus castus*: results of a double-blind comparison with a placebo. *Ceska Gynekol.* 63(5):388–392.

Hirobe C, et al. (1997). Cytotoxic flavonoids from *Vitex agnus-castus*. *Phytochemistry.* 46(3):521–524.

Hobbs C. (1998). *Vitex, The Women's Herb.* (2nd ed.). Loveland, CO: Interweave Press.

Jarry H, et al. (1994). In vitro prolactin but not LH and FSH release is inhibited by compounds in extracts of *Agnus castus*: direct evidence for a dopaminergic principle by the dopamine receptor assay. *Experimental & Clinical Endocrinology.* 102:448–454.

Kustrak KJ, et al. (1992). The composition of the essential oil of *Vitex agnus castus*. *Planta Medica.* 58(Suppl. 1):A681.

Lauritzen D, et al. (1997). Treatment of premenstrual tension syndrome with *Vitex agnus-castus*. Controlled, double-blind study versus pyridoxine. *Phytomedicine.* 4(3):183–189.

Loch EG, et al. (2000). Treatment of premenstrual syndrome with a phytopharmaceutical formulation containing *Vitex agnus-castus*. *Journal of Women's Health & Gender-Based Medicine.* 9(3):315–320.

Milewicz A, et al. (1993). *Vitex agnus castus* extract in the treatment of luteal phase defects due to a latent hyperprolactinemia. Results of a randomized placebo-controlled double-blind study. *Arzneimittelforschung.* 45:752–756.

Mills S, Bone K. (1999). *Principles and Practice of Phytotherapy.* Edinburgh: Churchill Livingstone.

Review of Natural Products. (1998). St. Louis: Facts and Comparisons.

Snow J. (1996). Vitex. *Protocol Journal of Botanical Medicine.* 1(4):20–23.

Weiss RF, Fintelmann V. (2000). *Herbal Medicine.* (2nd ed.). Stuttgart: Thieme.

🌿 NAME: Cinnamon (*Cinnamomum verum*)

Common Names: Ceylon cinnamon, true cinnamon; Chinese cinnamon, which has similar uses, is *Cinnamomum aromaticum*

Family: *Lauraceae*

Description of Plant: A small evergreen tree native to southern India and Sri Lanka, now cultivated in India, Sri Lanka, Malaysia, and Madagascar

Medicinal Part: Bark and occasionally leaves and buds

Constituents and Action (if known)

- Volatile oils (aldehydes): halt growth of *Aspergillus* (Tantaoui-Elaraki & Beraoud, 1994) and *Escherichia coli* (De et al., 1999); antifungal, antiviral, bactericidal effects (Leung & Foster, 1996)
  - Cinnamaldehyde (60%–80%): antiulcer activity
  - Terpenes (eugenol and others): anesthetic and antiseptic activity
  - Cinnamyl alcohol and acetate, limonene
- Condensed tannins
- Methylene chloride extracts: have inhibitory effect on *Helicobacter pylori* (Tabak et al., 1999)
- Cinnamon extract has antioxidant activity (Mancini-Filho et al., 1988)

Nutritional Ingredients: Used as a spice and flavoring

Traditional Use

- Antibacterial, antifungal, carminative, antihemorrhagic
- Flavoring agent for unpleasant-tasting medicines
- Essential oil used to treat GI upset, dysmenorrhea, hemorrhages (with oil of erigeron) (menorrhagia, hemoptysis, hematuria, nose bleeds)
- Used to treat diarrhea, dysentery, vomiting, and nausea

Current Use

- May be useful for treating gastric ulcers and inhibiting *H. pylori* (Tabak et al., 1999)
- Soothes the GI system; useful for flatulence, nausea, bloating, borborygmus, mild gastric upset, poor fat digestion
- Adjunct therapy for insulin resistance (syndrome X) and adult-onset insulin-resistant diabetes. Cinnamon increases the use of endogenous insulin (Khan, 1990).

Available Forms, Dosage, and Administration Guidelines

- Used in combination with other herbs; rarely used alone
- *Bark:* Unless otherwise prescribed, 2 to 4 g/day of ground bark

- *Infusion or decoction:* 0.25 to 0.5 tsp powdered bark in 8 oz hot water, steep covered 30 minutes; take 2 to 4 oz three times daily
- *Fluid extract* (1:1: 10 to 25 gtt (0.5–1.3 mL), three times daily
- *Tincture* (1:5, 70% alcohol): 40 to 80 gtt (2–4 mL), three times daily
- *Essential oil:* 1 to 2 gtt three times daily

Pharmacokinetics—If Available (form or route when known): Not known

Toxicity: Large amounts increase heart rate and intestinal motility, followed by sleepiness and depression (Bisset, 1994).

Contraindications: None known

Side Effects: Skin irritation from contact with cinnamon powder, oral lesions from chewing cinnamon gum

Long-Term Safety: As a spice, long-term use is safe.

Use in Pregnancy/Lactation/Children: Use as a spice is fine; avoid large doses.

Drug/Herb Interactions and Rationale (if known): None known

Special Notes: Cinnamon has been found to kill *E. coli* 0157, the potentially fatal bacteria that causes serious food poisoning. Along with cloves and garlic, cinnamon added to meats and unpasteurized apple cider killed 99.5% of the bacteria.

BIBLIOGRAPHY

Bisset NG. (Ed.). (1994). *Herbal Drugs and Phytopharmaceuticals.* Stuttgart: Medpharm Scientific Publishers.

Blumenthal M, et al. (2000). *Herbal Medicine: Expanded Commission E Monographs.* Austin, TX: American Botanical Council.

De M, et al. (1999). Antimicrobial screening of some Indian spices. *Phytotherapy Research.* 13(7):616–618.

Khan A, et al. (1990). Insulin potentiating factor and chromium content of selected foods and spices. *Biological Trace Elements Research.* 24:183–188.

Lawrence Review of Natural Products. (1995). St. Louis: Facts and Comparisons.

Leung AY, Foster S. (1996). *Encyclopedia of Common Natural Ingredients Used in Food, Drugs and Cosmetics.* (2nd ed.). New York: John Wiley & Sons.

Mancini-Filho J, et al. (1988). Antioxidant activity of cinnamon (*Cinnamomum zeylanicum*, Brene) extracts. *Boll Chim Farm.* 137(11):443–447.

Tabak M, et al. (1999). Cinnamon extracts' inhibitory effect on *Helicobacter pylori. Journal of Ethnopharmacology.* 67(3):269–277.

Tantaoui-Elaraki A, Beraoud L. (1994). Inhibition of growth and aflatoxin production in *Aspergillus parasiticus* by essential oils of selected plant materials. *Journal of Environmental Pathology, Toxicology, & Oncology.* 13(1):67.

NAME: Coltsfoot (*Tussilago farfara*)

Common Names: Bullfoot, coughwort, foalswort

Family: *Asteraceae*

Description of Plant: Creeping weedy perennial that flowers before leafing out. Flowers are yellow, followed by a white dandelion-like puffball.

Medicinal Part: Leaf, flowers

Constituents and Action (if known)
- Mucilage (6%–10%)
- Tannins (5%)
- Triterpenes: beta-amyrin, arnidol, faradiol
- Pyrrolizidine alkaloids: trace amounts of tussilagine, isotussilagine, senkirkine, senecionin in some samples
- Flavonoids

History: Painted pictures of coltsfoot leaves were used as a sign of an herbalist in medieval France.

Nutritional Ingredients: The leaves, burned to ash, have been used as a salt substitute.

Traditional Use
- Expectorant, pectoral, demulcent
- Dry coughs, bronchitis, bronchial catarrh, asthma, sore throat, chest colds, tonsillitis
- Irritation of the bladder

Current Use: Dry, irritable, ticklish coughs; chronic irritation of the mouth and throat with hoarseness

Available Forms, Dosage, and Administration Guidelines: *Tea:* 1 tsp dried herb in 8 oz water, steep 20 minutes; take 4 oz three times daily

Pharmacokinetics—If Available (form or route when known): Not known

Toxicity: Contains trace amounts of pyrrolizidine alkaloids, a cumulative liver poison associated with veno-occlusive disease. FDA classifies it as an herb of "undefined safety."

Contraindications: Pregnancy, breast-feeding, use in children, liver disease

Side Effects: None known

Long-Term Safety: The German Commission E warns against use for more than 28 days per year. Short-term use only.

Use in Pregnancy/Lactation/Children: Do not use.

Drug/Herb Interactions and Rationale (if known): None known

Special Notes
• The tea would be the safest preparation because the trace amounts of the pyrrolizidine alkaloids are poorly water-soluble.
• Source of the herb is important: two common adulterants, Western coltsfoot (petasites) and *Adenostyles alliariae*, contain dangerous levels of pyrrolizidine alkaloids.
• In Chinese medicine, the flowers (kuan dong hua) are also used for coughs and wheezing.

BIBLIOGRAPHY
Bisset NG, Wichtl M. (1994). *Herbal Drugs and Phytopharmaceuticals.* Boca Raton, FL: CRC Press.
DerMarderosian AH, Liberti LE. (1988). *Natural Products Medicine.* Philadelphia: GF Stickley Co.
Gruenwald J. (1998). *PDR for Herbal Medicines.* Montvale, NJ: Medical Economics Co.

Schultz V, et al. (1998). *Rational Phytotherapy: A Physician's Guide to Herbal Medicine* (3rd ed.). Berlin: Springer-Verlag.

Sperl W, et al. (1995). Reversible hepatic veno-occlusive disease in an infant after consumption of pyrrolizidine-containing herbal tea. *European Journal of Pediatrics.* 154(2):112–116.

 NAME: Cranberry (*Vaccinium macrocarpon*)

Common Names: Trailing swamp cranberry, small cranberry, southern mountain cranberry, marsh apple

Family: *Ericaceae*

Description of Plant: Small trailing evergreen vine producing pink-purple flowers from May to August; loves water; grows well in acidic bogs but also in acidic mountain forests

Medicinal Part: Ripe fruit

Constituents and Action (if known)

- Anthocyanins or proanthocyanidins: high-molecular-weight anthocyanins (flavonoids) prevent *Escherichia coli* from adhering to bladder wall (Howell et al., 1998; Ofek et al., 1991; Zafiri et al., 1989; Zopf & Roth, 1996) as well as the teeth and gums (Weiss et al., 1998)
- Organic acids (citric, malic, guinic, benzoic, glucuronic): slow biotransformation of acids, which increases excretion of hippuric acid, which acidifies the urine. Quinic and benzoic acids break down and form hippuric acid in urine) (Avorn et al., 1994; Der Marderosian, 1977; Kahn et al., 1967; Walsh, 1992).
- Catechin
- Triterpenoids
- Fructose: prevents adhesion of type 1 *E. coli* to the urinary tract (Zafiri, et al., 1989)
- Carbohydrates (10%), ascorbic acid (10 mg)

Nutritional Ingredients: Can be used to make relish or sauces and juice. The bitter and sour taste of cranberries makes added sweeteners a necessity. Unsweetened cranberries are low in calories (209 calories/lb), are a good source of fiber, and are high in vitamin C and flavonoids.

Traditional Use

- To reduce fever (used as a refrigerant)
- To acidify the urine and treat urinary tract infections, urinary calculi
- To prevent and treat scurvy
- To soothe swollen glands and wounds (poultice)

Current Use

- Lowers incidence of and prevent urinary tract infections (Avorn et al., 1994; Gibson et al., 1991; Howell et al., 1998)
- Decreases incidence of urinary stones
- Decreases symptoms in chronic pyelonephritis (6 oz juice twice daily)
- Reduces odor in urine in incontinent patients (Walsh, 1992)
- Unsweetened juice may prevent coaggregation of gum bacteria and reduce plaque formation (Weiss et al., 1998).

Available Forms, Dosage, and Administration Guidelines

Preparations: Whole fruit, raw or jellied; juice, fruit concentrate, capsules

Typical Dosage

- *Capsules:* One capsule morning and night, but up to nine 300- to 500-mg capsules a day. For intensive use, up to 15 capsules.
- *Food:* 3 to 10 oz fresh fruit a day
- *Juice:* 5 to 20 oz cranberry juice cocktail a day (make sure juice contains real cranberry; most contain 10% to 33% cranberry)
- Or follow manufacturer's or practitioner's recommendations.

Pharmacokinetics—If Available (form or route when known): None known

Toxicity: None known

Contraindications: Do not use in urinary obstruction.

Side Effects: None with normal doses; large doses (3–4 L/day) may result in diarrhea

Long-Term Safety: Very safe

Use in Pregnancy/Lactation/Children: None known; safe

Drug/Herb Interactions and Rationale (if known): None known

Special Notes

- Should not be used as a substitute for anti-infectives when a urinary tract infection is present
- Persons with diabetes should use sugar-free juices.
- Always drink at least six to eight glasses of water per day.

BIBLIOGRAPHY

Avorn J, et al. (1994). Reduction of bacteriuria and pyuria after ingestion of cranberry juice. *Journal of the American Medical Association.* 271:751.

Der Marderosian AH. (1997). Cranberry juice. *Drug Therapy.* 7:151.

Gibson L, et al. (1991). Effectiveness of cranberry juice in preventing urinary tract infections in long-term care facility patients. *Journal of Naturopathic Medicine.* 2:45–47.

Howell AB, et al. (1998). Inhibition of the adherence of P-fimbriated *Escherichia coli* to uroepithelial-cell surfaces by proanthocyanidin extracts from cranberries. *New England Journal of Medicine.* 339(15):1085–1086.

Kahn DH, et al. (1967). Effect of cranberry juice on urine. *Journal of the American Dietetic Association.* 51:251.

McCaleb R, et al. (2000). *Encyclopedia of Popular Herbs.* Roseville, CA: Prima Publishers.

Ofek I, et al. (1991). Anti-*Escherichia coli* adhesion activity of cranberry and blueberry juices. *New England Journal of Medicine.* 324:1599.

Walsh BA. (1992). Urostomy and urinary pH. *Journal of ET Nursing.* 19:110.

Weiss EI, et al. (1998). Inhibiting interspecies coaggregation of plaque bacteria with a cranberry juice constituent. *Journal of the American Dental Association.* 129(12):1719–1123.

Zafiri D, et al. (1989). Inhibitory activity of cranberry juice on adherence of type 1 and type P fimbriated *Escherichia coli* to eucaryotic cells. *Antimicrobial Agents & Chemotherapy.* 33:92–98.

Zopf D, Roth S. (1996). Oligosaccharide anti-infective agents. *Lancet.* 347:1017–1021.

NAME: Dandelion (*Taraxacum officinale*)

Common Names: Lion's tooth, priest's crown, *pissenlit* (French), *diente de leon* (Spanish)

Family: *Asteraceae*

Description of Plant
- Member of the aster family, closely related to chicory
- Perennial; grows 12 inches high
- Spatula-like leaves are deeply toothed, shiny, and hairless.
- Yellow flowers bloom much of the year and are light-sensitive, opening in the morning and closing in the evening and in wet weather.

Medicinal Part: Root and leaf, dried or fresh. Fresh root preparations are more potent than dried root.

Constituents and Action (if known)
Leaf
- Sesquiterpene lactones (eudesmanolides): increase bile secretions (Duke, 1992; Newall et al., 1996); may contribute to mild anti-inflammatory activity (Leung & Foster, 1996; Newall et al., 1996); contribute to the allergenic component of dandelion; may cause mild gastrointestinal discomfort (Bisset, 1994); diuretic effect, may reduce blood pressure (Bisset, 1994)
- Triterpenes
  ○ Taxarerol: antiulcer and dyspepsia effects (Duke, 1992)
  ○ Taraxol, beta-amyrin
- Carotenoids (lutein, violaxanthin)
- Flavonoids (apigenin, luteolin)
- Phenolic acids (caffeic and chlorogenic acids)
- Phytosterols (sitosterol, stigmasterol, taraxastecol)
- Minerals

Root
- Triterpenes
- Lactopictine (taraxacin)
- Taraxol
- Inulin (2% in spring, 40% in autumn): a source of fruto-oligo-saccharides

Nutritional Ingredients
- Rich source of vitamins A, D, B complex, C (contains more vitamin A than an equal serving of carrots, up to 14,000 IU per 100 g)
- Rich source of minerals: iron, silicon, magnesium, sodium, potassium, zinc, manganese, calcium, copper, and phosphorus
- Substantial amounts of choline, a nutrient for the liver
- Rich source of fiber and fruto-oligo-saccharides

Traditional Use
- Both leaf and root have been used for centuries to treat liver and gallbladder conditions as well as digestive problems. The root and to a lesser degree the leaves, are used as cholagogues, bitter tonics, aperients, and liver tonics. The leaf is a nonirritating diuretic and has been used for dysuria, edema, obesity, and hypertension.
- Topical application of milky latex to warts

Current Use
Herb
- As a nonirritating, potassium-sparing diuretic, dandelion leaf contains high levels of K+ (Blumenthal, 2000; ESCOP, 1997)
- For the prevention of urinary calculi

Root
- As a mild laxative (aperient), especially with clay-colored stools
- Stimulates digestion and appetite (root and leaf); used for anorexia, inadequate bile secretion, dysbiosis, impaired hepatic and biliary function, and digestive torpor (flatulence, bloating, constipation)
- Anti-inflammatory properties: indicated for rheumatic conditions (Bradley, 1992)

Nutritional Use: Tender leaves can be used in salads or lightly cooked as a nutritious vegetable; flowers can be used to make wine; root can be roasted and used to make a coffee-like beverage.

Available Forms, Dosage, and Administration Guidelines
- *Food:* Eat young leaves raw or lightly cooked in the spring.

- *Dried leaf:* 4 to 10 g by infusion three times a day.
- *Dried root:* 2 to 8 g by infusion or decoction three times a day
- *Tea:* Steep 1 to 2 tsp cut and sifted dried root in a cup of hot water for 30 to 40 minutes; take twice a day, in morning and evening.
- *Tinctures:* leaf (1:5, 30% alcohol): 40–80 gtt (2 to 4 mL) three times a day; fresh root (1:2, 30% alcohol): 100–140 gtt (5 to 10 mL) three times a day
- *Powdered solid extract* (4:1): 250 to 500 mg/day

Pharmacokinetics—If Available (form or route when known): None known

Toxicity: None reported

Contraindications: Do not use with obstruction of the bile ducts, gallbladder, empyema and ileus; may exacerbate these conditions (Newall et al., 1996).

Side Effects: Milky latex in leaves may cause contact dermatitis; bitterness may exacerbate hyperacidity.

Long-Term Safety: Safe

Use in Pregnancy/Lactation/Children: Long-time use as food; no adverse reactions expected

Drug/Herb Interactions and Rationale (if known)
- Use cautiously with antihypertensives because the leaf is a diuretic. Treat it as you would a prescription diuretic.
- Avoid concurrent use of diuretics because there is a strong possibility of potentiating effects (but not K+ loss, because dandelion contains K+).

BIBLIOGRAPHY
Bartram T. (1995). *Encyclopedia of Herbal Medicine.* Dorset, UK: Grace Publishers.
Bisset NG. (Ed.). (1994). *Herbal Drugs and Phytopharmaceuticals.* Boca Raton, FL: CRC Press.
Blumenthal M, et al. (2000). *Herbal Medicine: Expanded Commission E Monographs.* Austin, TX: American Botanical Council.
Bradley P. (Ed.). (1992). *British Herbal Compendium,* Vol. I. Dorset: British Herbal Medicine Association.

Duke JA. (1992). *Handbook of Biologically Active Phytochemicals and Their Activities*. Boca Raton, FL: CRC Press.

ESCOP Monographs On the Medicinal Uses of Plant Drugs. (1996–1999). Exeter: ESCOP.

Foster S. (1998). *101 Medicinal Herbs*. Loveland, CO: Interweave Press.

Hobbs C. (1989). *Taraxacum officinale*: a monograph and literature review. In: *Eclectic Dispensatory*. Portland, OR: Eclectic Medical Publications.

Lawrence Review of Natural Products. (1998). St. Louis: Facts & Comparisons.

Leung A, Foster S. (1996). *Encyclopedia of Common Natural Ingredients*. (2nd ed.). New York: John Wiley & Sons.

Newall C, et al. (1996). *Herbal Medicines*. London: Pharmaceutical Press.

Swanston-Flatt SK, et al. (1989). Glycaemic effects of traditional European plant treatments for diabetes. Studies in normal and streptozotocin diabetic mice. *Diabetes Research*. 10(2):69–73.

 NAME: Dan Shen (*Salvia miltiorrhiza*)

Common Names: Red root sage, tan sheng (Wade-Giles)

Family: *Lamiaceae*

Description of Plant: A small perennial in the mint family with reddish-purple flowers. The best roots are cultivated and are a rich purple-black color inside with a red outer bark.

Medicinal Part: Root

Constituents and Action (if known)
- Diterpene quinones: tanshiones, 1, IIA (0.5%): reduce calcium uptake by myocardium; IIB is an anti-inflammatory anticoagulant with cytotoxic activity against human carcinoma lines in vitro
- Cryptotanshinone, isotanshinones 1, IIA, IIB
- Salvianolic acids A,B,C: inhibited peroxidation of rat liver microsomes (Bone, 1996)
- Baicalin

Nutritional Ingredients: None

Traditional Use

- Antibacterial, antihepatotoxin, antioxidant, renal protective, emmenagogue, anti-inflammatory, mild sedative
- In traditional Chinese medicine, used to "move blood"—for instance, promoting menstrual flow, removing blood stasis and pain (dysmenorrhea, abdominal pain, hepatomegaly and angina). It is also used for insomnia and palpitations and topically for bruises.

Current Use

- Cardiovascular disease: studies have shown the benefits of this herb for angina pectoris, hypertension, and angiitis. It is not cardiotonic but potentiates other cardiotonic herbs such as astragalus and *Angelica sinensis*. In a controlled study, dan shen reduced lipid peroxidation, and in 20 patients with hyperviscosity syndrome all symptoms disappeared (Bone, 1996).
- Antihepatotoxin: the decoction of the herb decreased elevated levels of serum glutamic-pyruvic transaminase (SGPT) and pathologic changes in rabbits with acute liver damage caused by carbon tetrachloride. The herb also restored normal liver function and prevented liver fibrosis in clinical studies (You-ping, 1998).
- May be useful in protecting the kidney from renotoxic drugs
- Increases maturation of osteoblasts and fibroblasts; may be useful in promoting healing of fractures

Available Forms, Dosage, and Administration Guidelines

Preparations: Dried herb, capsules, tea, tincture

Typical Dosage

- *Dried root:* 2 to 6 g per day
- *Capsules:* Two 500-mg capsules, one to three times per day
- *Tea:* 1 tsp dried root in 8 oz hot water, decoct 10 minutes, steep 30 minutes; take two cups per day
- *Tincture* (1:5, 35% alcohol): 30 to 80 gtt (1.5–4 mL) three times a day

Pharmacokinetics—If Available (form or route when known): Not known

Toxicity: Intraperitoneal and intragastric administration in mice in substantial doses showed no toxicity.

Contraindications: Bleeding disorders, pregnancy

Side Effects: A few patients taking this herb may experience dry mouth, dizziness, numbness of the hands, and GI disturbance. These symptoms usually disappear without disrupting treatment.

Long-Term Safety: Safe in normal therapeutic dosages

Use in Pregnancy/Lactation/Children: Avoid in pregnancy and lactation; use in older children with professional supervision.

Drug/Herb Interactions and Rationale (if known): May potentiate the actions of barbiturates, blood-thinning medications (warfarin), and cardiac glycosides (digoxin)

Special Notes
• Much of the research done on dan shen has been with isolated constituents and with injectable forms of the drug. These studies have little relevance to oral use of this herb.
• As with most Chinese herbs, this herb is rarely used by itself. It is almost always combined with other herbs based on traditional Chinese formulas.

BIBLIOGRAPHY
Bone K. (1996). *Clinical Applications of Ayurvedic and Chinese Herbs.* Queensland, Australia: Phytotherapy Press.
Foster S, Yue Chong XI. (1992). *Herbal Emissaries.* Rochester, VT: Healing Arts Press.
Hu L, et al. (1996). Experimental study of the protective effects of astragalus and *Salvia miltiorrhiza bunge* on glycerol-induced acute renal failure in rabbits. *Chung Hua Wai Ko Tsa Chih.* 34(5):311–314.
Tang W, Eisenbrand G. (1992). *Chinese Drugs of Plant Origin.* Berlin: Springer-Verlag.
Wasser S, et al. (1998). *Salvia miltiorrhiza* reduces experimentally-induced hepatic fibrosis in rats. *Journal of Hepatology.* 29(5):760–771.
Wu YJ, et al. (1998). Increase of vitamin E content in LDL and reduction of atherosclerosis in cholesterol-fed rabbits by a water-

soluble antioxidant-rich fraction of *Salvia miltiorrhiza*.
Arteriosclerosis & Thrombosis Vascular Biology. 18(3):481–486.
You-ping Z. (1998). *Chinese Materia Medica: Chemistry, Pharmacology and Applications.* Amsterdam: Harwood.

🌿 NAME: Devil's Claw (*Harpagophytum procumbens*)

Common Names: Grapple plant, wood spider

Family: *Pediliaceae*

Description of Plant: Shrubby vine native to southwest Africa; fruit has grapples that attach to animal fur

Medicinal Part: Root

Constituents and Action (if known)
- Iridoid glucosides (0.5%–3%)
  ○ Harpagoside is found in twice the concentration in secondary roots: anti-inflammatory activity (Vanhaelen et al., 1981; Whitehouse et al., 1983), negative chronotropic and positive inotropic effects by altering calcium influx into smooth muscle
- Procombide (Bendall et al., 1979)
- Harpagide

Nutritional Ingredients: None known

Traditional Use
- Internal: bitter tonic for indigestion; reduces fever; used as blood purifier; relieves rheumatic and arthritic pain, low back pain and headaches
- External: treats boils, sores, ulcers

Current Use
- Anti-inflammatory for arthritis (Chrubasik et al., 1996) and tendinitis (Bradley, 1992)
- Improves appetite, decreases indigestion and heartburn

Available Forms, Dosage, and Administration Guidelines
Preparations: Dried secondary tubers, cut and sifted or powdered; capsules, tablets, tinctures, tea. Some products are

standardized to harpagoside content. Possible gastric degradation of this herb may explain the conflicting results of studies. Recommendations for enteric-coated tablets designed to break down in the bowel may enhance activity of this herb.

Typical Dosage

- *Capsules:* Up to six 400- to 500-mg capsules a day
- *Tea:* For indigestion, steep 0.25 tsp of dried tuber in a cup of hot water for 10 to 15 minutes.
- *Tincture* (1:5, 25% alcohol): 20 to 40 gtt (1–2 mL) three times a day
- Or follow manufacturer's or practitioner's recommendations

Pharmacokinetics—If Available (form or route when known): None known

Toxicity: None known

Contraindications: Gastric and duodenal ulcers

Side Effects: Mild and infrequent gastrointestinal symptoms and headaches

Long-Term Safety: Unknown

Use in Pregnancy/Lactation/Children: Unknown; should be used under practitioner's guidance. Self-medication during pregnancy or breast-feeding is not advised.

Drug/Herb Interactions and Rationale (if known): Theoretical possibility of interaction with antiarrhythmic medications

Special Notes: Current research suggests anti-inflammatory and analgesic activity. Because of conflicting results, additional research is needed.

BIBLIOGRAPHY

Bendall M, et al. (1979). The structure of procumbide. *Australian Journal of Chemistry.* 32(9):2085.

Blumenthal M, et al. (2000). *Herbal Medicine, Expanded Commission E Monographs.* Austin, TX: American Botanical Council.

Bradley P. (Ed.). (1992). *British Herbal Compendium,* Vol. I. Bournemouth: British Herbal Medicine Association.

Chrubasik S, et al. (1996). Effectiveness of *Harpagophytum procumbens* in treatment of acute low back pain. *Phytomedicine.* 3(1):1–10.

ESCOP Monographs On the Medicinal Uses of Plant Drugs.
  (1996–1999). Exeter: ESCOP.
Review of Natural Products. (1996). St. Louis: Facts and Comparisons.
Vanhaelen M, et al. (1981). Biological activity of *Harpagophytum
  procumbens* D.C. Part 1: Preparation and structure of harpagogenin.
  Journal Pharmacie Belgique. 36:38.
Wegner T. (1999). Therapy of degenerative diseases of the
  musculoskeletal system with South African devil's claw. *Wiener
  Medizinische Wochenschrift.* 149(8-10):254–257.
Whitehouse LW, et al. (1983). Devil's claw (*Harpagophytum
  procumbens*): no evidence for anti-inflammatory activity in the
  treatment of arthritic disease. *Canadian Medical Association Journal.*
  129(3):249.

 NAME: Dong quai (*Angelica sinensis*)

Common Names: Tang kuei, Chinese angelica, dang-gui

Family: *Apiaceae*

Description of Plant: An aromatic member of the parsley
family; thrives in cool, shaded mountain woods in southern
and western China

Medicinal Part: Prepared root and rhizomes

Constituents and Action (if known)

- Coumarins (osthol, psoralen, bergapten, flurcoumarin,
  angelol, angelicone): vasodilatory and antispasmodic
  properties, central nervous system stimulant, may inhibit IgE
  titers so may have immunosuppressive activity, increase
  spleen function, anti-inflammatory, analgesic, antipyretic
  activity, uterine stimulant
- Essential oils (0.4%–0.7%)
  - *N*-butylidene phthalide: inhibitory effect on uterus (Duke
    & Foster, 1999), vasodilatory action lowers blood pressure
    but duration of action is short
  - Ligustilide: antiasthmatic and antispasmodic activity in
    vivo (Tang & Eisenbrand, 1992)
- Ferulic acid: inhibited rat platelet aggregation and serotonin
  release in vivo and in vitro (Tang & Eisenbrand, 1992)
- Psoralens: increases sensitivity to sun

Nutritional Ingredients: Vitamin B_{12} and folinic acid (the active form of folic acid); increases oxygen use in liver and glutamic acid and cysteine oxidation

Traditional Use

- One of the most frequently used women's herbs in the world. Has been used by the Chinese for thousands of years as a tonic for the female reproductive system, the blood, liver, and the heart.
- Used to nourish the blood and increase circulation. Blood (*xue*) deficiency syndromes include symptoms such as a pale complexion, pale tongue and nails, dizziness, palpitations, feeling cold, and anemia.
- Used in formulas for menstrual, menopausal, and cardiac conditions; also used to treat headache, neuralgia, constipation, Raynaud's disease, herpes zoster, and arthralgias

Current Use

- Useful female reproductive tonic; used in combination with herbs such as chaste tree or black cohosh for menstrual and menopausal symptoms
- Cardiovascular effects: increases number of red blood cells and platelets; stimulates hematopoiesis in the bone marrow; can prolong the refractory period and correct experimentally induced atrial fibrillation. In animal studies (rats and rabbits), dong quai prevented experimental coronary arteriosclerosis.
- Successfully used to treat Buerger's disease and constrictive aortitis. Often combined with dan shen (salvia) to treat angina, peripheral vascular disorders, and stroke.
- Used in traditional Chinese medicine, often with astragalus, to treat hematologic immune disorders such as thrombocytopenic purpura and to reduce the immunosuppressive effects of cortisone
- Adjunctive therapy for liver disease: reduced thymol turbidity in 88 cases of chronic hepatitis or liver cirrhosis. Use with milk thistle, turmeric, or schisandra berry.

Available Forms, Dosage, and Administration Guidelines

Preparations: Dried root, whole, sliced, or powdered; capsules, tablets, tinctures, combination products

Typical Dosage
- *Root:* 2 to 6 g per day
- *Capsules:* Up to six 500- to 600-mg capsules a day
- *Tincture* (1:5, 70% alcohol): 40 to 80 gtt (2–4 mL) up to three times a day
- Or follow manufacturer's or practitioner's recommendations.
- *Tea:* 1 tsp dried root in 12 oz water, lightly decoct (covered) for 20 minutes, let steep 1 hour; take 8 oz two or three times per day.
- In Chinese and Japanese medicine, dong quai is always used in conjunction with other herbs.

Pharmacokinetics—If Available (form or route when known): None known

Toxicity: Handling the fresh plant may cause photodermatitis in sensitive people.

Contraindications: Do not use with heavy menses (may increase bleeding) or with bleeding, fibroids, or diarrhea. If breast tenderness or soreness occurs, discontinue use. Do not use in bleeding disorders.

Side Effects: Possible photosensitization, menorrhagia, diarrhea

Long-Term Safety: Long-term history of safe use; no safety issues expected

Use in Pregnancy/Lactation/Children: Not used in the first trimester; used cautiously in traditional Chinese medicine during the remainder of the pregnancy only by trained professionals

Drug/Herb Interactions and Rationale (if known): With warfarin and other anticoagulant drugs, dong quai may increase the bleeding time. If using concurrently, obtain prothrombin time and International Normalized Ratio (INR) to rule out interactions.

Special Notes
- When recently studied alone, dong quai had no effect on reducing menopausal symptoms (Bates, 1997). However,

dong quai is never prescribed alone in the Orient but always administered in combination with other herbs.

- Dong quai does *not* have estrogenic effects (Hirata et al., 1997).
- High-quality root heads have substantially greater concentrations of active constituents. Ligustilide in high-grade roots has been found to be 10 times the level found in normal commercial-grade root heads.

BIBLIOGRAPHY

Bates B. (Aug. 1, 1997). Dong quai shown not effective for menopause. *Internal Medicine News.*

Bone K. (1996). *Clinical Applications of Ayurvedic and Chinese Herbs.* Queensland: Phytotherapy Press.

Duke JA, Foster S. (1999). *Handbook of Medicinal Herbs.* Boca Raton, FL: CRC Press.

Hirata JD, et al. (1997). Does dong quai have estrogenic effects in postmenopausal women? A double-blind, placebo-controlled trial. *Fertility & Sterility.* 68(6):981–986.

Mills S, Bone K. (1999). *Principles and Practice of Phytotherapy.* Edinburgh: Churchill Livingstone.

Tang W, Eisenbrand G. (1992). *Chinese Drugs of Plant Origin.* Berlin: Springer-Verlag.

You-Ping Z. (1998). *Chinese Materia Medica: Chemistry, Pharmacology and Applications.* Amsterdam: Harwood.

E

NAME: Echinacea (*Echinacea angustifolia, Echinacea purpurea, Echinacea pallida*)

Common Names: American coneflower, Kansas snake root, purple coneflower, Missouri snake root

Family: *Asteraceae*

Description of Plant

- The Echinacea genus contains nine species and two varieties.
- Perennial herb, part of the daisy family, native to Midwest North America, from Saskatchewan to Texas
- Height, 1.5 to 3 feet

- Most species have purple flowers.
- Chewing the cone of *E. purpurea* or the root of *E. angustifolia* causes tingling and numbing of the lips and tongue.

Medicinal Part: The aerial portion (*E. purpurea*) and the root (*E. pallida, E. augustifolia, E. purpurea*)

Constituents and Action (if known)

- As with many medicinal plants, no active single ingredient has been identified as being responsible for the medicinal value. Echinacea's numerous constituents all contribute to its activity.
- Caffeic acid derivatives: increase phagocytosis (most active in flowering heads)
  ○ Echinacosides (*E. pallida, E. angustifolia*), chlorogenic acid (*E. purpurea, E. angustifolia*), chicoric acid (*E. purpurea*)
  ○ Stimulate phagocytosis, increase leukocyte activity (Melchart et al., 1994, 1998; Schoneberger, 1992)
  ○ May offer photoprotection from sun damage when applied topically (Facino et al., 1995)
  ○ Has weak activity against *Escherichia coli, Pseudomonas aeruginosa, Staphylococcus aureus*, and *Streptococci* spp.
  ○ Increase macrophage activity, increase T-cell activity and interferon
  ○ Inhibit hyaluronidase activity, thus limiting degenerative inflammatory disease and the spread of viruses (Mills & Bone, 1999)
- Lipophilic components
  ○ Alkylamides: enhance phagocytosis, inhibit edema, and enhance wound healing (Mills & Bone, 1999)
  ○ Echinacein (pungent component): a complex isobutylamide
  ○ *E. angustifolia* roots or *E. purpurea* flower heads contain unsaturated alkyl ketones or isobutylamides: inhibit leukemic cells.
- Polyacetylenes (polyynes) found in *E. pallida* roots: ketoalkynes and ketoalkenes
- *D*-acidic arabinogalactan polysaccharide
  ○ As an injectable, stimulates B-lymphocyte proliferation, T lymphocytes, beta-interferon, and tumor necrosis factor;

particularly high in roots of *E. purpurea*; is not active
orally (Parnham, 1996)

○ Decreases activity of herpes simplex virus-1 and influenza
virus A

Nutritional Ingredients: None known

Traditional Use

- Native Americans used echinacea to treat wounds, burns,
abscesses, insect bites, sore throats, toothaches, and joint
pains, and as an antidote for poisonous snake bites.
- In 1870 it was introduced as "Meyer's Blood Purifier" for all
matter of ailments. Eclectic physician John King and
pharmacist John Uri Lloyd reluctantly tested this patent
medicine and were surprised to discover a valuable and
active medicine.
- Eclectic physicians used echinacea for patients with blood
dyscrasias, a tendency toward infections, sepsis, boils,
staphylococcal infections, and putrid sore throat.

Current Use

- To prevent and treat the common cold (may decrease the
chances of getting a cold and decrease its severity). Echinacea
has been officially approved in Germany for treating colds,
influenza, and upper respiratory infections.
- To serve as supportive treatment for otitis media, sinusitis,
bronchitis, cystitis, prostatitis, tonsillitis, and laryngitis
- To treat infections, particularly candida (does not treat source
of infection)
- To enhance wound healing (topically)
- To help prevent skin photodamage from ultraviolet sunlight
(topically)
- Used in Germany along with chemotherapy in the treatment
of cancer
- May enhance white blood cell count in persons undergoing
chemotherapy

**Available Forms, Dosage, and Administration
Guidelines**

- Research needs to be done to determine the most effective
preparations, differences between the species, and the parts
of the plant to use.

- Take at first sign of infection (may need to take 1 g three times a day).

Preparations

- Dried whole herb or root; capsules, expressed juice of fresh flowering plant, flex-tabs, tablets, tinctures
- Some products are standardized to echinacoside, although the compound has not been found to stimulate the immune system, nor does it represent therapeutic activity.
- The most research has been done in Germany with a product now produced in the United States under the brand name Echinaguard (Nature's Way).
- Look for tinctures made with a 50% alcohol content, because active constituents are better extracted in this menstruum.

Typical Dosage

- *Capsules:* Up to nine 300- to 400-mg capsules a day
- *Tincture:* (1:2, 50% alcohol) 60 to 90 gtt (3–5 mL) four to six times a day. This is equivalent to 1 to 2 g of dried root a day. Use as needed at the onset of symptoms of cold or flu.
- *Freeze-dried plant:* 325 to 650 mg three times a day
- *Juice* (of aerial portion of *E. purpurea* stabilized in 22% ethanol): 2 to 3 mL (0.5–0.75 tsp) three times a day
- *Fluid extract* (1:1): 1 to 2 mL (0.25–0.5 tsp) three times a day
- *Solid (dry powdered) extract* (6.5:1): 300 mg three times a day

Pharmacokinetics—If Available (form or route when known): None known

Toxicity: None known

Contraindications

- Autoimmune diseases such as multiple sclerosis and rheumatoid arthritis. This is based on the speculation that stimulating an overactive immune system will worsen symptoms, but there is no research evidence to confirm this. In fact, the herb is commonly used by British and Australian herbalists to treat autoimmune diseases as an immune amphoteric.
- If patients have allergies to *Asteraceae* family pollen (chrysanthemum, chamomile, ragweed, daisy), avoid

products made from echinacea flowers. The leaf juice or root products should not provoke an allergic response.

Side Effects: Transitory tingling or numbing of the mouth, throat, and lips

Long-Term Safety: Safe

Use in Pregnancy/Lactation/Children: No data available. Regular use in Germany by millions of people, including pregnant and breast-feeding women and children, has not produced any known side effects or toxicity.

Drug/Herb Interactions and Rationale (if known): None

Special Notes
- In North America, *E. angustifolia* is the most popular species of echinacea, even though there is much more research showing effectiveness for *E. purpurea* and *E. pallida.*
- Echinacea species are being overharvested in the wild. Use products made from the cultivated herb.
- Most effective when started at first sign of infection. Take in sufficient amounts; split total daily dosage into four to six doses per day.
- Recent research showed no benefit when taken for a 3-month period to prevent colds, but cold symptoms and duration were reduced when taken at the start of a cold (Melchart et al., 1995).
- Some authors have stated that hepatotoxicity may be caused by long-term use of echinacea. Echinacea does contain minute amounts of pyrrolizidine alkaloids, but they are the nontoxic saturated variety. There is no evidence or known possibility of hepatic damage resulting from the use of this herb.
- Another echinacea myth is that it is best or works only when taken short term (7–14 days). This is due to a mistranslated German study that showed that the effects gradually wear off if you stop taking echinacea. Unfortunately, the improper translation stated that the effects wear off if you continue to take echinacea. The eclectic physicians who introduced echinacea into Western clinical practice and used this medicine extensively for 50 years believed it was more effective the longer it was used (Bergner, 1994).

BIBLIOGRAPHY

Barnes J. (1998). Lack of evidence of efficacy of Echinacea in URTI. *Pharmacy Journal.* 260–267.

Bauer R, Wagner H. (1991). *Echinacea* species as potential immunostimulatory drugs. *Econ Med Plant Res.* 5:253–321.

Bauer R, et al. (1988). TLC and HPLC Analysis of Echinacea pallida and E angustifolia Roots. *Planta Med;* 54:426.

Bergner, P. (1994). Echinacea myth: Phagocytosis is not diminished after ten days. *Medical Herbalism.* 6(1)1.

Bodinet C, et al. (1993). Host resistance-increasing activity of root extracts from Echinacea species. *Planta Medica.* 59:A672–A673.

Bone K. (1997). Echinacea: what makes it work? *Modern Phytotherapist.* 3(2):19–23.

Braunig B, et al. (1992). *Echinacea pupurea* radix for strengthening the immune response in flu-like infections. *Z Phytother* 13, 7-13, 1992.

Burger RA, et al. (1997). Echinacea-induced cytokine production by human macrophages. *International Journal of Immunopharmacology.* 19(7):371–379.

Dorn M, et al. (1997). Placebo-controlled, double-blind study of *Echinaceae pallidae* radix in upper respiratory tract infections. *Complementary Therapeutic Medicine.* 3:40–42.

Facino R. (1995). Echinacea in preventing skin damage. *Planta Medica.* 61:510–514.

Facino RM, et al. (1995). Echinacoside and caffeoyl conjugates protect collagen from free radical-induced degradation; a potential use of Echinacea extracts in the prevention of skin photodamage. *IL Farmaco.* 61(6):510–514.

Melchart D, et al. (1994). Immunomodulation with *Echinacea:* a systematic review of controlled clinical trials. *Phytomedicine.* 1:245–254.

Melchart D, et al. (1995). Results of five randomized studies on the immunomodulatory activity of preparations of Echinacea. *Journal of Alternative & Complementary Medicine.* 1:145–160.

Melchart D, et al. (1998). Echinacea root extracts for the prevention of upper respiratory tract infections: a double-blind, placebo-controlled randomized trial. *Archives of Family Medicine.* 6:541–545.

Mills S, Bone K. (1999). *Principles and Practice of Phytotherapy.* Edinburgh: Churchill Livingstone.

Mullins RJ. (1998). Echinacea-associated anaphylaxis. *Medical Journal of Aust.* 168(4):170–171.

Myers S, Wohlmuth H. (1998). Echinacea-associated anaphylaxis. *Medical Journal of Aust.* 168(11):583–584.

Parnham MJ. (1996). Benefit-risk assessment of the squeezed sap of the purple coneflower (*Echinacea purpurea*) for long-term oral immunostimulation. *Phytomedicine*. 3(1):95–102.

The Review of Natural Products. (1997–1998). Facts and Comparisons. Wolters-Kluwer Co., St. Louis, MO.

Schoneberger D. (1992). The influence of immune stimulating effects of pressed juice from *Echinacea purpurea* on the course and severity of colds. *Forum Immunologie*. 8:2–12.

Wagner H & Proksch A. (1985). Immunostimulatory drugs of fungi and higher plants. In: *Economic and Medicinal Plant Research, vol. 1* (Farnsworth N, Hikino H. & Wagner H, eds.) Orlando, FL: Academic Press, pp 113–155.

 NAME: Evening Primrose (*Oenothera biennis*)

Common Names: King's cure-all

Family: *Onagraceae*

Description of Plant: Native to North America and Europe; yellow-flowered biennial herb growing up to 4.5 feet tall

Medicinal Part: Oil from seeds

Constituents and Action (if known)

- Essential fatty acids
  - Gamma-linolenic acid (GLA): reduces inflammation by reducing prostaglandin E_1 (Fan & Chapkin, 1998), reduces hypertension and platelet activity
  - May enhance oxygen free radical production and lipid peroxidation in glioma tumor cells, thus slowing their growth (Das et al., 1995)
  - Linoleic acid (LA): cannot be produced by the human body; body must convert LA to GLA. Deficiencies of LA are associated with diabetes, cancer, viral infections, and hypercholesterolemia and affect prostaglandin E_1 and E_2 synthesis.
  - Oleic acid
  - Palmitic acid
  - Stearic acid

Nutritional Ingredients: Seeds were used for food by native Americans and are high in omega-6 oils. Root and young leaves may be used as a vegetable but they have a peculiar, bitter flavor.

Traditional Use

- Whole plant used as poultice for bruises
- Leaf and root bark used for spastic coughs, irritable bowel syndrome; antispasmodic
- Tea made from seed for sore throats and gastrointestinal irritation
- Decoction of root used to treat hemorrhoids

Current Use

- Reduces symptoms of asthma
- Reduces symptoms of migraines
- Reduces inflammation in arthritis, but no evidence that it can modify disease
- Decreases premenstrual symptoms (O'Brien & Massil, 1990)
- The oil, applied topically, softens the cervix; start using in the last 3 weeks of pregnancy.
- Reduces symptoms of allergic-induced eczema
- Reduces symptoms of uremic pruritus (Yoshimoto-Furuie et al., 1999)
- Increases fat content of breast milk when taken during lactation
- Reduces symptoms of atopic dermatitis and eczema (McCaleb et al., 2000)
- Preliminary research shows a reduction of symptoms in diabetic neuropathy (Keen et al., 1993)
- May reduce hyperactivity in children with ADHD, but large doses are necessary
- May be lethal to cancer cells (high levels of fatty acids) but not normal cells. More research needed.

Available Forms, Dosage, and Administration Guidelines

Preparations: Expressed oil from seeds; capsules

Typical Dosage

- Dosage is based on a GLA content of 8%.
- *Capsules:* Up to 12 gel-caps of the oil a day (3–6 g/day)

- *Oil:* 0.5 tsp a day
- Or follow manufacturer's or practitioner's recommendations
- For ADHD, 5 to 8 g/day in divided doses

Pharmacokinetics—If Available (form or route when known): None known

Toxicity: None known

Contraindications: Seizure disorder; may exacerbate seizures

Side Effects: A few patients taking large doses experienced abdominal discomfort, nausea, or headache.

Long-Term Safety: Safe for long-term use when used appropriately

Use in Pregnancy/Lactation/Children
- Safe oral doses do not start or affect labor.
- Children: use only under supervision of a qualified practitioner

Drug/Herb Interactions and Rationale (if known): Do not use concurrently with phenothiazines: may increase risk of seizures.

Special Notes
- Research on six healthy volunteers could not determine any change in prostaglandin level (Martens-Lobenhoffer & Meyer, 1998).
- Black currant seed oil and borage seed oil contain greater quantities of GLA at a lower cost, but research on the usefulness of these oils is lacking.
- Patients taking omega-6 supplements should also supplement their intake of omega-3 fatty acids (fish or flaxseed oil). Omega-6 fatty acids in excess can contribute to inflammatory processes and impede absorption of omega-3 fatty acids. A good ratio is 4:1 (omega-6 fatty acids to omega-3 fatty acids).

BIBLIOGRAPHY

Das UN, et al. (1995). Local application of gamma-linolenic acid in the treatment of human gliomas. *Cancer Letters*. 94:147–155.

Fan YY, Chapkin RS. (1998). Importance of dietary gamma-linolenic acid in human health and nutrition. *Journal of Nutrition.* 128(9):1411–1414.

Keen H, et al. (1993). Treatment of diabetic neuropathy with gamma-linolenic acid. *Diabetes Care.* 16(1):8–15.

Martens-Lobenhoffer J, Meyer FP. (1998). Pharmacokinetic data of gamma-linolenic acid in healthy volunteers after the administration of evening primrose oil (Epogam). *International Journal of Clinical Pharmacology Therapeutics.* 36(7):363–366.

McCaleb R, et al. (2000). *Encyclopedia of Popular Herbs.* Roseville, CA: Prima Publishers.

O'Brien PM, Massil H. (1990). Premenstrual syndrome: clinical studies on essential fatty acids. In: Horrobin DF. (ed.). *Omega 6 Essential Fatty Acids: Pathophysiology and Role in Clinical Medicine.* New York: Wiley-Liss.

Yoshimoto-Furuie K, et al. (1999). Effects of oral supplementation with evening primrose oil for six weeks on plasma essential fatty acids and uremic skin symptoms in hemodialysis patients. *Nephron.* 81(2):151–159.

NAME: Eyebright (*Euphrasia officinale*)

Common Names: Meadow eyebright, red eyebright

Family: *Scrophulariaceae*

Description of Plant: Annual; grows about 4 inches to 1 foot high, blooms from July to September; partially parasitic on grasses, grows in Northern regions (Canada, northern Europe, Maine)

Medicinal Part: Fresh or dried herb (preparations made from the fresh herb are vastly superior)

Constituents and Action (if known)

- Iridoid glycosides: aucubin (anti-inflammatory [Recio et al., 1994]), catalpol, euphroside, ixoroside, aucubigenin (aglycone of aucubin): antibacterial activity against *Micrococcus aureus, Escherichia coli, Bacillis subtilis, Mycobacterium phlei*, and to a lesser degree antifungal, with the greatest activity against *Penicillium italicum* (Mills & Bone, 1999). Antiviral activity: hepatitis B and hepatoprotective activity (Chang & Yamaura, 1993; Mills & Bone, 1999).

- Tannins: astringent, anti-inflammatory (Mills & Bone, 1999)
- Flavonoids (quercetin, apigenin): anti-inflammatory (Mills & Bone, 1999)
- Volatile oils

Nutritional Ingredients: None known

Traditional Use
- Topically for eye infections and irritation (especially conjunctivitis and blepharitis)
- To treat coughs and sore throats
- As a homeopathic remedy to treat conjunctivitis
- To treat allergies, postnasal drip, sinus headaches, and sinus infections
- Part of British herbal tobacco smoked for chronic bronchial infections and colds
- Topical: eye fatigue, conjunctivitis (homeopathic remedy) (Bisset, 1994)
- Internal: allergic rhinitis, sinusitis, otitis media, postnasal drip, red, itchy eyes associated with hay fever

Available Forms, Dosage, and Administration Guidelines
Preparations: Dried herb, whole, cut and sifted, or powdered; capsules, tablets, fresh plant tinctures, eye wash, other preparations
Typical Dosage
- *Capsules:* Up to five 400- to 500-mg capsules a day
- *Tea:* Steep 1 to 2 tsp in a cup of hot water for 10 to 15 minutes; take three times a day.
- May be used externally as an eye wash or compress
- *Fresh plant tincture* (1:2, 35% alcohol): 30 to 40 gtt (1.5–2 mL) up to four times a day
- Or follow manufacturer's or practitioner's recommendations

Pharmacokinetics—If Available (form or route when known): None known

Toxicity: None known

Contraindications: None known

Side Effects: None

Long-Term Safety: Unknown; no adverse effects expected

Use in Pregnancy/Lactation/Children: No research available; no adverse effects expected

Drug/Herb Interactions and Rationale (if known): Unknown

Special Notes
- Topical ophthalmic preparations should be made into sterile saline solutions.
- No controlled studies are available to determine efficacy for its various uses. Long-term clinical use by eclectic and naturopathic physicians and herbalists and the astringent, anti-inflammatory, antiviral, and antibacterial activity of its constituents suggest efficacy.

BIBLIOGRAPHY

Bisset NG (ed). (1994). *Herbal Drugs and Phytopharmaceuticals.* Stuttgart: Medpharm Scientific Publishers.

Chang IM, Yamaura Y. (1993). Aucubin: a new antidote for poisonous Amanita mushrooms. *Phytotherapy Research.* 7:53–56.

Lawrence Review of Natural Products. (1996). St. Louis: Facts and Comparisons.

Mills S, Bone K. (1999). *Principles and Practice of Phytotherapy.* Edinburgh: Churchill Livingstone.

Recio M, et al. (1994). Structural considerations on the iridoids as antiinflammatory agents. *Planta Medica.* 60:232–234.

F

 NAME: False Unicorn (*Chamaelirium luteum*)

Common Names: Helonias root, devil's bit, rattlesnake, blazing star, fairy-wand

Family: *Liliaceae*

Description of Plant: Lily native to the United States. A threatened species because of overharvesting and loss of habitat. Male and female flowers bloom on separate plants.

Medicinal Part: Root, collected in autumn

Constituents and Action (if known)
- Steroidal saponins, 10% from root: chamaelirin
- Diosgenin
- Fatty acids: oleic, linoleic, stearic acid (Cataline et al., 1942)
- Other actions: may act by increasing human chorionic gonadotropin (Brandt, 1996)

Nutritional Ingredients: None known

Traditional Use
- Used as a uterine and female reproductive tonic: amenorrhea, dysmenorrhea (with pelvic congestion and a feeling of fullness), infertility, morning sickness; was an ingredient in a well-known eclectic formula called "mother's cordial." This formula was given in the last 2 to 3 weeks of pregnancy to promote a healthy delivery.
- Appetite stimulant
- Diuretic

Current Use
- Female reproductive amphoteric
- Menstrual and uterine problems, such as premenstrual symptoms, amenorrhea, dysmenorrhea, menorrhagia
- Infertility, with anovulatory cycles

Available Forms, Dosage, and Administration Guidelines
Preparations: Dried root, chopped for decoction, tincture
Typical Dosage
- *Tincture* (1:5, 60% alcohol): 20 to 30 gtt (1–1.5 mL) three or four times a day
- *Decoction:* 0.5 tsp dried root to 8 oz boiling water, gently decoct 15 minutes, steep 45 minutes; take 4 oz (half-cup) twice a day

Pharmacokinetics—If Available (form or route when known): None known

Toxicity: None reported

Contraindications: None known

Side Effects: Large doses may cause nausea and vomiting.

Long-Term Safety: No adverse effects expected

Use in Pregnancy/Lactation/Children: Traditionally used during pregnancy, but safety cannot be confirmed. No research on use during breast-feeding, so avoid.

Drug/Herb Interactions and Rationale (if known): None known

Special Notes
- Because of its threatened status, this plant should be used only when absolutely indicated. Other herbs such as chaste tree, black cohosh, or dong quai can be used for many of the same complaints.
- Often adulterated in commerce with true unicorn root (*Aletris farinosa*), which has a decidedly different activity.

BIBLIOGRAPHY

Brandt D. (1996). A clinician's view. *HerbalGram.* 36:75.

Cataline EL, et al. (1942). The phytochemistry of Helonias I. Preliminary examination of the drug. *Journal of the American Pharmaceutical Association.* 31:519.

Grieve M. (1996). *A Modern Herbal.* New York: Barnes & Noble, Inc.

Mills S, Bone K. (1999). *Principles and Practice of Phytotherapy.* Edinburgh: Churchill Livingstone.

Review of Natural Products. (1999). St. Louis: Facts and Comparisons.

 NAME: Fenugreek (*Trigonella foenum-graecum*)

Common Names: Bird's foot, Greek hayseed, trigonella

Family: *Fabeaceae*

Description of Plant: Member of the pea family. Annual native to the Mediterranean region, the Ukraine, and India; now commonly cultivated in India, Morocco, Turkey, and China.

Medicinal Part: Dried ripe seeds

Constituents and Action (if known)

- Galactomannans: mucilagin coats stomach and can relieve constipation because it adds fiber; may also be responsible for lowering cholesterol
- Pyridine alkaloids: trigonelline, gentianine, and carpaine can be degraded to nicotinic acid during roasting. This change is associated with the flavor of the seed and may also lower cholesterol (Bordia et al., 1997).
- Steroidal sapogenins
  - Diosgenin, yamogenin, tigogenin, neotigogenin, sarsasapogenin, and yuccagen can lower plasma cholesterol, glucose, and glucagon levels; may increase food consumption (Khosla et al., 1995)
  - Graecunins—saponins (actual glycosides of diosgenin, gitogenin, and trigogenin, fenugrin B, and coumarin compounds): may cause side effect of bleeding (Petit et al., 1995; Sauvaire et al., 1991)
  - Fenugreekine, a saponin, may possess cardiotonic, diuretic, antiviral, and antihypertensive properties (Dinesh et al., 1994a).
- Flavonoids
  - Vitexin, isovitexin, apigenin, luteolin, orientin, quercetin
  - Protein (20%–30%) and free amino acids (lysine, tryptophan, histidine, arginine)
  - Minerals and lipids

Nutritional Ingredients: Vitamins A, B_1, C; minerals (calcium, iron). Seeds are rich in protein and have been used as animal forage. Used as a flavoring for maple syrup substitutes. Used for centuries as a cooking spice (curries in India, bread in Egypt, coffee substitute in Africa).

Traditional Use

- Demulcent, emollient, nutritive, hypoglycemic agent
- Used topically to treat boils, cellulitis, leg ulcers, eczema
- For chronic coughs, bronchitis
- To stimulate milk flow in nursing mothers
- As a tea for gastric irritation (gastritis, dyspepsia, anorexia, ulcers, mouth sores)

Current Use

- Lowers glucose levels in insulin-dependent diabetes (Sharma et al., 1996)
- Lowers cholesterol levels, triglycerides, low-density lipids, high-density lipoproteins (Bordia et al., 1997)
- Decreases symptoms of gastritis (tea is particularly soothing) and lack of appetite (Blumenthal et al., 2000)

Available Forms, Dosage, and Administration Guidelines

Preparations: Seed, whole or powdered; capsules, tablets, tinctures, tea

Typical Dosage
- *Seed:* 1.5 tsp a day.
- *Capsules:* Up to six 600- to 700-mg capsules a day
- *Tea:* 1 to 2 tsp freshly powdered seed to 8 oz room-temperature water, steep 1 hour; take two or three cups per day
- *Tincture* (1:5, 25% alcohol): 60 to 120 gtt (3–6 mL) three times a day
- *Powdered drug:* 50 g to 0.25 L water, and apply topically
- *External use:* Soak 10 tsp powdered seed in hot water to make a poultice.
- Or follow manufacturer's or practitioner's recommendations.

Pharmacokinetics—If Available (form or route when known): None known

Toxicity: None

Contraindications: None known

Side Effects: Intestinal gas and diarrhea; possible hypoglycemia; repeated topical applications may cause rashes

Long-Term Safety: Used as a spice in the Middle East; no adverse effects expected

Use in Pregnancy/Lactation/Children: Do not use in pregnancy; may stimulate uterus. Traditionally used to promote milk flow in nursing mothers. Safety data unavailable.

Drug/Herb Interactions and Rationale (if known): May interfere with antidiabetic medications. If given concurrently, monitor blood sugar levels. Separate all drugs by 2 hours to prevent binding. May enhance anticoagulant effect of anticoagulants; monitor International Normalized Ratio (INR) if given concurrently.

Special Notes: In persons with diabetes, fenugreek seems to lower cholesterol and blood glucose levels. This effect is not noted in persons without diabetes. More research must be done to establish efficacy.

BIBLIOGRAPHY

Blumenthal M, et al. (2000). *Herbal Medicine: Expanded Commission E Monographs.* Austin, TX: American Botanical Council.

Bordia A, et al. (1997). Effect of ginger (*Zingiber officinale* Rosc.) and fenugreek (*Trigonella foenum graecum* L.) on blood lipids, blood sugar and platelet aggregation in patients with coronary artery disease. *Prostaglandins, Leukotrienes and Essential Fatty Acids.* 58(5):379–384.

Dinesh P, et al. (1994a). Hypocholesterolemic effect of hypoglycaemic principle of fenugreek (*Trigonella foenum graecum*) seeds. *Indian Journal of Clinical Biochemistry.* 9:13–16.

Dinesh P, et al. (1994b). Effects of the hypoglycemic principle from *Trigonella foenum graecum.* Proceedings of the XVIth International Congress of Biochemistry and Molecular Biology, New Delhi, 1994.

Khosla P, et al. (1995). Effect of *Trigonella foenum graecum* (fenugreek) on blood glucose in normal and diabetic rats. *Indian Journal of Physiology & Pharmacology.* 39(2):173.

Petit PR, et al. (1995). Steroid saponins from fenugreek seeds: extraction, purification, and pharmacological investigation on feeding behavior and plasma cholesterol. *Steroids.* 60(10):674.

Sauvaire Y, et al. (1991). Implication of steroid saponins and sapogenins in the hypocholesterolemic effect of fenugreek. *Lipids.* 26(3):191.

Sharma RD, et al. (1996). Hypolipidaemic effect of fenugreek seeds: a chronic study in non-insulin dependent diabetic patients. *Physiotherapy Research.* 10:332–334.

 NAME: Feverfew (*Tanacetum parthenium*)

Common Names: Featherfew, bachelor's button, midsummer daisy, nosebleed

Family: *Asteraceae*

Description of Plant: A member of the daisy family native to central and southern Europe. Short bushy perennial that grows 1 to 3 feet tall. Commonly cultivated in England, North America, and Latin America. Flowers are daisy-like, with a yellow center and 10 to 20 white rays; blooms July to October.

Medicinal Part: Leaves and flowers (fresh or dried)

Constituents and Action (if known)

- Sesquiterpene lactones
  - Parthenolides lower serotonin levels (very unstable in feverfew) (Heptinstall et al., 1992; Johnson et al., 1985; Murphy et al., 1988; Vickers, 1985).
  - Parthenolides were believed to be the active constituents, but recent research has shown this to be untrue (Awang, 1998a).
  - Interact with protein kinase C pathway, inhibiting granule secretion from platelets, which causes an antimigraine effect, and from polymorphs, which has an antiarthritic activity (Mills & Bone, 1999)
  - Secotana partholides A
  - Artecatin
  - 3 beta-hydroxyparthenolide
- Flavonoids (Knight, 1995): luteolin, apigenin
- Eudesmanolides: antibacterial activity; inhibited *Staphylococcus aureus, Escherichia coli, Salmonella* spp.
- Monoterpenes (trans chrysanthenyl): possible anti-inflammatory activity (Awang, 1998b), insecticidal activity (Hobbs, 1990)
- Essential oils: bactericidal, fungicidal (Mills & Bone, 1999)
- Other actions: anti-inflammatory; inhibits platelet phospholipase A, which prevents the release of arachidonic acid activity (Groenewegen & Heptinstall, 1992; Mills & Bone, 1999); inhibits histamine release; inactivates polymorphonuclear leukocytes; inhibits leukotrienes and prostaglandins

Nutritional Ingredients: None known

Traditional Use

- Anthelmintic, antipyretic, anti-inflammatory, bitter tonic, emmenagogue (high doses)

- Use dates back thousands of years (Greeks and early Europeans) for the treatment of headaches (including migraines), arthritis, menstrual cramps, digestive upsets, and respiratory conditions such as asthma
- Antipyretic: hot tea used to break high fevers

Current Use
- Beneficial in migraine headaches (reduces severity and frequency)
- Is approved in Canada for migraine prevention as long as it contains 0.2% parthenolide (this is not a guarantee of therapeutic activity)
- Reduces inflammation in arthritis if taken regularly (Pattrick et al., 1989)
- Relieves menstrual pain
- Possible benefit for psoriasis and arthritis (Mills & Bone, 1999)
- Insect repellent
- Balm for insect bites

Available Forms, Dosage, and Administration Guidelines
Preparations: Fresh or dried leaves; capsules, tablets, tinctures. Some products are standardized to 0.2% parthenolide, even though other constituents may be responsible for the herb's action.

Typical Dosage
- *Capsules:* Capsules with 25 mg of freeze-dried leaves
- *Fresh herb:* Eat two average-sized leaves a day
- *Tincture* (1:2 or 1:5, 30% alcohol): 20 to 40 gtt (1–2 mL) three times per day
- Or follow manufacturer's or practitioner's recommendations
- Need to take for 1 to 2 weeks before result is seen

Pharmacokinetics—If Available (form or route when known): None known

Toxicity: None known

Contraindications: Hypersensitivity to members of the *Asteraceae* family (ragweed, chamomile, chrysanthemums, and so forth)

Side Effects

- With regular use, rebound migraine headaches and joint stiffness may occur after stopping: "post-feverfew syndrome" (de Weerdt et al., 1996; Johnson et al., 1985)
- Mouth ulcerations, sore tongue, and lip swelling have occurred, especially when consuming the fresh leaves.
- Contact dermatitis associated with handling the plant
- Allergic reaction (allergy to *Asteraceae*)

Long-Term Safety: Safe, but when stopped, increased number of headaches may develop

Use in Pregnancy/Lactation/Children: Do not use in pregnancy (may cause uterine contractions), and in breast-feeding women or in children younger than 2

Drug/Herb Interactions and Rationale (if known): Use anticoagulants with caution; may increase bleeding. Monitor coagulation time.

Special Notes: Long-term use is more effective for reducing the severity and number of migraines. Slow withdrawal may reduce the likelihood and severity of post-feverfew syndrome. Herbalists believe that the plant is most effective when harvested when in flower.

BIBLIOGRAPHY

Awang D. (1998a). Parthenocide: the demise of a facile theory of feverfew activity. *Journal of Herbs, Spices and Medicinal Plants.* 5(4):95–98.

Awang D. (1998b). Prescribing therapeutic feverfew (*Tanacetum parthenium*). *Integrative Medicine.* 1(1):11–13.

Awang DVC. (1993). Feverfew fever. *HerbalGram.* 29:34.

Barsby RWJ, et al. (1993). Feverfew and vascular smooth muscle: extracts from fresh and dried plants show opposing pharmacological profiles, dependent upon sesquiterpene lactone content. *Planta Medica.* 59:20–25.

de Weerdt CJ, et al (1996). Randomized double-blind placebo controlled trial of a feverfew preparation. *Phytomedicine.* 3(3):225.

Groenewegen WA, Heptinstall S. (1992). A comparison of the effects of an extract of feverfew and parthenolide, a component of feverfew, on human platelet activity in vitro. *Journal of Pharmacy & Pharmacology.* 43:391–395.

Heptinstall S, et al. (1985). Extracts from feverfew inhibit granule secretion in blood platelets and polymorphonuclear leucocytes. *Lancet.* 8437:1071–1074.

Heptinstall S, et al. (1992). Parthenolide content and bioactivity of feverfew (*Tanacetum parthenium* [L] Schultz-Bip.). Estimation of commercial and authenticated feverfew products. *Journal of Pharmacy & Pharmacology.* 44:391–395.

Hobbs C. (Winter 1990). Feverfew. *National Headache Foundation Newsletter,* p. 10.

Johnson S. (1984). *Feverfew: A Traditional Herbal Remedy for Migraine and Arthritis* (p. 19). London: Sheldon Press.

Johnson ES, et al. (1985). Efficacy of feverfew as prophylactic treatment of migraine. *British Medical Journal.* 291:569.

Knight DW. (1995). Feverfew: chemistry and biological activity. *Natural Products Report.* 12(3):271–276.

Lawrence Review of Natural Products. (1994). St. Louis: Facts and Comparisons.

Mills S, Bone K. (1999). *Principles and Practice of Phytotherapy.* Edinburgh: Churchill Livingstone.

Murch S, et al. (1997). Melatonin in feverfew and other medicinal plants. *Lancet.* 350:1598–1599.

Murphy JJ, et al. (1988). Randomized double-blind placebo-controlled trial of feverfew in migraine prevention. *Lancet.* 8(601):189–192.

Palevitch D, et al. (1997). Feverfew (*Tanacetum parthenium*) as a prophylactic treatment for migraine: a double-blind placebo-controlled study. *Phytotherapy Research.* 11:508–511.

Pattrick M, et al. (1989). Feverfew in rheumatoid arthritis: a double-blind, placebo-controlled study. *Annals of Rheumatic Disease.* 48:547.

Vickers HR. (1985). Feverfew and migraine. *British Medical Journal.* 291:827.

Vogler BK, et al. (1998). Feverfew as a preventive treatment for migraine: a systematic review. *Cephalalgia.* 18(10):704–708.

Williams CA, et al. (1999). The flavonoids of *Tanacetum partheneum* and *T. vulgare* and their anti-inflammatory properties. *Phytochemistry.* 51(3):417–423.

 NAME: Flax (*Linum usitatissimum*)

Common Names: Flaxseed, linseed

Family: *Linaceae*

Description of Plant: One of the world's oldest cultivated (10,000 years) plants. Grown for its fiber (linen), seed oil (linseed oil), and seeds. Cultivated throughout the world (India, China, Turkey, Argentina, Morocco).

Medicinal Part: Seeds and oil

Constituents and Action (if known)

- Essential fatty acids
  - Omega-3, essential fatty acids (linolenic, lenoleic, oleic acids): responsible for anti-inflammatory properties and cholesterol-lowering properties (Bierenbaum et al., 1993; Caughey et al., 1996; Cunnane et al., 1993; Gerster, 1998; Prasad, 1997; Prasad et al., 1998); lower thrombin-stimulated platelet aggregation (Bierenbaum et al., 1993; Ferretti & Flanagan, 1996; Tetta et al., 1990); may slow renal failure and decrease renal transplant rejection (Clark, 1994; Parbtani & Clark, 1996)
- Lignans, including secoisolariciresinol diglucoside, are phytochemicals shown to have weak estrogenic and antiestrogen properties. They assist with control of menopausal signs and changes (Haggans et al., 1999; Thompson et al., 1996). Anticarcinogenic, possibly of benefit in treating SLE, hyperlipidemia, and rheumatoid arthritis. May have anticancer effects by lowering tumor necrosis factor (Caughey et al., 1996; Thompson et al., 1997).
- Mucilage (3%–10%)

Nutritional Ingredients: Flaxseed is a source of both dietary lignans (phytochemicals) and omega-3 fatty acids. Seed is 25% protein.

Traditional Use

- Emollient, demulcent, bulk laxative
- Seeds used by early Romans for colds, urinary tract inflammation, lung conditions, and as a laxative
- Poultice of the seeds, mixed with oil or water, applied to inflamed skin, boils, styes, and dry, itching skin
- Decoctions used for sore throats

- Seeds have been used to remove foreign objects from the eye. The seed is placed in the eye, the foreign object adheres to it, and then both are removed (Evans, 1989).

Current Use
- Fiber and stool softener
- Bulk laxative for chronic constipation. The moistened seeds decrease transit time, increase stool weight, stimulate peristalsis, and protect and soothe mucosa.
- Laxative-dependent constipation
- May assist in weight loss when taken before meals because it provides a feeling of fullness
- Lowers plasma lipids: cholesterol (9%), triglycerides, low-density lipoproteins (18%) (Cunnane et al., 1993)
- May reduce the need for anticholesterol drugs
- Decreases pain from inflammatory bowel disease
- Acts as a phytoestrogen to reduce premenstrual symptoms and signs and changes of menopause
- May reduce risk of breast, ovarian, and prostate cancer if used regularly (Thompson, 1998)
- Reduces pathogenesis of degenerative nephritis in autoimmune disease such as lupus (Clark, 1994)
- Provides insoluble fiber in diet, which can reduce blood cholesterol by binding to bile acids in the intestinal tract, and interferes with the reabsorption of soluble fiber
- Decreases platelet stickiness
- May reduce the incidence and progression of cancer by reducing tumor necrosis factor levels

Available Forms, Dosage, and Administration Guidelines
Preparation: Seed, whole or powdered; expressed oil of seed
Typical Dosage
- *Seed:* Soak 1–4 tbsp whole or cracked seed in 1 cup water for several hours and drink; take up to three times a day.
- *Ground:* Grind flaxseeds in coffee grinder and take 1 tsp twice a day, up to 4 tbsp twice daily. Flaxseeds begin to oxidize in 20 minutes, so use fresh ground. Sprinkle on food or mix in liquid.
- *Soft geltab:* 1,000 mg four times a day

- *Oil:* 1 to 4 tbsp a day. Very temperature-sensitive, so store in refrigerator, do not heat, and use in recipes that do not require cooking.
- Or follow manufacturer's or practitioner's recommendations.

Pharmacokinetics—If Available (form or route when known): None known

Toxicity: None known

Contraindications: Persons with diverticulosis should not ingest seeds because they can get trapped in the diverticula and cause inflammation. Also contraindicated in persons with small bowel disease and inflammation, colicky bowel conditions, and bowel obstruction.

Side Effects: Seed ingestion can produce diarrhea, flatulence, nausea; allergic reaction.

Long-Term Safety: Safe

Use in Pregnancy/Lactation/Children: In pregnancy, flaxseed is a common food; no adverse effects are expected. For breast-feeding women and children, use appears safe, and no adverse effects are expected.

Drug/Herb Interactions and Rationale (if known)
- Separate from all other drugs by at least 2 hours. Because of its mucilaginous properties, flaxseed can bind with drugs, rendering them unabsorbable (especially cardiac glycosides).
- Avoid concurrent use with laxatives and stool softeners because it may potentiate the laxative effect.

Special Notes: Differences in flaxseed are found in various growing locations, variety, and harvest year. Drink enough fluid to minimize flatulence and prevent constipation. Never ingest immature seeds, because they contain cyanogenic nitrates and glucosides, which may cause unsteady gait, tachycardia, weakness.

BIBLIOGRAPHY
Bierenbaum ML, et al. (1993). Reducing atherogenic risk in hyperlipemic humans with flax seed supplementation: a preliminary report. *Journal of the American College of Nutrition.* 12:501–504.

Blumenthal M, et al. (2000). *Herbal Medicine: Expanded Commission E Monographs.* Austin, TX: American Botanical Council.

Caughey GE, et al. (1996). The effect on human tumor necrosis factor alpha and interleukin 1 beta production on diets enriched in n-3 fatty acids from vegetable oil or fish oil. *American Journal of Clinical Nutrition.* 63(1):116–122.

Clark WF. (1994). Treatment of lupus nephritis; immunosuppression, general therapy, dialysis and transplantation. *Canadian Journal of Investigative Medicine.* 17:588.

Cunnane SC, et al. (1993). High alpha-linolenic acid flaxseed (*Linum usitatissimum*): some nutritional properties in humans. *British Journal of Nutrition.* 69:443.

ESCOP Monographs on the Medicinal Uses of Plant Drugs. (1997). Exeter: ESCOP.

Ferretti A, Flanagan VP. (1996). Antithromboxane activity of dietary alpha-linolenic acid: a pilot study. *Prostaglandins Leukotrienes & Essential Fatty Acids.* 54(6):451–455.

Gerster H. (1998). Can adults adequately convert alpha-linolenic acid (18:3n-3) to eicosapentaenoic acid (20:5n-3) and docosahexaenoic acid (22:6n-3)? *International Journal of Vitamin & Nutrition Research.* 68(3):159–173.

Haggans CJ, et al. (1999). Effect of flaxseed consumption on urinary estrogen metabolites in postmenopausal women. *Nutrition & Cancer.* 33(2):188–195.

Haggerty W. (1999). Flax, ancient herb and modern medicine. *HerbalGram.* 45:51–56.

Kurzer MS, Xu X. (1997). Dietary phytoestrogens. *Annual Review of Nutrition.* 17:353–381.

Lawrence Review of Natural Products. (1999). St. Louis: Facts and Comparisons.

Nesbitt PD, et al. (1999). Human metabolism of mammalian lignan precursors in raw and processed flaxseed. *American Journal of Clinical Nutrition.* 69(3):549–555.

Nesbitt PD, Thompson LU. (1997). Lignans in homemade and commercial products containing flaxseed. *Nutrition & Cancer.* 29(3):222–227.

Parbtani A, Clark WF. (1996). Flaxseed and its components in renal disease. *Flaxseed in Human Nutrition.* Champaign, IL: AOCS Press.

Prasad K. (1997). Dietary flaxseed in prevention of hypercholesterolemic atherosclerosis. *Atherosclerosis.* 32(1):69–76.

Prasad K, et al. (1998). Reduction of hypercholesterolemic atherosclerosis by CDC-flaxseed with very low alpha-linolenic acid. *Atherosclerosis.* 136(2):367–375.

Tetta C, et al. (1990). Release of platelet activating factor in systemic lupus erythematosus. *International Archives of Allergy & Applied Immunology.* 91:244.

Thompson LU. (1998). Experimental studies on lignans and cancer. *Bailliere's Clinical Endocrinology & Metabolism.* 12(4):691–705.

Thompson LU, et al. (1996). Flaxseed and its lignan and oil components reduce mammary tumor growth at a late stage of carcinogenesis. *Carcinogenesis.* 17(6):1373–1376.

Thompson LU, et al. (1997). Variability in anticancer lignan levels in flaxseed. *Nutrition & Cancer.* 27(1):26–30.

G

NAME: Garlic (*Allium sativum*)

Common Names: *Knoblaunch* (German), stinking rose, *da suan* (Chinese)

Family: *Lilliaceae*

Description of Plant

- A pungent member of the lily family that is cultivated worldwide. The largest commercial production of garlic is in central California.
- The odor of garlic is caused mainly by the enzymatic breakdown of alliin into allicin. Once cooked, there is less odor and less physiologic effect.

Medicinal Part: Bulb

Constituents and Action (if known)

- Garlic contains hundreds of constituents, with at least 23 sulphur compounds having been identified.
- Thiosulfanates (sulfur compounds; 1% dry weight)
  - Allicin is one of the most active ingredients, and its breakdown produces other sulphur compounds such as allyl sulphides, ajoenes, oligosulphides, and vinyldithiines. Allicin has extensive antimicrobial activity, inhibiting the growth of many bacteria (*Helicobacter pylori*) and fungus (*Candida albicans*) and localized yeast infections (Jonkers et al., 1999). It interferes with the hepatic metabolism of

cholesterol, thus reducing serum cholesterol levels (Berthold et al., 1998; Koscielny et al., 1999;). It tends to lower low-density lipoproteins and raise high-density lipoproteins, which transports cholesterol to the liver (Isaacsohn et al., 1998). It may protect endothelial tissue from oxidized low-density lipoprotein injury (Ide & Lau, 1999; Munday et al., 1999). It reduces serum triglycerides by as much as 13% (Silagy & Neil, 1994a). It reduces blood pressure (Silagy & Neil, 1994b). It improves peripheral arterial disease. It may modestly reduce blood glucose.

- Ajoene has weak antifungal activity and reduces platelet stickiness, but only for a few hours (Legnani et al., 1993). It interferes with the hepatic metabolism of cholesterol, thus reducing serum cholesterol. It has antiviral activity against HIV (Shoji et al., 1993).
- Diallyl sulfide and other sulfur components have antitumor activity and may raise levels of glutathione S-transferase, which contributes to detoxification of carcinogens. It has antiviral properties and inhibits herpes simplex, HIV, and cytomegalovirus (Hughes & Lawson, 1991).
- Y-glutamyl-s-trans-propenyl cysteine

Other actions
- Antioxidant activity
- May mediate nitric oxide synthase activation, which helps restore endothelial function, which in turn improves the elasticity of blood vessels and reduces atherosclerotic heart disease (ASHD) and blood pressure
- Inhibits inflammatory prostaglandins

Nutritional Ingredients: Garlic is a common food and spice used in Chinese, French, Thai, Cajun, Italian, and many other world cuisines. Garlic is a minor source of selenium, chromium, potassium, germanium, calcium, iron, and vitamins A, C, and B complex.

History: Sanskrit records document the use of garlic 5,000 years ago. The Chinese have used it for at least 3,000 years. Hippocrates and Aristotle wrote about garlic to treat many medical conditions.

Traditional Use

- Antibacterial and antiviral for the lungs: pneumonia, bronchitis, coughs
- Traditionally, garlic has been and is still used today in Chinese, Ayurvedic, and naturopathic medicine as an antibacterial and antiviral agent, an expectorant, and a wound dressing. It is used to reduce mildly elevated blood pressure and to treat colds, gastric ulcers, bacterial diarrhea, sinus infections, vaginal yeast infections, and otitis media.
- Louis Pasteur confirmed the antibacterial activity of garlic in 1858.
- Used topically, garlic relieves wasp and bee stings.

Current Use

- Antibacterial and viral properties: fresh garlic is an effective treatment for antibiotic-resistant pneumonia as well as viral lung and sinus infections and colds. It is also useful for treating *Helicobacter pylori* infections causing gastric or duodenal ulcers, and traveler's diarrhea (Ankri & Mirelman, 1999).
- Lowers high blood pressure; used in the treatment of mild Hypertension (Blumenthal et al., 2000)
- Reduces ASHD and peripheral arterial vascular disease
- May prevent blood clots because it inhibits platelet aggregation and thins the blood
- Reduces cholesterol and triglyceride levels (hypolipidemia). The majority of more than 100 studies show that garlic can reduce low-density lipoproteins (mean decrease 16%), lower total cholesterol (mean decrease serum cholesterol 10.6%), and reduce triglycerides (average decrease 13.4%) (Koch & Lawson, 1996).
- Cancer prevention: more than 220 studies have correlated ingestion of garlic (raw and cooked) with lower rates of stomach, intestinal, and other cancers. One study concluded that garlic and other alliums inhibited the formation of carcinogenic nitroso compounds (Lamm & Riggs, 2000).
- Decreases atherosclerosis: garlic is approved in Europe for its cardiovascular effect to lower blood lipids and decrease atherosclerotic heart disease changes in the blood vessels. In a 4-year randomized double-blind clinical trial, patients took either garlic tablets (900 mg/day) or placebo. After 4 years,

the garlic group had a 2.6% reduction in plaque volume and the placebo group had an increase of 15.6% (Blumenthal et al., 2000).

Available Forms, Dosage, and Administration Guidelines

Preparations: Fresh or dried cloves, capsules, "odorless" tablets, tinctures, aged garlic extracts

Typical Dosage

- *Capsules:* Up to three 500- to 600-mg capsules a day, or follow manufacturer's recommendations. Look for products that deliver at least 5,000 micrograms of allicin daily. Do not use the odorless variety; research on its effectiveness is contradictory.
- *Food:* One clove of fresh garlic per day. As for garlic constituents, the whole is greater than any of the parts. Whole fresh garlic is more active than any single constituent. Mince a clove of garlic, let it stand 10 to 15 minutes, and then mix with yogurt, applesauce, honey, or some other carrier agent. Do not chew. This method will help prevent respiratory and body odor. Consuming parsley after eating garlic also helps control "garlic breath." One to 1.5 fresh cloves (1.8–2.7 g) equals 10 g fresh garlic, 18 mg garlic oil, or 600 to 900 mg garlic powder. Drying alters the active ingredients of garlic, including allicin (Krest & Keusgen, 1999a).
- Lipid-lowering effect: 600 to 900 mg, 4 g fresh garlic, or 10 mg garlic oil gel caps, 2–3 per day

Pharmacokinetics—If Available (form or route when known): Unknown

Toxicity: In average doses, no toxicity. In humans, daily administration of high doses of garlic essential oil (120 mg), equal to 60 g fresh garlic per day, for a 3-month period, did not produce any abnormal findings.

Contraindications: Some concerns have been raised about the consumption of garlic before surgery. Studies have shown a very transient inhibition of platelet aggregation (only a few hours), so patients need not worry about reduced clotting. Persons with garlic or allium allergies should avoid using garlic.

Side Effects: Heartburn, nausea, flatulence, GI disturbances, allergic reactions, body and breath odor, headache (rare). Topically, may cause skin irritation. May increase bleeding tendencies.

Long-Term Safety: Very safe

Use in Pregnancy/Lactation/Children: Normal doses are fine. Use caution when consuming abnormally large amounts of fresh garlic or garlic preparations. Excessive garlic intake can cause colic in breast-feeding infants.

Drug/Herb Interactions and Rationale (if known)

- Use caution with anticoagulants: may increase risk of bleeding. Five to 20 cloves of garlic equal 1 aspirin (650 mg). Check prothrombin time and INR.
- May enhance activity of antiplatelet products; concurrent use not recommended.

Special Notes: Do not cook at high temperatures or for very long: garlic loses its medicinal value when it loses volatile compounds. When cooking with fresh garlic, cut, chop, or crush the clove 10 to 15 minutes before it is to be used. Alliin, inactive in the whole garlic clove, is activated by the enzyme allinase. Alliin in turn becomes the active ingredient allicin.

BIBLIOGRAPHY

Ankri S, Mirelman D. (1999). Antimicrobial properties of allicin from garlic. *Microbes & Infection.* 1(2):125–129.

Aydin A, et al. (2000). Garlic oil and *Helicobacter pylori* infection. *American Journal of Gastroenterology.* 95(2):563–564.

Berthold HK, et al. (1998). Effect of a garlic oil preparation on serum lipoproteins and cholesterol metabolism. A randomized controlled trial. *Journal of the American Medical Association.* 279:1900–1902.

Blumenthal M, et al. (2000). *Herbal Medicine: Expanded Commission E Monographs.* Austin, TX: American Botanical Council.

Breithaupt-Grogler K, et al. (1997). Protective effect of chronic garlic intake on elastic properties of aorta in the elderly. *Circulation.* 98(8):2649–2655.

Dirsch VM, et al. (1998). Effect of allicin and ajoene, two compounds of garlic, on inducible nitric oxide synthase. *Atherosclerosis.* 139(2):333–339.

Dorant E, et al. (1993). Garlic and its significance for the prevention of cancer in humans: a critical view. *British Journal of Cancer.* 67:424–429.

Dorant E, et al. (1996). Consumption of onions and a reduced risk of stomach carcinoma. *Gastroenterology.* 110(1):12–20.

Ernst E. (1997). Can allium vegetables prevent cancer? *Phytomedicine.* 4(1):79–83.

ESCOP Monographs on the Medicinal Uses of Plant Drugs: Allii sativi Bulbs. (1997). Exeter: ESCOP.

Ho C, Huang M. (eds.). (1995). Food phytochemicals for cancer prevention II: teas, spices, and herbs (ACS Symposium Series 547). *Trends in Food Science Technology.* 6:216–217.

Hughes BG, Lawson LD. (1991). Antimicrobial effects of *Allium sativum* L. (garlic), *Alium ampeloprasum* L. (elephant garlic), and *Allium cepa* L. (onion) garlic compounds and commercial garlic supplement products. *Phytotherapy Research.* 5:154–158.

Ide N, Lau BH. (1999). Aged garlic extract attenuates intracellular oxidative stress. *Phytomedicine.* 6(2):125–131.

Isaacsohn JL, et al. (1998). Garlic powder and plasma lipids and lipoproteins. A multicenter randomized, placebo-controlled trial. *Journal of the American Medical Association.* 158:1189–1194.

Jonkers D, et al. (1999). Antibacterial effect of garlic and omeprazole on *Helicobacter pylori. Journal of Antimicrobial Chemotherapy.* 43(6):837–839.

Koch HP. (1993). Garlic: fact or fiction? *Phytotherapy Research.* 7:278–280.

Koch HP, Lawson LD. (1996). *The Science and Therapeutic Application of Allium sativum L and Related Species.* Baltimore: Williams & Wilkins.

Koscielny J, et al. (1999). The antiatherosclerotic effect of Allium sativum. *Atherosclerosis.* 144(1):237–249.

Krest I, Keusgen M. (1999a). Quality of herbal remedies from *Allium sativum*: differences between alliinase from garlic powder and fresh garlic. *Planta Medica.* 65(2):139–143.

Krest I, Keusgen M. (1999b). Stabilization and pharmaceutical use of alliinase. *Pharmazie.* 54(4):289–293.

Lamm DL, Riggs DR. (2000). The potential application of *Allium sativum* (garlic) for the treatment of bladder cancer. *Urologic Clinics of North America.* 27(1):157–162.

Legnani C, et al. (1993). Effects of a dried garlic preparation on fibrinolysis and platelet aggregation in healthy subjects. *Arzneimittel-Forschung.* 43:119–122.

Munday JS, et al. (1999). Daily supplementation with aged garlic extract, but not raw garlic, protects low density lipoprotein against in vitro oxidation. *Atherosclerosis*. 143(2):399–404.

Nai-lan G, et al. (1993). Demonstrations of the anti-viral activity of garlic extract against human cytomegalovirus in vitro. *Chinese Medical Journal*. 106:93–96.

Sasaki J, et al. (1999). Antibacterial activity of garlic powder against *Escherichia coli* 0-157. *Journal of Nutrition Science & Vitaminology*. 45(6):785–790.

Shoji S, et al. (1993). Allyl compounds selectively killed human immunodeficiency virus (type 1), infected cells. *Biochemisty Biophysical Research Communications*. 194:610–621.

Silagy C, Neil A. (1994a). Garlic as a lipid lowering agent: a meta-analysis. *Journal of the Royal College of Physicians of London*. 28:39–45.

Silagy C, Neil AW. (1994b). A meta-analysis of the effect of garlic on blood pressure. *Journal of Hypertension*. 12:463–468.

Simons LA, et al. (1995). On the effects of garlic on plasma lipids and lipoproteins in mild hypercholesterolemia. *Atherosclerosis*. 113:219–225.

✿ NAME: Ginger (*Zingiber officinale*)

Common Names: Jamaica ginger, ginger root

Family: *Zingiberaceae*

Description of Plant

- An erect perennial herb with thick tuberous rhizomes underground and stems that grow to 2 to 4 feet. Linear-lanceolate leaves are 6 to 12 inches long.
- Grows in the tropics; major producers are Jamaica, India, China, Thailand, Mexico, and Australia

Medicinal Part: Rhizome

Constituents and Action (if known)

- Essential oils (1%–3%): give ginger its characteristic aroma; may inhibit bacteria (Inouye et al., 1984)
  - Monoterpenes (geranial, neral)
  - Sesquiterpenes (zingiberene, sesquiphellandrene, beta-bisabolene)

- Antiemetic activity (Bone & Wilkinson, 1990; Fischer-Rasmussen et al., 1991; Grontved et al., 1988; Mowrey & Clayson, 1982; Phillips et al., 1993; Stewart et al., 1991; Suekawa et al., 1984)
- Pungent principals (1%–2.5%)
  - Gingerols (gradually decompose into shogaols during storage) inhibit prostaglandins and leukotrienes; may reduce inflammation and pain of arthritis (Srivastava & Mustafa, 1992); account for pungent effects and flavor; cardiotonic effects and inotropic effect (Shoji et al., 1982); decrease thromboxanes and platelet activity (Srivastava, 1989); inhibits nonsteroidal anti-inflammatory agent injury to stomach (Yoshikawa et al., 1992)
  - Shogaols: cardiotonic, antipyretic, antitussive activity; enhances gastrointestinal motility (Suekawa et al., 1984; Yamahura et al., 1990)
- Diaryheptanoids: may reduce inflammation and pain of arthritis, inhibit inflammatory prostaglandins
- Zerumbome and epoxide: antineoplastic activity (used for cancer treatment in China) (Babbar, 1982)
- Methanolic extracts: inotropic effects
- Other actions: improves production and secretion of bile from liver (Yamahura et al., 1985)

Nutritional Ingredients: As a spice, used to flavor food and drinks. Frequently used in Chinese, Thai, and Indian cuisine. Roots can also be candied.

Traditional Use
- Antiemetic, carminative, expectorant, emmenagogue, anti-inflammatory, diaphoretic, circulatory stimulant
- Commonly used in traditional Chinese medicine for thousands of years. Fresh ginger (shen jiang) and dry ginger (gan jiang) are used slightly differently. The fresh rhizome is used for damp coughs, colds, influenza, diarrhea, and nausea. The dry root is used for deficient (cold) bleeding, arthralgias, and cold hands and feet and is considered more effective for digestive upsets, such as nausea, gas, and vomiting.

- In China, ginger root and stem are used as pesticides against aphids and fungal spores.

Current Use

- Anti-inflammatory for arthralgias: studies have shown that patients with osteoarthritis and rheumatoid arthritis and chronic muscular pain experienced relief from pain and swelling with no adverse effects.
- Lowers fevers and decreases the severity of colds: diaphoretic, antipyretic (lowered fevers 38% in rats), antirhinoviral activity (in vitro)
- Decreases motion sickness, vomiting, and morning sickness: numerous studies have confirmed ginger's ability to reduce seasickness, motion sickness, postsurgical nausea, vomiting, and hyperemesis gravidarum. The herb compared very favorably with conventional medications without the side effects associated with metoclopramide.
- May protect against ulcers from stress, alcohol, aspirin
- Relieves dizziness and vestibular disorders

Available Forms, Dosage, and Administration Guidelines

Preparations: Fresh or dried root; capsules, tablets, tinctures

Typical Dosage

- *Capsules:* Up to eight 500- to 600-mg capsules a day
- *Fresh root:* 500 to 1,000 mg three times a day
- *Dried ground root:* 0.5 to 1 tsp a day
- *Fresh tincture* (1:2, 60% alcohol): 20 to 40 gtt (1–2 mL) in water three times a day
- *Dry tincture* (1:5, 60% alcohol): 15 to 30 gtt (0.8–1.5 mL) in water three times a day
- Or follow manufacturer's or practitioner's recommendations.
- For migraine headache: Two capsules at beginning of migraine to decrease nausea
- Motion sickness: Take 0.5 g powdered ginger or 0.5 tsp fresh ginger every 15 minutes for an hour before traveling; continue this dosage during the trip if any signs of illness occur.
- Nausea from chemotherapy or surgery: A week before chemotherapy, take 2 g powdered ginger daily. Persons who are already receiving chemotherapy have a sensitive digestive

tract and should start with 250 mg powdered ginger daily, gradually increasing to a level that is comfortable and effective.

- As a digestive tonic: 1 g powdered ginger before or after a meal. Digestive tea can be made by simmering about 1 tsp fresh grated ginger in a cup of water for 15 minutes, then strain.
- Ulcers, heart disease, and inflammatory ailments: Seek the counsel of a trained herbalist or a medical practitioner schooled in the use of botanicals. Dramatic benefits can require high doses; research has found that the greatest relief of arthritis pain, for example, occurred with a daily intake of up to 7 g powdered ginger and 50 g fresh rhizome.
- Colds and flu: Take 0.5 to 1 g powdered ginger in capsules per hour for 2 to 3 days

Pharmacokinetics—If Available (form or route when known): Onset, 25 minutes; duration, 4 hours

Toxicity: Nontoxic at normal levels. Long history of use as food, beverage, and spice.

Contraindications: None known

Side Effects: Topical applications may produce irritation in some patients. Gastrointestinal discomfort may occur if taken on an empty stomach or in large doses.

Long-Term Safety: Very safe

Use in Pregnancy/Lactation/Children: No adverse effects expected. Clinical trials using ginger for morning sickness have produced no adverse effects.

Drug/Herb Interactions and Rationale (if known): If given with anticoagulants, may enhance bleeding. Use together with caution. Obtain prothrombin time and International Normalized Ratio (INR) to rule out any herb/drug interactions.

Special Notes: There has been concern that taking ginger before surgery might increase the risk of bleeding because constituents have shown antiplatelet activity. Numerous studies have been performed in which ginger was given just before surgery to reduce postsurgical nausea. In none of these studies was increased bleeding noted (Visalyaputra et al., 1998).

BIBLIOGRAPHY

Babbar OP. (1982). Protective patterns of different interferons: possible efficacy of chick embryo and plant interferons against microbial infections and malignancies of animals. *Indian Journal of Experimental Biology.* 20:572.

Bensky D, Gamble A. (1993). *Chinese Herbal Medicine: Materia Medica.* Seattle: Eastland Press

Bliddal H, et al. (2000). A randomized, placebo-controlled, cross-over study of ginger extracts and ibuprofen in osteoarthritis. *Osteoarthritis & Cartilage.* 8(1):9–12.

Blumenthal M, et al. (2000). *Herbal Medicine: Expanded Commission E Monographs.* Austin, TX: American Botanical Council.

Bone ME, Wilkinson DJ. (1990). Ginger root: a new antiemetic. *Anaesthesia.* 45:669–671.

ESCOP Monographs on the Medicinal Uses of Plant Drugs, Zigiberis Rhizoma. (1996). Exeter: ESCOP.

Fischer-Rasmussen W, et al. (1991). Ginger treatment of hyperemesis gravidarum. *European Journal of Obstetrics & Gynecology.* 38(1):19.

Fulder S. (Fall 1996). Ginger as an anti-nausea remedy in pregnancy. The issue of safety. *HerbalGram.* 38:47–50.

Grontved A, et al. (1988). Ginger root against seasickness. *Acta Otolaryngology.* 105:45–49.

Inouye S, et al. (1984). Inhibitory effect of volatile constituents of plants on the proliferation of bacteria. Antibacterial activity of plant volatiles. *Microbial Biochemistry.* 100:232.

Kiuchi F, et al. (1992). Inhibition of prostaglandin and leukotriene biosynthesis by gingerols and diarylheptanoids. *Chemical & Pharmaceutical Bulletin.* 40:387–391.

Lawrence Review of Natural Products. (1998). St. Louis: Facts and Comparisons.

Mills S, Bone K. (1999). *Principles and Practice of Phytotherapy.* Edinburgh: Churchill Livingstone.

Mowrey DB, Clayson DE. (1982). Motion sickness, ginger and psychophysics. *Lancet.* 1:655.

Phillips S, et al. (1993). *Zingiber officinale* (ginger): an antiemetic for day case surgery. *Anaesthesia.* 48:715–717.

Sharma SS, Gupta YK. (1998). Reversal of cisplatin-induced delay in gastric emptying in rats by ginger (*Zingiber officinale*). *Journal of Ethnopharmacology.* 62(1):49–55.

Shoji N, et al. (1982). Cardiotonic principles of ginger(*Zingiber officinale* Roscoe). *Journal of Pharmaceutical Science.* 71(10):1174.

Srivastava KC. (1989). Effect of onion and ginger consumption on platelet thromboxane production in humans. *Prostaglandins, Leukotrienes & Essential Fatty Acids*. 35:183–185.

Srivastava KC, Mustafa T. (1992). Ginger (*Zingiber officinale*) in rheumatism and musculoskeletal disorders. *Medical Hypotheses*. 39:342–348.

Stewart JJ, et al. (1991). Effects of ginger on motion sickness susceptibility and gastric function. *Pharmacology*. 42:111–120.

Suekawa M, et al. (1984). Pharmacological studies on ginger. I. Pharmacological actions of pungent constituents, (6)-gingerol and (6)-shogaol. *Journal of Pharmacobio-dynamics*. 7:836–848.

Surh YJ, et al. (1998). Chemoprotective properties of some pungent ingredients present in red pepper and ginger. *Mutation Research*. 402(1-2):259–267.

Visalyaputra S, et al. (1998). The efficacy of ginger root in the prevention of postoperative nausea and vomiting after outpatient gynaecological laparoscopy. *Anaesthesia*. 53(5):506–510.

Yamahura J, et al. (1990). Gastrointestinal mobility enhancing effect of ginger and its active constituents. *Chemical & Pharmaceutical Bulletin*. 38:430–431.

Yamahura J, et al. (1985). Cholagagic effect of ginger and its active constituents. *Journal of Ethnopharmacology*. 13:217–225.

Yoshikawa M, et al. (1992). 6-Gingesulfonic acid, a new anti-ulcer principle, and ginger glycolipids A, B, and C, three new monoacyldigalactosylglycerols, from *Zingiberis rhizoma* originating in Taiwan. *Chemical & Pharmaceutical Bulletin*. 40:2239–2241.

 NAME: Ginkgo (*Ginkgo biloba*)

Common Names: Maidenhair tree

Family: *Ginkgoaceae*

Description of Plant

- Slow-growing, deciduous tree that can grow to 125 feet, 3 to 4 feet in diameter, and live up to 1,000 years
- Male and female trees look slightly different and bear different flowers.
  ◦ Male: upright flowers develop on leaf axis
  ◦ Female: wider shape, wider crown, flowers have two terminal "naked" ovules on a stalk

- Female trees produce a small, yellow-to-orange fruit with thick fleshy layers that gives off a foul odor when mature. The fruit "hides" the highly prized inner seed.

Medicinal Part: Leaf. Highest concentration of active compounds may be present in autumn. It is thought that when chlorophyll fades, flavonoids are more available, but this is not proven.

Constituents and Action (if known)

- Terpene lactones (ginkgolide B and bilobalide): inhibit platelet-activating factor, which is elevated in inflammatory and allergic reactions, improve oxygen and glucose uptake at the cellular level, improve memory, enhance mental accuracy, increase circulation to extremities, reduce infarct size in brain, and may increase neuronal growth factors.
  - Ginkgolides A, B, C, J (20 carbon-diterpene): reduce the percentage of damaged neurons after ischemia, neuroprotective; reduce cholesterol transport, resulting in decreased corticosteroid synthesis; increase circulation; control mast cell degranulation.
  - Bilobalide (15 carbon sesquiterpene): protects neurons from injury from ischemic damage, may stimulate regeneration of damaged nerve cells
- Flavonoids (bilobetin, ginkgetin, and about 40 others): neutralize free radicals and antagonize lipid peroxidation
- Flavonols (quercetin, kaensysferol, isorhamnetin): inhibit platelet activity, antioxidant activity
- Sesquiterpenes
- Organic acids (vanillic acid, ascorbic acid, p-coumaric)
- Other actions: vasoregulating effects, relaxes blood vessels and strengthens vessel walls, therefore effective in persons who bruise easily; inhibits lipid peroxidation of membranes; moderates cerebral energy metabolism; increases activity of brain waves (different ginkgo products act in different parts of brain)

Nutritional Ingredients: Processed seeds have been used in Chinese medicine and in foods for centuries

Traditional Use: The tree was first cultivated in the Orient, then introduced into Europe in the early 1700s and brought to the United States in the 1780s. Little traditional use of the leaves. The processed nuts have been used as a food (congee) and as a medicine for coughs, asthma, frequent urination, and damp heat leukorrhea.

Current Use
- Cerebral insufficiency (difficulty in concentration and memory, absent-mindedness, confusion, lack of energy, dizziness): improves cerebral blood flow
- Possible reduction of muscle damage in patients with chronic disease (Parkinson's, MS) by improving blood flow
- Relieves tinnitus (ringing of ears) and may improve hearing (Holgers et al., 1994)
- Slows macular degeneration and protects retina, particularly in diabetic retinopathy
- Improves alpha-wave activity in brain
- Stimulates production of prostacyclins, which may prevent heart attacks
- Improves peripheral vascular insufficiency (Raynaud's disease, intermittent claudication): increases walking distance and decreases leg pain) (Peters et al., 1998)
- Stabilizes symptoms of Alzheimer's disease/dementia for 6 to 8 months (Maurer et al., 1997; 1998)
- Reduces asthma symptoms through reduction of platelet-activating factor. Studies show significant clinical improvement in adults.
- Relieves vertigo associated with vestibular dysfunction
- Helps improve penile blood flow for patients with impotence caused by atherosclerosis, diabetes, and selective serotonin reuptake inhibitor use
- Prevented acute altitude sickness at moderate elevations (5,400 m)
- One controlled double-blind study showed substantial improvement in premenstrual symptoms, including breast tenderness, anxiety, and depression.

Available Forms, Dosage, and Administration Guidelines
Preparations: A highly concentrated leaf extract (50:1), standardized to 24% flavonoid glycosides (ginkgo flavone glycosides), 6% terpenoids (ginkgolides and bilobalide), with

the controversial ginkgolic acid removed. Ginkgo must be used for 6 to 8 weeks before results are evident.

Typical Dosage

- *Capsules:* three capsules containing at least 40 mg standardized extract a day, or follow manufacturer's or practitioner's recommendations
- *Tincture:* 1:2, 70% alcohol—40 to 60 gtt (2–3 mL) three times a day; 1:5, 70% alcohol—60 to 100 gtt (3–5 mL) three times a day
- *Standardized extract of 24% glycosides, 6% terpene lactones, and at least 0.8% ginkgolide B:* 40 to 80 mg three times a day
- For dementia: 120 to 240 mg/day, divided into two or three doses
- For peripheral vascular disease, vertigo, tinnitus: 120 to 160 mg/day, divided into two or three doses
- Should be taken for at least 8 weeks before efficacy is evaluated

Pharmacokinetics—If Available (form or route when known)

- Onset: readily
- Peak: 2 to 3 hours
- Duration: unknown
- Half-life: 5 hours
- Excretion: exhaled air, urine, feces

Toxicity: Very safe; seizures when unprocessed seeds and fruit are ingested

Contraindications: Vasodilative headaches

Side Effects: Minimal and transient GI upset, headache, dizziness, allergic reactions. The fruit pulp and raw seeds are toxic and are not used in medicinal preparation. Fruit can cause an allergic reaction (like poison ivy) when touched.

Long-Term Safety: Safe

Use in Pregnancy/Lactation/Children: No trials available. Regular use in Europe has shown no adverse reactions.

Drug/Herb Interactions and Rationale (if known): Use cautiously with aspirin and coumarin; may increase bleeding tendencies. Obtain prothrombin time and INR to rule out possible potentiation.

Special Notes: Standardized ginkgo extracts are regulated as drugs in Germany. In China, ginkgo is available in tablet and injectable forms. The seeds, often sold in Oriental grocery stores, should be boiled before consumption to remove toxic compounds. Ginkgo is one of the most researched herbs in the world: more than 400 research papers have been published. Several studies have shown effectiveness in treating dementia, peripheral vascular disease, and tinnitus but did not compare ginkgo with traditional drug therapy.

BIBLIOGRAPHY

Bruno C, et al. (1993). Regeneration of motor nerves in bilobalide-treated rats. *Planta Medica.* 59:302–307.

Cohen B, et al. (1995). Decreased brain choline uptake in older adults. *Journal of the American Medical Association.* 274(11):902–907.

DeSmet P, et al. (1997). *Ginkgo Biloba.* Berlin: Springer-Verlag.

Eisenburg D. (1993). Herbal and magical medicine: traditional healing today. *New England Journal of Medicine.* 328:215–216.

Ferradini C, et al. (1993). *Ginkgo Biloba Extract (IGb761) as a Free Radical Scavenger.* Amsterdam: Elsevier.

Hofferberth B. (1994). The efficacy of EGb 761 in patients with senile dementia of the Alzheimer type, a double-blind placebo-controlled study on different levels of investigation. *Human Psychopharmacology.* 9:215–222.

Holgers KM, et al. (1994). *Ginkgo biloba* extract for the treatment of tinnitus. *Audiology.* 33:85–92.

Hoyer S. (1995). Possibilities and limits of therapy of cognition disorders in the elderly. *Z Gerontol Geriatr.* 28(6):457–462.

Huguet F. (1994). Decreased cerebral 5-HTIA receptors during aging: reversal by ginkgo biloba extract (EGb 761). *Journal of Pharmacy & Pharmacology.* 46:316–318.

Itil T. (1995). Natural substances in psychiatry (ginkgo biloba in dementia). *Psychopharmacology Bulletin.* 31:147–158.

Itil T. (June 1996). Early diagnosis and treatment of memory disturbances. *American Journal of Electromedicine.* pp. 81–85.

Itil TM, et al. (1996). Central nervous system effects of ginkgo biloba, a plant extract. *American Journal of Therapeutics.* 3(1):63–73.

Kanowski S. (1996). Proof of efficacy of the ginkgo biloba special extract EGb 761 in outpatients suffering from mild to moderate primary degenerative dementia. *Pharmacopsychiatry.* 29(2):47–56.

Kanowski S, et al. (1997). Proof of efficacy of the ginkgo biloba special extract EGb 761 in outpatients suffering from mild to moderate primary degenerative dementia of the Alzheimer type or multi-infarct dementia. *Phytomedicine.* 4(1):3–13.

Kim YS, et al. (1998). Antiplatelet and antithrombotic effects of a combination of ticlopidine and Ginkgo biloba ext. *Thrombosis Research.* 91(1):33–38.

Kleijnen J, Knipschild P. (1992). *Ginkgo biloba* for cerebral insufficiency. *British Journal of Clinical Pharmacology.* 34(4):352–358.

Kobuchi H, et al. (1997). Ginkgo biloba extract (EGb 761): Inhibitory effect of nitric oxide production in the macrophage cell line RAW 264.7. *Biochemisty & Pharmacology.* 53:897–903.

Koltai M, et al. (1991). Platelet activating factor (PAF). A review of its effects, antagonists and possible future clinical implications. *Drugs.* 42:9–29.

Krieglstein J. (1994). Neuroprotective properties of ginkgo biloba constituents. *Zeitschrift Phytotherapie.* 15:92–96.

LeBars PL, et al. (1997). A placebo-controlled, double-blind randomized trial of an extract of *Ginkgo biloba* for dementia. *Journal of the American Medical Association.* 278(16):1327–1332.

Li CL, Wong YY. (1997). The bioavailability of ginkgolides in *Ginkgo biloba* extracts. *Planta Medica.* 63(6):563–565.

Mancini M, et al. (1993). Clinical and therapeutic effects of *Ginkgo biloba* extract versus placebo in the treatment of psychorganic senile dementia of arteriosclerotic origin. *Gazetta Medicale Italiana.* 152:69–80.

Maurer K, et al. (1997). Clinical efficacy of *Ginkgo biloba* special extract EGb 761 in dementia of the Alzheimer type. *J Psychiatric Research.* 31(6):645–655.

Maurer K, et al. (1998). Clinical efficacy of *Ginkgo biloba* special extract EGb 761 in dementia of the Alzheimer type. *Phytomedicine.* 5(6):417–424.

Mills S, Bone K. (1999). *Principles and Practice of Phytotherapy.* Edinburgh: Churchill Livingstone.

Nemecz G, Combest WL. (1997). *Ginkgo biloba. U.S. Pharmacist.* 22:144–151.

Newall C, et al. (1996). *Herbal Medicines.* London: Pharmaceutical Press.

Oyama Y, et al. (1996). *Ginkgo biloba* extract protects brain neurons against oxidative stress. *Brain Research.* 712(2):349–352.

Perry N, et al. (1996). European herbs with cholinergic activities: potential in dementia therapy. *International Journal of Geriatric Psychiatry.* 11(12):1063–1069.

Peters H, et al. (1998). Demonstration of the efficacy of ginkgo biloba special extract EGb 761 on intermittent claudication—a placebo-controlled, double-blind multicenter trial. *Vasa.* 27(2):106–110.

Sastre J, et al. (1998). A *Ginkgo biloba* extract (EGb 761) prevents mitochondrial aging by protecting against oxidative stress. *Free Radicals Biology Medicine.* 24(2):298–304.

Schatzberg AM. (1998). Ginkgo biloba for dementia. *Journal of Family Practice.* 46(1):20.

Snowden DA. (1997). Brain infarction and the clinical expression of Alzheimer disease. *Journal of the American Medical Association.* 277:813–817.

Vester J. (1994). Efficacy of ginkgo biloba in 90 outpatients with cerebral insufficiency caused by old age. *Phytomedicine.* 1:9–16.

Wesnes KA, et al. (1997). The cognitive, subjective, and physical effects of a *Ginkgo biloba/Panax ginseng* combination in healthy volunteers with neurasthenic complaints. *Psychopharmacology Bulletin.* 33(4):677–683.

 NAME: Goldenseal (*Hydrastis canadensis*)

Common Names: Ground raspberry, Indian dye, yellow Indian paint, yellow root paint, yellow puccoon, jaundice root

Family: *Ranunculaceae*

Description of Plant
- Small perennial (10–12 inches) found in rich woods from Vermont to Arkansas
- Dark-red berries in April and May
- Rhizomes are gold-yellow and knotted in appearance
- Plant has been harvested almost to the point of extinction in the wild. Since the early 1990s, commercial farming has been started to reduce reliance on the wild plants.

Medicinal Part: Root, rhizome

Constituents and Action (if known)
- Isoquinoline alkaloids: hydrastine (3.2%–4%), berberine (2%–4.5%), hydrastinine, and canadine (0.5%–1%)

- ○ Hydrastine: antibacterial, constricts blood vessels, may elevate blood pressure, stimulates bile secretion, may reduce gastric inflammation
- ○ Berberine: stimulates bile and bilirubin secretion; antibacterial and antifungal activity and some antineoplastic activity (in mice it shrinks tumors) (Castleman, 1991)
- ○ Enhance apoptosis
- ○ Effective against many bacteria that cause diarrhea (Kuo et al., 1995), inhibit enterotoxins (Mills & Bone, 1999)
- ○ May lower blood pressure
- ○ Reduce anticoagulation effect of heparin (Preininger, 1975)
- ○ Antitubercular activity (Gentry et al., 1998)
- Volatile oil

Nutritional Ingredients: None known

Traditional Use

- Antibacterial, cholagogue, antihemorrhagic, mucous membrane tonic, bitter tonic, anti-inflammatory
- To treat inflammation of mucous membranes: boggy atonic mucosa with excess secretions and a tendency toward infection, such as gingivitis, pyorrhea, gastric and duodenal ulcers, ulceration of the cervix
- As a bitter tonic to improve appetite and treat dyspepsia
- As a cholagogue for liver disorders with inadequate bile secretion
- Antibacterial and antifungal agent for strep throat, conjunctivitis, vaginal candidiasis, tonsillitis, and otitis media

Current Use

- Effective as a mouthwash for treating minor oral problems (pyorrhea and gingivitis)
- As a topical or local antibacterial, antifungal, and mucous membrane amphoteric: erosion of the cervix vaginal pack, conjunctivitis, gastric and duodenal ulcers, aphthous ulcers, thrush, vaginal candidiasis, strep throat, rectal fissures (suppository)

- Enhances primary IgM response (rats) (Rehman et al., 1999)

Available Forms, Dosage, and Administration Guidelines

Preparations: Dried root, whole or powdered; leaf, capsules, extracts, ointments, salves, tablets, tinctures

Typical Dosage

- *Capsules:* Up to six 500- to 600-mg capsules a day
- *Tincture* (1:5, 60% alcohol): 20 to 40 gtt (1–2 mL) three times a day
- *Dried rhizome:* 0.5 to 1 g three times a day
- Or follow manufacturer's or practitioner's recommendations

Pharmacokinetics—If Available (form or route when known): None known

Toxicity: Excessive doses can cause jaundice and mild elevation of liver enzymes. The oral LD_{50} for goldenseal extract in mice is 1,620 mg/kg. Isolated berberine sulfate at doses of more than 0.5 g can cause GI irritation, nose bleeds, dizziness, renal irritation, and dyspnea.

Contraindications: Hypertension (theoretical concern); diarrhea, GI cramping, and pain; mouth ulcerations; nausea and vomiting

Long-Term Safety: Unknown

Use in Pregnancy/Lactation/Children: Do not use in pregnancy (Hoffmann, 1987).

Drug/Herb Interactions and Rationale (if known)

- Use cautiously with heparin.
- May interfere or enhance hypotensive effects of antihypertensive agents; use cautiously.

Special Notes

- Much of the Goldenseal used in the United States is used inappropriately. If this herb were used only for truly useful therapies, the demand for this endangered plant would diminish dramatically. It is used to mask the appearance of illicit drugs on urine drug screens in humans and in racehorses; however, this belief is false and originates from a fictional literary work that depicts the plant to be useful for hiding opiate ingestion.

- It is also used as an "herbal antibiotic," which it is not. Goldenseal's antibacterial activity affects only tissues with which it comes into contact: mucous membranes, gastric mucosa, and the urinary tract. It has no profound systemic antibiotic activity.

- Many other herbs can be used as substitutes
  - Mucous membrane tonics: yerba manza, yellow root, Chinese coptis, myrrh, calendula
  - Cholagogues and bitter tonics: barberry, Oregon grape root, artichoke leaf, gentian
  - Antibacterials: garlic, thyme, Chinese coptis, usnea.

BIBLIOGRAPHY

Castleman M. (1991). *The Healing Herbs.* Emmaus, PA: Rodale Press.

Gentry EJ, et al. (1998). Antitubercular natural products: berberine from the roots of commercial *Hydrastis canadensis* powder. Isolation of inactive 8-oxotetrahydrothalifendine, canadine, beta-hydrastine, and two new quinic acid esters, hycandinic acid esters-1 and -2. *Journal of Natural Products.* 61(10):1187–1193.

Hoffmann D. (1987). *The Herbal Handbook.* Rochester, VT: Healing Arts Press.

Kuo CL, et al. (1995). Berberine complexes with DNA in the berberine-induced apoptosis in human leukemic HL-60 cells. *Cancer Letters.* 93:193–200.

Lawrence Review of Natural Products. (1994). St. Louis: Facts and Comparisons.

Mills S, Bone K. (1999). *Principles and Practice of Phytotherapy.* Edinburgh: Churchill Livingstone.

Preininger V. (1975). The pharmacology and toxicology of the Papaveraceae alkaloids. In Maske RHF, Holmes HL. *The Alkaloids,* vol. 15. New York: Academic Press.

Rehman J, et al. (1999). Increased production of antigen-specific immunoglobulins G and M following in vivo treatment with the medicinal plants *Echinacea angustifolia* and *Hydrastis canadensis.* *Immunology Letters* 68(2-3):391–395.

Snow JM. (1997). *Hydrastis canadensis* L. (Ranunculaceae). *Protocol Journal of Botanical Medicine.* 2(2):25–27.

NAME: Gotu Kola (*Centella asiatica*)

Common Names: Indian pennywort, Brahmi, gotu cola

Family: *Apiaceae*

Description of Plant
- Weedy, creeping, low-growing herb native to tropical areas of India, Sri Lanka, and Southeast Asia
- Member of the parsley family. Has round-lobed leaves and tiny pink flowers.

Medicinal Part: Fresh and dried aerial parts

Constituents and Action (if known)
- Triterpenoids: responsible for wound healing and anti-inflammatory properties, strengthen varicose veins (Alpaia et al., 1990; Babu et al., 1995)
  - Asiatic acid
  - Madecassic acid
  - Asiaticoside A, B: randomized double-blind study versus placebo with topical application in 94 patients with chronic venous insufficiency showed subjective (reduction of edema, leg pain, heaviness of legs) and objective (plethysmographic measurements of vein tone) improvements (Gruenwald et al., 1998)
  - Oxyasiaticoside: inhibited tuberculosis bacilli in vivo (Emboden, 1985)
  - Madecassoside
- Volatile oils: camphor, cineole
- Flavonoids (quercetin)
- Isothankuniside
- Polyacetylenes
- Gotu kola is not related to the dried seeds of *cola nitide* (kola nuts, kola, cola), and it does not contain caffeine.

Nutritional Ingredients: Used in making a soft drink in Thailand

Traditional Use
- Anxiolytic, memory and brain tonic, nervine, antispasmodic, vulnerary, sedative, antibacterial, anti-inflammatory

- In India's traditional Ayurveda medicine, it was used as a calming and rejuvenating herb, especially for nerve and brain cells. It is used to increase intelligence, longevity, and memory, retarding aging and senility. Also used to reduce anxiety, treat petit mal epilepsy, for rheumatic pain, as a diuretic, and for varicose veins. Often used as a wash topically for skin infections, leprosy, and burns.
- In Chinese medicine, was often used interchangeably with several other species of low-growing, round-leaved plants under the name of *Zhi xue cao*. Used for treating dermatitis, wounds, sores, dysentery, tuberculosis, jaundice, hematuria, and hemoptysis and as a nerve tonic.

Current Use

- Oral: reduces stress and fatigue, improves memory, improves learning ability, reduces anxiety and depression (Alpaia et al., 1990; DeLucia & Sertie, 1997; Pointel et al., 1987)
- Topical: relieves inflammation, rebuilds damaged skin, promotes wound and burn healing, shows promise in treating psoriasis and varicose veins (Gruenwald et al., 1998)
- Reduced formation of ulcers in animal studies
- Clinical herbalists and naturopathic physicians use it orally for skin and connective tissue conditions where the tissue is red, hot, and inflamed. Often used with sarsaparilla for psoriatic arthritis, rheumatoid arthritis, scleroderma, psoriasis, and eczema (Winston, 1999).

Available Forms, Dosage, and Administration Guidelines

Preparations: Dried herb, cut and sifted or powdered; capsules, tablets, tinctures, teas. In other countries, standardized to asiaticoside.

Typical Dosage

- *Capsules:* Up to eight 400- to 500-mg capsules a day
- *Tea:* Steep 1 tsp dried herb in 1 cup of hot water for 10 to 15 minutes; take 4 oz three times a day
- *Tincture* (1:2, 30% alcohol): 30 to 60 gtt (1.5–3 mL) up to three times a day
- Or follow manufacturer's or practitioner's recommendations

Pharmacokinetics—If Available (form or route when known): None known

Toxicity: Topical solutions rarely cause contact dermatitis.

Contraindications: None known

Side Effects: None known

Long-Term Safety: Long-term use as a beverage and medicine in India, China, and other East Asian countries suggests reasonable safety.

Use in Pregnancy/Lactation/Children: Not known; best avoided in pregnant and breast-feeding women

Drug/Herb Interactions and Rationale (if known): None known. Can potentiate action of anxiolytic medications.

Special Notes: Gotu kola is also known as Brahmi, as is another herb, *Bacopa monnieri*. There is much confusion and debate in Ayurvedic medicine as to which herb is the true Brahmi of ancient Indian medical literature.

BIBLIOGRAPHY

Alpaia MR, et al. (1990). Effects of *Centella asiatica* extract on mucopolysaccharide metabolism in subjects with varicose veins. *International Clinical Pharmaceutical Research.* 10(4):229.

Babu TD, et al. (1995). Cytotoxic and anti-tumor properties of certain Taxa of *Umbelliferae* with special reference to *Centella asiatica* (L.) Urban. *Journal of Ethnopharmacology.* 48:53.

Chakraborty T, et al. (1996). Preliminary evidence of antifilarial effect of *Centella asiatica* on canine dirofilariasis. *Fitoterapia.* 67(2):110–112.

DeLucia R, Sertie JAA. (1997). Pharmacological and toxicological studies on *Centella asiatica* extract. *Fitoterapia.* 68(5):413–416.

Emboden W. (1985). The ethnopharmacology of *Centella asiatica* (L.) Urban (Apiaceae). *Journal of Ethnobiology.* 5(2):101–107.

Gruenwald J, et al. (eds.). (1998). *PDR for Herbal Medicines.* Montvale, NJ: Medical Economics.

Lawrence Review of Natural Products. (1996). St. Louis: Facts and Comparisons.

Nalini K, et al. (1992). Effect of *Centella asiatica* fresh leaf aqueous extract on learning and memory and biogenic amine turnover in albino rats. *Fitoterapia.* 63(3):232–236.

Pointel JP, et al. (1987). Titrated extract of *Centella asiatica* (TECA) in the treatment of venous insufficiency of the lower limbs. *Angiology.* 38(1 Pt 1):46.

Shukla A, et al. (1999). In vitro and in vivo wound healing activity of asiaticoside isolated from *Centella asiatica. Journal of Ethnopharmacology.* 65(1):1–12.

Srivastava R, et al. (1997). Antibacterial activity of *Centella asiatica. Fitoterapia.* 68(5):466–467.

Winston D. (1999). *Herbal Therapeutics.* Broadway, NJ: Herbal Therapeutics, Inc. Research Library.

 NAME: Grape Seed Extract

Common Names: Red grape seed extract

Family: *Vitaceae*

Description of Plant: The common grape is cultivated throughout the world. The leaves are used as a food, the fruits as a food and to make wine, and the seeds as a source of procyanidolic oligomers (PCOs). Another source of PCOs (also known as procyanidins) is a product called pycnogenol, which is made from the bark of maritime pine trees.

Medicinal Part: Red grape seed, ground into oil

Constituents and Action (if known)
- Flavonoids called proanthocyanidins (Maffei Facino et al., 1994; Masquelier et al., 1979; Tixier et al., 1984)
  - Antioxidant
  - Oxygen free radical scavenger. Vitamin E scavenges in lipid and fatty body environments; vitamin C scavenges in aqueous and watery environments. Pycnogenol scavenges in both environments and does so more efficiently (Fitzpatrick et al., 1998; Tixier et al., 1984).
  - Improve circulation (Mollmann & Rohdewald, 1983; Sarrat, 1981)
  - Reduce inflammation (Ames et al., 1993)
  - Protect collagen from natural degradation (Fitzpatrick et al., 1998)

- ○ Inhibit xanthine oxidase activity (the enzyme that triggers the oxy radical cascade) (Fitzpatrick et al., 1998; Maffei Facino et al., 1994)
- ○ Improve capillary permeability and decrease fragility (Fitzpatrick et al., 1998; Sarrat, 1981)
- ○ Inhibit platelet activity without increasing bleeding time (Putter et al., 1999)
- Essential fatty acids and tocopherols: protect liver (Oshima et al., 1995), protect vitamin E from oxidation (Virgili et al., 1998)
- Tannins: enhance cell renewal in intestinal tract (Vallet et al., 1994)

Traditional Use: None

Current Use
- Reduces inflammation in joints, prevents changes in synovial fluid and collagen
- Inhibits tumor promotion
- Improves circulation (particularly in peripheral vascular disease), reduces capillary fragility associated with hypertension, diabetes, and obesity
- Slows macular degeneration, diabetic retinopathy, and retinitis pigmentosa; improves nearsightedness
- Possibly protects against cancer and heart disease
- Possibly equal to aspirin in its effect on platelet activity, but unlike aspirin does not affect clotting
- Reduces postsurgical swelling and edema
- Protects the gastric mucosa from inflammation and irritation associated with disease (ulcers, gastritis) and pharmaceuticals (acetaminophen)

Available Forms, Dosage, and Administration Guidelines: Buy products with the active chemical PCOs, also known as oligomeric procyanidins. Products are usually standardized to contain 92% to 95% PCOs. Recommended dosage is 50 to 100 mg PCOs per day for the healthy patient, 150 to 300 mg PCOs per day to treat illness. Follow manufacturer's or practitioner's recommendations.

Pharmacokinetics—If Available (form or route when known): Not known

Toxicity: None known

Contraindications: None known

Side Effects: Gastric upset, rash (rare)

Long-Term Safety: Safe

Use in Pregnancy/Lactation/Children: Unknown

Drug/Herb Interactions and Rationale (if known): None known

BIBLIOGRAPHY

Ames BN, et al. (1993). Oxidants, antioxidants and the degenerative diseases of aging. *Proceedings of the National Academy of Sciences USA.* 90:7915–7922.

Bagchi M, et al. (1997a). *Protective effects of vitamins C and E, and a grape seed proanthocyanidin extract (GSPE) on smokeless tobacco-induced oxidative stress and apoptopic cell death in human oral keratinocytes.* Paper presented at the Fourth Annual Meeting of the Oxygen Society, San Francisco, Nov. 22, 1997.

Bagchi D, et al. (1997b). Comparative in vitro and in vivo free radical scavenging abilities of grape seed proanthocyanidins and selected antioxidants. *FASEB Journal.* 11(3):4.

Bagchi D, et al. (1998). Protective effects of grape seed proanthocyanidins and selected antioxidants against TPA-induced hepatic and brain lipid peroxidation and DNA fragmentation, and peritoneal macrophage activation in mice. *General Pharmacology.* 30(5):771–776.

Facino R, et al. (1998). Photoprotective action of procyanidins from Vitis vinifera seeds on UV-induced damage: in vitro and in vivo studies. *Fitoterapia.* 69(5):39–50.

Fitzpatrick DF, et al. (1998). Endothelium-dependent vascular effects of Pycnogenol. *Journal of Cardiovascular Pharmacology.* 32(4):509–515.

Foster S. (1998). *101 Medicinal Herbs.* Loveland, CO: Interweave Press.

Lawrence Review of Natural Products. (1991–1995). St. Louis: Facts and Comparisons.

Maffei-Facino R, et al. (1994). Free radicals scavenging action and anti-enzyme activities of procyanidins from *Vitis vinifera.* A mechanism for their capillary protective action. *Arzneimittel-Forschung.* 44(5):592.

Masquelier J, et al. (1979). Flavonoids and pycnogenols. *International Journal of Vitaminology & Nutrition Research.* 49:307.

McCaleb RS, et al. (2000). *Encyclopedia of Popular Herbs*. Roseville, CA: Prima Publishers.

Mollmann H, Rohdewald P. (1983). A naturally occurring bioflavonoid complex (pycnogenol) with capillary-protective action. *Therapiewoche*. 33:4967.

Oshima Y, et al. (1995). Powerful hepatoprotective and hepatotoxic plant oligostilbenes, isolated from the Oriental medicinal plant *Vitis coigetiae* (Vitaceae). *Experientia*. 51(1):63.

Packer L, et al. (1999). Antioxidant activity and biologic properties of a procyanidin-rich extract from pine (*Pinus maritima*) bar, pycnogenol. *Free Radical Biology & Medicine*. 27(5-6):704–724.

Putter M, et al. (1999). Inhibition of smoking-induced platelet aggregation by aspirin and pycnogenol. *Thrombosis Research*. 95(4):155–161

Sarrat L. (1981). Therapeutic approach to functional disorders of lower extremities. *Bordeaux Medical Journal*. 14:685.

Schwitters B, Masquelier J. (1995). *OPC in Practice*. Rome: Alfa Omega.

Tixier JM, et al. (1984). Evidence by in vivo and in vitro studies that binding of pycnogenols to elastin affects its rate of degradation by elastases. *Biochemical & Pharmacology*. 33:3933.

Vallet J, et al. (1994). Dietary grape seed tannins: effects of nutritional balance and on some enzymic activities along the crypt-villus axis of rat small intestine. *Annals of Nutrition & Metabolism*. 38(2):75.

Virgili F, et al. (1998). Procyanidins extracted from pine bark protect alpha-tocopherol in ECV 304 endothelial cells challenged by activated RAW 264.7 macrophages: role of nitric oxide and peroxynitrite. *FEBS Letters*. 431(3):315–318.

 NAME: Green Tea (*Camellia sinensis*)

Common Names: Ceylon tea, Assam tea

Family: *Theaceae*

Description of Plant

- Tea plants are cultivated in India, Sri Lanka, and China.
- An evergreen shrub with white flowers, usually kept pruned to 2 to 4 feet tall
- Parts used include the leaf bud and the two adjacent young leaves, together with the stem. Older leaves are inferior.

- Green tea is prepared from the dried tea leaves. For black tea, the leaves are withered, rolled, enzymatically fermented, and then dried. Oolong tea is semifermented, about halfway between green and black.

Medicinal Part: Leaves

Constituents and Action (if known)

- Polyphenols (35% of dry weight of tea leaves)
  ○ Free radical scavengers (Prior & Cao, 1999; Yang, CS et al., 1998)
  ○ Anticancer activity (Kuroda & Hara, 1999; Yang, CS, 1998): inhibit cytochrome P-450 activation of carcinogens
  ○ Decreased cardiovascular disease: delay lipid peroxidation (Yokozawa et al., 1997); increase high-density lipoproteins, decrease low-density lipoproteins (Watanabe et al 1998; Yang et al., 1997); however, Tsubono et al. (1997) did not confirm this finding
  ○ Antioxidant: green and black tea both have antioxidant activity, but black tea has a lower level of polyphenols and is only 20% as active. Milk totally inactivates the antioxidant value of both teas but not the catechin content (Vanhet Hof et al., 1998).
  ○ Inhibit the growth of *Streptococcus* in mouth to prevent plaque formation (Rasheed & Haider, 1998)
  ○ Enhance activity of B and T lymphocytes and natural killer cells
- Epigallocatechin gallate
  ○ Antioxidant 100 times more effective than vitamin C and 25 times more effective than vitamin E (Katiyar et al., 1999; Pietta et al., 1998)
  ○ Applied topically, protects skin from ultraviolet light by up to 61%, so may prevent skin cancer
- Catechins: cancer-preventing activity; apoptosis-increasing activity (Hibasami et al., 1998)
  ○ Inhibit MRSA (Hamilton-Miller & Shah, 1999; Yam et al., 1997)
  ○ Tea and curcumin (turmeric) or the anticancer drug doxorubicin are additive in their antitumor effect (Sadzuka et al., 1998).
  ○ May support P53 gene, which suppresses cancer development

- Flavonols: lower gastrointestinal cancer risk (Constable et al., 1996)
- Catechols: reduce carcinogenic activity (Ji et al., 1997)
- Tannins: lower risk of dental caries; lowers risk of chromosomal mutations so lowers cancer risk; astringent for wounds, skin disorders, and eye problems (use as a poultice for baggy or tired eyes)
- Theophylline, theobromine, and other methylxanthines (caffeine): may cause nervousness, anxiety, tachycardia, and heartburn, but may also help various headaches and enhance water excretion. Caffeine increases sex hormone binding globulin, which can lower estradiol levels, thus lowering the risk of breast cancer (Nagata et al., 1998).
- Lignans and isoflavonoids: anticancer, antimutagenic, antiatherosclerosis effects
- Volatile oils (hexenal, henenol, aldehydes, phenols, geraniol)
- Protein (15%–20%)

Nutritional Ingredients: B vitamins, ascorbic acid (in green tea only)

History: The word tea can be traced back to 1655, when the Dutch introduced the word and beverage to England.

Traditional Use
- Used for more than 4,000 years as a beverage
- Chinese believe green tea is a cure for cancer and a longevity tonic.
- Used to increase concentration and mental clarity
- Used as a diuretic
- Topically, a cold wash is used for minor burns.

Current Use
- The world's second most widely consumed beverage; only water is consumed more frequently
- Diuretic
- Green tea has many proposed anticancer mechanisms: antioxidative reactions, enzyme activities, inhibition of lipid peroxidation, irradiation, inhibition of cellular proliferation, and anti-inflammatory activity (Fujiki et al., 1999; Katiyar et al., 1999; Tanaka et al., 1998). This suggests green tea may be useful as an unconventional therapy for breast cancer–

cancer onset in tea drinkers is delayed by years; may inhibit metastasis.
- Consumption of green tea lowers risk of prostate cancer (Gupta & Ahmad, 1999; Gupta et al., 1999).
- Green tea may enhance the P450 cytochrome system in the liver and protect against the heterocyclic amino mutagens found in cooked meat (Dashwood et al., 1999).
- Green tea tablets and capsules do not appear to have a cancer protection effect (Yang, CS, 1998).
- Protects the liver against oxidative damage
- Improves cardiovascular health: lowers low-density lipoproteins and increases high-density lipoproteins, decreases clotting tendencies
- Promotes healthy teeth by inhibiting growth of streptococci and other bacteria that cause plaque; is a source of natural fluoride.
- Boosts immune function
- Antioxidant: green tea can lower the oxidative stress in body related to cigarette smoking (Klaunig et al., 1999)

Available Forms, Dosage, and Administration Guidelines: One cup or more a day; steep tea in hot water for 1 to 2 minutes. It is unknown whether green tea extract (pill form) confers the same degree of protection; buy tablets standardized for polyphenol content.

Pharmacokinetics—If Available (form or route When Known): Peak antioxidant effect occurs 30 to 50 minutes after ingestion.

Toxicity
- May be associated with tea-induced asthma
- Extremely large intake of tea daily may be linked with increased risk of esophageal cancer.

Contraindications: Daily consumption of an average of 250 mL tea by infants has been shown to impair iron metabolism.

Side Effects: Hyperactivity in children; may deplete calcium from the bones; increased urination

Long-Term Safety: Safe

Use in Pregnancy/Lactation/Children: Caffeine is best avoided during pregnancy, but recent studies show no effect on the fetus. Thousands of years of human use suggest reasonable safety. Do not give to infants.

Drug/Herb Interactions and Rationale (if known):
Methylxanthine component of tea decreases the absorption of Ca^{++}. Separate by at least 2 hours.

Special Notes
- Separate milk from tea by at least 1 hour: milk complexes with polyphenols and renders them resistant to gastric breakdown and absorption, possibly by increasing the gastric pH.
- Tea contains caffeine (green tea, 10 mg/cup; black tea, 40 mg/cup).
- Never drink tea too hot because it may change the DNA structure in the esophagus and predispose it to esophageal cancer.
- Antimicrobial activity of tea decreases with the amount of oxidation. Thus, green tea is the highest in microbial activity and black tea is the lowest (Chou et al., 1999).
- Green tea may ultimately be able to lower the risk of chronic disease (Weisburger, 1999).
- Tea made from instant powders probably offers few benefits because active ingredients are lost in the processing (Constable et al., 1996).

BIBLIOGRAPHY

Chou CC, Lin LL, et al. (1999). Antimicrobial activity of tea as affected by the degree of fermentation and manufacturing season. *International Journal of Food Microbiology.* 48(2):125–130.

Constable A, et al. (1996). Antimutagenicity and catechin content of soluble instant teas. *Mutagenesis.* 11(2):189–194.

Dashwood RH, et al. (1999). Cancer chemopreventive mechanisms of tea against heterocyclic amine mutagens from cooked meat. *Proceedings of the Society for Experimental Biology & Medicine.* 220(4):239–243.

Fujiki H, et al. (1999). Mechanistic findings of green tea as cancer preventive for humans. *Proceedings of the Society for Experimental Biology & Medicine.* 220(4):225–228.

Gupta S, Ahmad N. (1999). Prostate cancer chemoprevention by green tea. *Seminars in Urology & Oncology.* 17(2):70–76.

Gupta S, et al. (1999). Prostate cancer chemoprevention by green tea: in vitro and in vivo inhibition of testosterone-mediated induction of ornithine decarboxylase. *Cancer Research.* 59(9):2115–2120.

Hamilton-Miller JM, Shah S. (1999). Disorganization of cell division of methicillin-resistant *Staphylococcus aureus* by a component of tea (*Camellia sinensis*): a study by electron microscopy. *FEMS Microbiology Letters.* 176(2):463–469.

Hibasami H, et al. (1998). Induction of apoptosis in human stomach cancer cells by green tea catechins. *Oncology Reports.* 5(2):527–529.

Ji B, et al. (1997). Green tea consumption and the risk of pancreatic and colorectal cancers. *International Journal of Cancer.* 70(3):255–258.

Katiyar S, et al. (1999). Polyphenolic antioxidant (-)-epigallocatechin-3-gallate from green tea reduces UVB-induced inflammatory responses and infiltration of leukocytes in human skin. *Photochemistry & Photobiology.* 69(2):148–153.

Klaunig JE, et al. (1999). The effect of tea consumption on oxidative stress in smokers and nonsmokers. *Proceedings of the Society for Experimental Biology & Medicine.* 220(4):249–254.

Kuroda Y, Hara Y. (1999). Antimutagenic and anticarcinogenic activity of tea polyphenols. *Mutation Research.* 436(1):69–97.

McCaleb R, et al. (2000). *Encyclopedia of Popular Herbs.* Roseville, CA: Prima Publishers.

Nagata C, et al. (1998). Association of coffee, green tea, and caffeine intakes with serum concentrations of estradiol and sex hormone-binding globulin in premenopausal Japanese women. *Nutrition & Cancer.* 30(1):21–24.

Pietta P, et al. (1998). Relationship between rate and extent of catechin absorption and plasma antioxidant status. *Biochemisty & Molecular Biology International.* 46(5):895–903.

Prior RL, Cao G. (1999). Antioxidant capacity and polyphenolic components of teas: implications for altering in vivo antioxidant status. *Proceedings of the Society for Experimental Biology & Medicine.* 220(4):255–261.

Rasheed A, Haider M. (1998). Antibacterial activity of *Camellia sinensis* extracts against dental caries. *Archives of Pharmaceutical Research.* 21(3):348–352.

Sadzuka Y, et al. (1998). Modulation of cancer chemotherapy by green tea. *Clinical Cancer Research.* 4(1):153–156.

Tanaka K, et al. (1998). Inhibition of N-nitrosation of secondary amines in vitro by tea extracts and catechins. *Mutation Research.* 412(1):91–98.

Tsubono Y, et al. (1997). Green tea intake in relation to serum lipid levels in middle-aged Japanese men and women. *Annals of Epidemiology.* 7(4):280–284.

Vanhet Hof KH, et al. (1998). Bioavailability of catechins from tea: the effect of milk. *European Journal of Clinical Nutrition.* 52(5):356–359.

Watanabe J, et al. (1998). Isolation and identification of acetyl-CoA carboxylase inhibitors from green tea. *Bioscience, Biotechnology, & Biochemistry.* 62(3):532–534.

Weisburger JH. (1999). Tea and health: the underlying mechanisms. *Proceedings of the Society for Experimental Biology & Medicine.* 220(4):271–275.

Yam T, et al. (1997). Microbiological activity of whole and fractionated crude extracts of tea and of tea components. *FEMS Microbiology Letters.* 152(1):169–174.

Yang CS, et al. (1998). Tea and tea polyphenols inhibit cell hyperproliferation, lung tumorigenesis, and tumor progression. *Experimental Lung Research.* 24(4):629–639.

Yang T, et al. (1997). Hypocholesterolemic effects of Chinese tea. *Pharmacologic Research.* 35(6):505–512.

Yokozawa T, et al. (1997). Influence of green tea and its 3 major components upon low-density lipoprotein oxidation. *Experimental Toxicology & Pathology.* 49(5):329–335.

NAME: Guarana (*Paullinia cupana*)

Common Names: Guarana paste or gum, Brazilian cocoa, Zoom (product name)

Family: *Sapindaceae*

Description of Plant
- Fast-growing, woody evergreen liana
- Native to the Amazonian region of Brazil and Venezuela
- Bears orange-yellow fruit containing up to three seeds each

Medicinal Part: Dried paste made from crushed seeds

Constituents and Action (if known)
- Methylxanthine alkaloids: caffeine (2.6%–5%) (coffee beans contain 1%–2% and dried tea leaves 1%–4%) (Bempong &

Houghton, 1992; Der Marderosian et al., 1988; Willard & McCormick, 1992). Guaranine, the methylxanthine found in guarana, is absorbed more slowly than caffeine from coffee or tea.

- Alkaloids (theophylline, theobromine): found only in bark, flowers, and leaves, not in seeds (Belliardo et al., 1985; Henman, 1982; *Review of Natural Products*, 2000)
- Tannins (12%; catachutannic acid, catechol): impart astringent taste, antioxidant properties (Yoshizawa et al., 1987), control diarrhea (Straten, 1994)
- Saponins (timbonise): antioxidant activity (Mattei et al., 1998; Yoshizawa et al., 1987), reduce absorption of guaranine (Straten, 1994)
- Other actions: inhibits platelet aggregation (Bydlowski et al., 1988, 1991)

Nutritional Ingredients: Classified as a food additive and dietary supplement; syrups, extracts used as flavoring and source of caffeine by soft drink industry

Traditional Use: Believed to be an aphrodisiac; used to treat migraines, diarrhea; used as a diuretic; used as a central nervous system stimulant to increase alertness and reduce fatigue

Current Use

- Diet aid (Breum et al., 1994); included in many thermogenic weight-loss formulas. Studies have shown the combination of ephedrine and caffeine has a synergistic effect of increasing the metabolic rate and reducing body weight. The widespread and unsupervised use of such products, especially in overdose, has caused adverse effects ranging from nervousness and increased blood pressure to death.
- Found in body-building products to increase energy and stamina
- Found in smoking cessation products to curb appetite and improve mood and energy
- May be beneficial for migraine headaches

Available Forms, Dosage, and Administration Guidelines

Preparations: Capsules and tablets

Typical Dosage

- *Capsules:* Two 500-mg capsules per day; daily dose should not exceed 3 g

Pharmacokinetics—If Available (form or route when known): Onset is more gradual than caffeine in coffee or tea; duration, 1 to 3 hours

Toxicity: None reported, but persons sensitive to caffeine should use with caution

Contraindications: Cardiovascular disease such as hypertension, angina, congestive heart failure; psychological disorders, especially mania

Side Effects: Increased diuresis, insomnia, nervousness, stomach upset; with excessive intake, diarrhea, headache, irritability, nausea, vomiting, hypertension, seizures, tremors, tachycardia, arrhythmias

Long-Term Safety: Unknown; tannin content may be carcinogenic with long-term use in humans (not proven by research)

Use in Pregnancy/Lactation/Children: Contraindicated

Drug/Herb Interactions and Rationale (if known)

- Do not use with respiratory drugs because of increased likelihood of side effects.
- Do not use with oral contraceptives, cimetidine, certain quinolone antibiotics, and verapamil: lowers caffeine clearance by 30% to 50%.
- Do not use with benzodiazepines: may be less effective.
- Do not use with monoamine oxidase inhibitors: increased blood pressure.
- Monitor patient carefully if used with beta-adrenergic agonists; may enhance response.
- Do not use with adenosine: may lower response.
- Do not use with lithium: may inhibit lithium clearance.

- Use with ma huang (ephedra) or ephedrine only under the supervision of a practitioner; guarana increases the central nervous system effects of ephedra.

Special Notes: The stimulating effect of guarana is associated with its level of caffeine. Reports in the media suggest that guarana may enhance cognitive function, but no scientific evidence exists (Galduroz & Carlini, 1996).

BIBLIOGRAPHY

Belliardo F, et al. (1985). HPLC determination of caffeine and theophylline in *Paullinia cupana* Kunth (guarana) and Cola spp. samples. *Z Lebensm Unters Forsch.* 180(5):398–401.

Bempong DK, Houghton PJ. (1992). Dissolution and absorption of caffeine from guarana. *Journal of Pharmacy & Pharmacology.* 44(9):769–771.

Breum L, et al. (1994). Comparison of an ephedrine/caffeine combination and dexfenfluramine in the treatment of obesity. A double-blind multi-centre trial in general practice. *International Journal of Obesity and Related Metabolic Disorders.* 18:99–103.

Bydlowski SP, et al. (1988). A novel property of an aqueous guarana extract (*Paullinia cupana*): inhibition of platelet aggregation in vitro and in vivo. *Brazilian Journal of Medical Research.* 21(3):535.

Bydlowski SP, et al. (1991). An aqueous extract of guarana (*Paullinia cupana*) decreases platelet thromboxane synthesis. *Brazilian Journal of Medical Research.* 24(4):421–424.

Der Marderosian AH, et al. (1988). *Natural Product Medicine.* Philadelphia: GF Stickly.

Galduroz JC, Carlini EA. (1996). The effects of long-term administration of guarana on the cognition of normal, elderly volunteers. *Revista Paulista de Medicina.* 114(1):1073–1078.

Henman AR. (1982). Guarana (*Paullinia cupana* var. sorbilis): ecological and social perspective on an economic plant of the central Amazon basin. *Journal of Ethnopharmacology.* 6(3):311–338.

Leung A, Foster S. (1996). *Encyclopedia of Common Natural Ingredients.* New York: John Wiley & Sons.

Mattei R, et al. (1998). Guarana (*Paullinia cupana*): toxic behavioral effects in laboratory animals and anti-oxidant activity in vitro. *Journal of Ethnopharmacology.* 60:111–116.

Review of Natural Products. (2000). St. Louis: Facts and Comparisons.

Straten M. (1994). *Guarana.* Saffron Walden, UK: CW Daniel Co.

Willard T, McCormick J. (1992). *Textbook of Advanced Herbology.* Calgary: Wild Rose College of Natural Healing, Ltd.

Yoshizawa S, et al. (1987). Antitumor promoting activity of *Epigallocatechin gallate,* the main constituent of tannin in green tea. *Phytotherapy Research.* 1:44–47.

 NAME: Guggul (*Commiphora mukul*)

Common Names: Guggal, gum guggulu, gum guggul, guggulipid, Indian bdellium

Family: *Burseraceae*

Description of Plant
- Small thorny shrub widely distributed in India
- Same genus as *Commiphora myrrha*, the myrrh of the Bible

Medicinal Part: Gum resin

Constituents and Action (if known)
- Lipid steroids (Z-guggulsterone, E-guggulsterone, and guggul extract): with lignans and diterpenoids, show lipid-lowering activity by increasing clearance and uptake and breakdown of low-density lipoprotein cholesterol by the liver and also reducing triglycerides (Agarwal et al., 1986; Das Gupta, 1990; Gopal & Saran, 1986; Nityanand et al., 1989); demonstrate thyroid-stimulating activity (Tripathi et al., 1984); protective effect on cardiac enzymes and on the cytochrome P-450 system against drug-induced necrosis (Kaul et al., 1989; Singh et al., 1990)

Additional Actions
- Mild effect on inhibiting platelet aggregation and promoting fibrinolysis
- Prevents formation of atherosclerosis and may cause regression of pre-existing atherosclerotic plaques
- Anti-inflammatory activity (Duwiejua et al., 1993, Sharma & Sharma, 1977)

Nutritional Ingredients: None known

Traditional Use: Used in traditional Ayurvedic medicine to treat arthritis, psoriasis, diabetes, gout, and obesity; currently used in Ayurvedic medicine to lower cholesterol

Current Use

- Protects against atherosclerosis, inhibits platelet aggregation, and may reduce risk of stroke and pulmonary embolism (Mester et al., 1979)
- Reduces both cholesterol (24%) and triglycerides (23%) (Nityanand et al., 1989) and increases high-density lipoprotein cholesterol (16%); activity begins in 2 to 4 weeks. Especially effective for type IIb and type IV hyperlipidemia (Agarwal et al., 1986).
- Reduces inflammation of nodulocystic acne
- Anti-inflammatory for arthritis
- Mildy stimulates thyroid activity, making this herb useful for mild hypothyroid conditions with obesity and hyperlipidemia

Available Forms, Dosage, and Administration

Guidelines: Always use processed gum guggal. Commercial guggulipid extracts are standardized to 2.5% guggulsterones. Normal dosage is 1,000 mg three times a day.

Pharmacokinetics—If Available (form or route when known): None known

Toxicity: None known

Contraindications: None known

Side Effects: Minor GI disturbance, mild headache, nausea, hiccups

Long-Term Safety: Appears to be safe; no adverse effects expected

Use in Pregnancy/Lactation/Children: Safe in pregnancy; unknown safety in breast-feeding women and children

Drug/Herb Interactions and Rationale (if known): Do not use with beta-blockers and calcium channel blockers such as diltiazem and propranolol: diminished efficacy and responsiveness (Dalvi et al., 1994).

Special Notes: Inhibition of platelet aggregation is reversible, so patients need only discontinue medication 1 to 2 days before surgery.

BIBLIOGRAPHY

Agarwal RC, et al. (1986). Clinical trial of gugulipid, a new hypolipidemic agent of plant origin in primary hyperlipidemia. *Indian Journal of Medical Research.* 84:626–634.

Dalvi SS, et al. (1994). Effect of gugulipid on bioavailability of diltiazem and propranolol. *Journal of the Association of Physicians of India.* 42(6):454–455.

Das Gupta R. (1990). A new hypolipidaemic agent. *Journal of the Association of Physicians of India.* 38(2):186.

Duwiejua M, et al. (1993). Antiinflammatory activity of resins from some species of the plant family *Burseraceae. Planta Medica.* 59:12.

Gopal K, Saran RK. (1986). Clinical trial of ethyl acetate extract of gum gugulu (gugulipid) in primary hyperlipidemia. *Journal of the Association of Physicians of India.* 34(4):249–251.

Kaul S, et al. (1989). Cardiac sarcolemma enzymes and liver microsomal cytochrome P450 in isoproterenol treated rats. *Indian Journal of Medical Research.* 90:62.

McCaleb R, et al. (2000). *Encyclopedia of Popular Herbs.* Roseville, CA: Prima Publishers.

Mester L, et al. (1979). Inhibition of platelet aggregation by gugulu steroids. *Planta Medica.* 37:367–369.

Nityanand S, et al. (1989). Clinical trials with gugulipid. A new hypolipidaemic agent. *Journal of the Association of Physicians of India.* 37(5):323–328.

Sharma JN, Sharma JN. (1977). Comparison of the anti-inflammatory activity of *Commiphora mukul* (an indigenous drug) with those of phenylbutazone and ibuprofen in experimental arthritis induced by mycobacterial adjuvant. *Arzneimittel-Forschung.* 28(2):1455–1458.

Singh V, et al. (1990). Stimulation of low-density lipoprotein receptor activity in liver membrane of guggulsterone-treated rats. *Pharmacologic Research.* 22:37.

Tripathi YB, et al. (1984). Thyroid-stimulating actions of z-guggulsterone obtained from *Commiphora mukul. Planta Medica.* 1:78.

NAME: Gymnema (*Gymnema sylvestre*)

Common Names: Gurmar (Hindi), meshasingi (Sanskrit)

Family: *Asclepiadaceae*

Description of Plant: Native climbing vine of India and Australia

Medicinal Part: Leaves

Constituents and Action (if known)
- Saponins (gymnemic acids [gymnenin])
  - Lower blood sugar similar to the way sulfonylureas act by stimulating release of endogenous insulin stores (Rahman & Zaman, 1989)
  - May block glucose receptors (Bone, 1996)
  - May act by increasing cell permeability for insulin (done in rats) (Persaud et al., 1999)
  - Diminish the ability to taste sweet substances and decrease appetite for up to 90 minutes
  - May lower glycogen content of tissue (done in rats) (Chattopadhyay, 1998)
  - Lowers cholesterol in hypertensive rats (Preuss et al., 1998)
  - May promote pancreatic function in persons with diabetes
- Polypeptide (gurmarin): reduces sweet taste on tongue
- The herb regulated blood sugar levels in alloxan diabetic rabbits and increased the activity of enzymes that stimulate the use of glucose by insulin-dependent pathways. Uptake of glucose into glycogen and protein was increased in the kidney, liver, and muscle (Bone, 1996).
- Liquid extract or tea inhibits the ability to taste bitter or sweet but does not interfere with the ability to taste sour, astringent, or pungent substances.

Nutritional Ingredients: None known

Traditional Use: Traditional treatment in Ayurvedic medicine for diabetes, obesity, coughs, dyspnea, and fevers, as a diuretic, and as an oral and topical remedy for snake bites

Current Use
- May be useful in reducing cravings for sweets for weight control.
- Used in management of blood sugar disorders. Two long-term human studies yielded interesting results. In the first study, use of gymnema in patients with insulin-dependent diabetes mellitus reduced insulin requirements and fasting

blood glucose, glycosylated hemoglobin, and glycosylated plasma protein levels. This study also showed what may be the enhancement of endogenous insulin production and perhaps pancreatic beta-cell regeneration (Bone, 1996). In the second study, conducted with patients with noninsulin-dependent diabetes, the results were very similar: both fasting and postprandial serum insulin levels increased compared with the control group taking conventional medication (Bone, 1996).

Available Forms, Dosage, and Administration Guidelines: Some patients may respond quickly, but it is best if taken for 6 to 12 months to maximize effects.

Typical Dosage
- *Leaf powder:* 2 to 4 g per day
  To lower blood sugar levels
- *Capsules:* Two 500-mg capsules twice a day
- *Tincture:* (1:5, 30% alcohol) 60 to 100 gtt (3–5 mL) twice a day

To reduce cravings for sweets and as an appetite suppressant
- *Tincture:* (1:5, 30% alcohol) 20 to 40 gtt (1–2 mL) in a small amount of water; swish in the mouth for 30 seconds. Repeat every 2 to 3 hours as needed.

Pharmacokinetics—If Available (form or route when known): None known

Toxicity: None known

Contraindications: None known

Side Effects: None known

Long-Term Safety: Not known

Use in Pregnancy/Lactation/Children: No studies available

Drug/Herb Interactions and Rationale (if known): In patients taking hyperglycemic drugs and insulin, monitor blood sugar levels carefully so dosage of drugs can be adjusted.

Special Notes: Most research has been done in rats and indicates a significant variation in the herb's ability to lower blood sugar. It appears to have no effects in the normal glycemic person (Chattopadhyay, 1999). More research needs to be done, but the herb looks very promising.

BIBLIOGRAPHY

Alschuler L. (1998). *Gymnema sylvestre*'s impact on blood sugar levels. *American Journal of Natural Medicine.* 5(9):26–30.

Baskaran K, et al. (1990). Antidiabetic effect of a leaf extract from *Gymnema sylvestre* in non-insulin dependent diabetes mellitus patients. *Journal of Ethnopharmacology.* 30:295–300.

Bone K. (1996). *Clinical Applications of Ayurvedic and Chinese Herbs.* Warwick: Phytotherapy Press.

Chattopadhyay RR. (1998). Possible mechanism of antihyperglycemic effect of *Gymnema sylvestre* leaf extract, part I. *General Pharmacology.* 31(3):495–496.

Chattopadhyay RR. (1999). A comparative evaluation of some blood sugar-lowering agents of plant origin. *Journal of Ethnopharmacology.* 67(3):367–372.

Ernst E. (1997). Plants with hypoglycemic activity in humans. *Phytomedicine.* 4(1):73–78.

Kapoor LD. (1990). *CRC Handbook of Ayurvedic Medicinal Plants.* Boca Raton: CRC Press.

Lawrence Review of Natural Products. (1989). St. Louis: Facts and Comparisons.

Persaud SJ, et al. (1999). *Gymnema sylvestre* stimulates insulin release in vitro by increased membrane permeability. *Journal of Endocrinology.* 163(2):207–212.

Preuss HG, et al. (1998). Comparative effects of chromium, vanadium and *Gymnema sylvestre* on sugar-induced blood pressure elevations in SHR. *Journal of the American College of Nutrition.* 17(2):116–123.

Rahman AU, Zaman K. (1989). Medicinal plants with hypoglycemic activity. *Journal of Ethnopharmacology.* 26:73.

H

 NAME: Hawthorn (*Crataegus monogyna, C. laevigata*)

Common Names: Maybush, Whitethorn

Family: *Rosaceae*

Description of Plant
- Small, spiny shrub or tree, native to Europe
- May be grown as a hedge but can grow to 15 to 18 feet
- Produces white flowers with pink anthers from April to June
- Spherical bright-red fruit contains one to three nuts

Medicinal Part: Blossoms, fruit, leaves. Many traditional preparations use only the ripe fruit.

Constituents and Action (if known)
- Flavonoids (0.044%–0.150% berries, 1.78%–2.1% leaves and flowers)
  - Increase contractility of heart, a positive inotropic effect; reduce peripheral vascular resistance, reduce afterload (similar to captopril), thus increasing cardiac output and cardiac performance (Ammon & Handel, 1981; Nasa et al., 1993; Wagner & Grevel, 1982), antioxidants (Upton, 1999)
  - Slightly inhibit Na+/K+ ATPase, might also be responsible for positive inotropic action (Loew, 1994)
  - Inhibit angiotensin-converting enzyme, thus reducing blood pressure
  - Hyperoside
  - Vitexin 2-0-rhamnoside; positive inotropic (Upton, 1999)
- Procyanidins (0.1%–6.9%): epicatechin: cardiotonic, positive inotropic, mild hypotensive, sedative (Upton, 1999)
- Oligomeric procyanidins (1.9%–3.26%): antioxidants, circulation enhancers (Upton, 1999)
- Triterpenid acids (0.3%–1.4%)
  - Ursolic acid: increased coronary blood flow (Mills & Bone, 1999)
  - Crateagolic acid: positive inotropic
  - Isovitexin
- Flavonal aglycones (quercetin, rutin): positive inotropic (Upton, 1999)
- Chlorogenic acid

Nutritional Ingredients: Flavonoids, vitamin C; fruits are made into jam; flowers have been used to make May wines

Traditional Use

- Nutritive, heart tonic, mild diuretic, nervine
- Use dates back to Dioscorides for stomach ailments and dropsy
- Used since the 1600s for heart problems, as a diuretic, and for urinary calculi
- The eclectic physicians used hawthorn for the aging or senile heart. Indications included angina, valvular deficiency, cardiac edema, palpitations, irregular and intermittent pulse, and dyspnea. They often recommended giving it with stronger cardiac medications such as cactus.

Current Use

- Reduces congestive heart failure (Gildor, 1998) but may not be effective used alone. Best in New York Heart Association stage I and II cardiac insufficiency (Leuchtgens, 1993; Reuter, 1994; Schmidt et al., 1994; Tauchert et al., 1994; Zapfe et al., 1993).
- Stabilizes angina (Hanack & Bruckel, 1983), improves myocardial and coronary circulation and myocardial tolerance of oxygen deficiency
- Reduces abnormal cardiac rhythms (premature ventricular contractions)
- Mild hypertension: mildly lowers blood pressure
- Atherosclerosis: prevents arterial degeneration
- Reduction of blood lipids: increased bile acid excretion, increased the binding of low-density lipoproteins to liver plasma membranes (Mills & Bone, 1999)
- Beneficial for attention deficit disorder and attention deficit hyperactive disorder as a solid extract
- Stabilizes collagen and antioxidant for inflammatory connective tissue disorders

Available Forms, Dosage, and Administration Guidelines

Preparations: Dried berries, leaves, flowers. Most research has been done on flowers and leaves. In Germany, only flowers and leaves are approved, not berries. Standardized in Europe to oligomeric procyanidins and flavonoids. To be effective, hawthorn may need to be administered for 2 weeks or more. Occasional dosing is of little value. Take regularly.

Typical Dosage

- *Capsules:* Up to nine 500- to 600-mg nonstandardized capsules a day. If standardized to either oligomeric procyanidins (18.75%) or total flavonoid content, usually calculated as vitexin (2.2%): 160 to 900 mg per day for at least 4 to 8 weeks.
- *Tea from berries:* Decoct 1 tsp dried berries in a cup of hot water for 10 to 15 minutes, steep an additional half-hour; take 8 oz three times a day.
- *Tea from blossoms:* 1 to 2 tsp in 8 oz hot water, infuse for 10 to 15 minutes; take two or three cups per day
- *Tincture* (1:5, 40% alcohol): 60 to 90 gtt (3–5 mL) up to three times a day, or follow manufacturer's or practitioner's recommendations
- *Fluid extract* (1:1): 1 to 2 mL three times a day
- *Freeze-dried berries:* 160-mg capsules, two to four per day
- *Solid extract* (native extract): 0.25 tsp twice a day

Pharmacokinetics—If Available (form or route when known): Oligomeric procyanidins: rapid absorption. Plasma half-life is 5 hours, indicating a prolonged presence in the blood (Mills & Bone, 1999).

Toxicity: None

Contraindications: Diastolic congestive heart failure

Side Effects: Products made with more than 50% leaf occasionally cause gastric upset.

Long-Term Safety: Safe for a lifetime of use

Use in Pregnancy/Lactation/Children: Safe

Drug/Herb Interactions and Rationale (if known)

- Use cautiously and under a physician's supervision with digitalis products: theoretical possibility of potentiation.
- Monitor blood pressure if used with antihypertensives, nitrates: increased risk of hypotension.
- Use cautiously with beta-blockers: may potentiate action.

Special Notes: Hawthorn is a cardiovascular trophorestorative and is appropriate for most adult patients as a nontoxic preventive therapy, as well as a mild but useful treatment for cardiovascular disease.

BIBLIOGRAPHY

Ammon HP, Handel M. (1981). *Crataegus*: toxicology and pharmacology. *Planta Medica*. 43:101–120.

ESCOP Monographs on the Medicinal Uses of Plant Drugs. (1999). Exeter: ESCOP.

Gildor A. (1998). *Crataegus oxycantha* and heart failure. *Circulation*. 98(19):2098.

Leuchtgens H. (1993). *Crataegus* special extract (WS 1442) in cardiac insufficiency. *Fortschritte der Medizin*. 111:352–354.

Loew D. (1994). Pharmacological and clinical results with *Crataegus* special extracts in cardiac insufficiency. *ESCOP Phytotelegram*. 6:20–26.

Mills S, Bone K. (1999). *Principles and Practice of Phytotherapy.* Edinburgh: Churchill Livingstone.

Nasa Y, et al. (1993). Protective effect of *Crataegus* extract on the cardiac mechanical dysfunction in isolated perfused working heart. *Arzneimittelforschung*. 43(9):945–949.

Reuter H. (1994). *Crataegus* as a herbal cardiac. *Zeitschrift Phytotherapie*. 15:73–81.

Schmidt U, et al. (1994). Efficacy of hawthorn (*Crataegus*) preparation of LI 132 in 78 patients with chronic congestive heart failure. *Phytomedicine*. 1:17–24.

Schussler M, et al. (1995). Myocardial effects of flavonoids from *Crataegus* species. *Arzneimittelforschung*. 45(8):842–845.

Schussler M, et al. (1995). Functional and antiischaemic effects of monoacetyl-vitex-inrhamnoside in different in vitro models. *General Pharmacology*. 26(7):1565–1570.

Tauchert M, et al. (1994). Effectiveness of hawthorn extract LI 132 compared with the ACE inhibitor captopril. *Munch Med*. 136(Suppl):S27–S33.

Upton R. (Ed.). (1999). *American Herbal Pharmacopoeia and Therapeutic Compendium.* Santa Cruz, CA: AHP.

Wagner H, Grevel J. (1982). Cardiotonic drugs IV: Cardiotonic amines from *Crataegus oxycantha*. *Planta Medica*. 45:98–101.

Zapfe G, et al. (1993). *Placebo-controlled multicenter study with Crataegus special extract WS 1442: clinical results in the treatment of NYHA II cardiac insufficiency.* Presented at the 5th Congress on Phytotherapy, June 11, 1993, Bonn, Germany.

NAME: Hops (*Humulus lupulus*)

Common Names: European hops, common hops, lupulin (resin)

Family: *Cannabaceae*

Description of Plant
- Climbing perennial plant with male and female flowers on separate plants
- May attain height of 25 feet
- Cultivated throughout the world
- The only other member of this plant family is cannabis

Medicinal Part: Strobiles (female influorescence) and lupulin (a yellow, sticky powder)

Constituents and Action (if known)
- Bitter principles (15%–25%) consisting of a soft resin and a hard resin
- Humulones (lipophilic soft resins): alpha-acids
- Lupolones (lipophilic soft resins): beta-acids
  - Have antimicrobial activity (Leung, 1996), inhibit the mouth muscles, inhibit tumor promotion in mouse skin (Yasukawa et al., 1995), inhibit arachidonic acid-induced inflammatory ear edema in mice (Yasukawa et al., 1995)
- Xanthohumols: inhibit dracylglycerol (the extramicrosomal hepatic enzyme) (Tabata et al., 1997), may have antiproliferative activity against breast and ovarian cancer (Miranda et al., 1999)
- Essential oils (myrcene, humulene, carophyllene): sedative and hypnotic effects
- Beta-bitter acid: estrogenic activity, but this still needs to be researched (Milligan et al., 1999)

Nutritional Ingredients: Major use as an ingredient and flavoring in beer

Traditional Use
- Diuretic
- Placed in small pillows next to bed to induce sleep

- Digestive bitter useful for nervous stomach and to treat GI tract spasms
- Sedative/anodyne for insomnia, anxiety, nervousness, tension headaches

Current Use: Insomnia, especially with difficulty falling asleep; restlessness, anxiety, and tension caused by stress, usually combined with other sedative botanicals such as valerian, California poppy, chamomile

Available Forms, Dosage, and Administration Guidelines
Typical Dosage
- *Tea:* 1 tsp dried herb to 8 oz hot water, steep 20 minutes; take 4 oz three times a day
- *Capsules:* Up to six 500-mg capsules per day
- *Tincture* (1:5, 60% alcohol): 30 to 60 gtt (1.5–3 mL) up to three times daily

Pharmacokinetics—If Available (form or route when known): None known

Toxicity: Safe in recommended doses

Contraindications: Clinical depression; hops allergies or sensitivities; estrogen-positive tumors because they may be stimulated (Zava et al., 1998), but reports of estrogenic activity in hops have been inconclusive (ESCOP, 1997)

Side Effects: Contact dermatitis to plant; sedation; bronchial irritation when ground herb dust is inhaled

Long-Term Safety: Has been consumed as a part of beer by a large percentage of the world's population for hundreds of years; no adverse response expected

Use in Pregnancy/Lactation/Children: No data; use cautiously

Drug/Herb Interactions and Rationale (if known)
- Use cautiously with central nervous system depressants (anticholinergics, antihistamines, anxiolytics, antidepressants, antipsychotics, alcohol): may cause additive effects

- Use cautiously with drugs metabolized by the cytochrome P-450 system: may cause decreased plasma levels of these drugs (theoretical concern)
- Avoid with phenothiazine-type antipsychotics: may cause additive effects on hyperthermia.

Special Notes: Long storage of hops (more than 1 year) causes the labile soft resin compounds to degrade into hard resin compounds, which are mostly inert.

BIBLIOGRAPHY

ESCOP Monographs on the Medicinal Uses of Plant Drugs. (1997). Exeter: ESCOP.

Goese M, et al. (1999). Biosynthesis of bitter acids in hops. A (13)C-NMR and (2)H-NMR study on the building blocks of humulone. *European Journal of Biochemistry.* 263(2):447–454.

Lawrence Review of Natural Products. (1991). St. Louis: Facts and Comparisons.

Leung AY, Foster S. (1996). *Encyclopedia of Common Natural Ingredients Used in Food, Drugs, and Cosmetics.* New York: John Wiley and Sons.

Milligan SR, et al. (1999). Identification of a potent phytoestrogen in hops (*Humulus lupulus* L.) and beer. *Journal of Clinical Endocrinology & Metabolism.* 84(6):2249–2252.

Miranda CL, et al. (1999). Antiproliferative and cytotoxic effects of prenylated flavonoids from hops (*Humulus lupulus*) in human cancer cell lines. *Food Chemistry & Toxicology.* 37(4):271–285.

Tabata N, et al. (1997). Xanthohumols, diacylglycerol acyltransferase inhibitors, from *Humulus lupulus. Phytochemistry.* 46(4):683–687.

Wichtl M, Bisset NG. (Eds.). (1994). *Herbal Drugs and Phytopharmaceuticals.* Stuttgart: Medpharm.

Yasukawa K, et al. (1995). Humulone, a bitter in the hop, inhibits tumor promotion by 12-P-tetradecanoylphorbol-13 acetate in two-stage carcinogenesis in mouse skin. *Oncology.* 52(2):156–158.

Zava DT, et al. (1998). Estrogen and progestin bioactivity of foods, herbs and spices. *Proceedings of the Society for Experimental Biology & Medicine.* 217:369–378.

NAME: Horse Chestnut (*Aesculus hippocastanum*)

Common Name: Buckeye (often associated with American species that are not used for medicine)

Family: *Hippocastanaceae*

Description of Plant
- Deciduous tree with gray-brown bark; may achieve height of 75 feet
- Cultivated worldwide; has palmate leaves with five to seven leaflets
- Has pink and white flowers that develop into a fruit with a leathery husk containing one to three dark seeds or nuts

Medicinal Part: Seeds

Constituents and Action (if known)
- Escin (Aescin), a complex mixture of triterpene glycosides (saponins): reduces capillary wall permeability, anti-inflammatory activity, potentiates contractile response to norepinephrine, increases venous tone, stabilizes endothelium (Bielanski & Piotrowski, 1999; Diehm et al., 1992; Rehn et al., 1996), reduces cutaneous capillary hyperpermeability induced by histamine or serotonin, thus reducing edema
- Condensed tannins
- Flavones (quercetin, kaempherol)
- Fatty acids

Nutritional Ingredients: None known

Traditional Use
- Hemorrhoids, rectal spasms, neuralgia
- Arthritis, rheumatism, neuralgias
- To relieve venous congestion with dull, aching pain and a feeling of fullness
- Lotions and creams have been used to speed healing of blunt sports injuries.

Current Use
- Improves vascular tone, so it is beneficial in chronic venous insufficiency, varicose veins, hemorrhoids, lymphedema, leg

edema, leg heaviness, and peripheral vascular disease (use with ginkgo, blueberry, or hawthorn)
- Reduces tissue injury in bruises, sprains, and postsurgical trauma
- Reduces nighttime leg cramps, itching, and leg edema
- Topical applications are beneficial for hemorrhoids, varicose veins, and trauma injuries.
- Injectable forms are available in Europe and are used to treat severe head trauma and deep vein thrombosis and to reduce swelling in surgery.

Available Forms, Dosage, and Administration Guidelines

Preparations: Capsules, tablets, tinctures, standardized products. Use products with dosage equivalent to 100 mg escin per day.

Typical Dosage

- *Tablets* (standardized to 40 mg escin): Two or three 200-mg tablets per day
- *Capsules* (dried herb): Two to four 500-mg capsules per day for a maximum of 1 to 2 g per day
- *Tincture* (1:5, 40% alcohol): 30 to 60 gtt (1.5–3 mL) three times a day

Pharmacokinetics—If available (form or route when known):

Saponins are large molecules with low bioavailability when taken orally. They can be hydrolyzed by the gut flora, and the sapogenins or liver metabolites may be the primary active form of escin.

Toxicity: Bark, leaves, and fruit capsules are potentially toxic. FDA classifies it as unsafe because of glycosides, saponins, and esculin. Signs of toxicity include muscle twitching, weakness, dilated pupils, vomiting, diarrhea, paralysis, stupor, and hepatic injury. The seed and its extract have a very low risk associated with oral or topical use in the recommended dosage.

Contraindications: Do not use topically on broken or ulcerated skin.

Side Effects: Rarely, nausea, stomach upset, urticaria

Long-Term Safety: Long-term use in Europe and many clinical studies show no problems associated with long-term use.

Use in Pregnancy/Lactation/Children: Horse chestnut seed extracts have been used in numerous clinical studies that included pregnant women. Some studies excluded women in their third trimester. No adverse effects have been reported, but do not use without a clinician's recommendation. Avoid use in breast-feeding woman and children.

Drug/Herb Interactions and Rationale (if known): None known

Special Notes: Many European companies are including this herb or its purified extract escin in cosmetics for sensitive skin, pimples, and sunburn.

BIBLIOGRAPHY

Bielanski TE, Piotrowski ZH. (1999). Horse-chestnut seed extract for chronic venous insufficiency. *Journal of Family Practice*. 48(3):171–172.

Blumenthal M, et al. (2000). *Herbal Medicine: Expanded Commission E Monographs*. Austin, TX: American Botanical Council.

Bombardelli E, et al. (1996). A review: *Aesculus hippocastanum L. Fitoterpia*. 67:483–511.

Diehm C, et al. (1992). Medical edema protection: clinical benefits in patients with deep vein incompetence. A placebo-controlled, double-blind study. *Vasa*. 21:188–192.

Diehm C, et al. (1996). Comparison of leg compression stocking and oral horse chestnut seed extract in patients with chronic venous insufficiency. *Lancet*. 347:292–294.

ESCOP Monographs on the Medicinal Uses of Plant Drugs. (1999). Exeter: ESCOP.

Greeske K, Pohlmann BK. (1996). Horse chestnut seed extract: an effective therapy principle in general practice. Drug therapy of chronic venous insufficiency. *Fortschritte der Medizin*. 114(15):196–200.

Lawrence Review of Natural Products. (1998). St. Louis: Facts and Comparisons.

Mills S, Bone K. (1999). *Principles and Practice of Phytotherapy*. Edinburgh: Churchill Livingstone.

Pittler MH, Ernst E. (1998). Horse-chestnut seed extract for chronic venous insufficiency. A criteria-based systematic review. *Archives of Dermatology*. 134(11):1356–1360.

Rehn D, et al. (1996). Comparative clinical efficacy and tolerability of oxerutins and horse chestnut extract in patients with chronic venous insufficiency. *Arzneimittelforschung.* 5:483–487.

Steiner M. (1991). Conservative therapy of chronic venous insufficiency. The extent of the edema-preventive effect of horse chestnut seed extract. *Vasa.* 33(Suppl):217.

NAME: Huang Qin (*Scutellaria baicalensis*)

Common Names: Scute root, baical scullcap

Family: *Lamiaceae*

Description of Plant

- A small perennial member of the mint family with blue-violet flowers
- Grows in dry, sandy soils in the mountains of northeast and southwest China

Medicinal Part: Root

Constituents and Action (if known)

- Flavones and flavone glycosides
  - Baicalein: antiallergic effect, inhibits histamine release from mast cells (Bensky & Gamble, 1992), choleretic, antioxidant, anti-inflammatory, antileukemic, renal protective (Bone, 1996)
  - Baicalin (6.4%–17%): central nervous system sedative, or antitumor
  - Wogonin: inhibited platelet aggregation
  - Wogonoside
  - Norwogonin
  - Scullcap flavone I, II
  - Scutellarein
- The extract inhibits phosphodiesterase, which increases cAMP and causes antiplatelet activity and hypotensive (vasodilation) effects (Bone, 1996).
- The herb has broad-spectrum antibacterial activity against *Staphylococcus aureus, Corynebacterium diphtheriae, Pseudomonas aeruginosa, Streptococcus pneumoniae,* and *Neisseria meningitidis.*

Nutritional Ingredients: None

Traditional Use: Antibacterial, antiallergic, diuretic, anti-inflammatory, antipyretic, hypotensive, choleretic. In traditional Chinese medicine, scute root clears damp heat conditions (diarrhea, dysentery, bronchitis with profuse yellow, green, or bloody sputum, urinary tract infections with painful urination, and hematuria). The root is also used topically for boils, as an adjunct for treating damp heat jaundice (hepatitis), to prevent miscarriage, and for liver fire symptoms (headache, red, painful eyes, red head or ears, and a persistent bitter taste in the mouth).

Current Use

- Hyperimmune response: useful for reducing histamine release from mast cells (allergic hives, allergic asthma, allergic rhinitis). Also can be useful with immune amphoterics such as reishi, grifola, or licorice for autoimmune conditions (rheumatoid arthritis, scleroderma, lupus).
- Chronic hepatitis: may be used with milk thistle, turmeric, schisandra to prevent and treat liver disease
- Useful with other antibacterial agents for acute respiratory, urinary tract, and bowel infections
- Mild hypertension has been effectively treated with huang qin.

Available Forms, Dosage, and Administration Guidelines

Typical Dosage

- *Dried herb:* 2 to 6 g per day
- *Tea:* 1 tsp dried root in 8 oz hot water, decoct 15 minutes, steep 40 minutes; take two or three cups per day
- *Tincture* (1:5, 45% alcohol): 30 to 80 gtt (1.5–4 mL) three times a day

Pharmacokinetics—If Available (form or route when known): Not known

Toxicity: Low potential for toxicity

Contraindications: Chronic low-grade (cold) diarrhea

Side Effects: Rarely, gastrointestinal disturbance and diarrhea

Long-Term Safety: Safe when used in normal therapeutic doses

Use in Pregnancy/Lactation/Children: Traditionally used to prevent miscarriage. Use under professional supervision only.

Drug/Herb Interactions and Rationale (if known): Theoretical interaction with blood thinners; use cautiously together

Special Notes: Like most Chinese herbs, it is rarely if ever used alone. It is combined with other herbs based on classic formulas.

BIBLIOGRAPHY

Bensky D, Gamble A. (1992). *Chinese Herbal Medicine: Materia Medica*. Seattle: Eastland Press.

Bone K. (1996). *Clinical Applications of Ayurvedic and Chinese Herbs*. Queensland, Australia: Phytotherapy Press.

Chung CP, et al. (1995). Pharmacological effects of methanolic extract from the root of *Scutellaria baicalensis* and its flavonoids on human gingival fibroblast. *Planta Medica.* 61(2):150–153.

Foster S. (1992). *Herbal Emissaries*. Rochester, VT: Healing Arts Press.

Gao Z, et al. (1999). Free radical scavenging and antioxidant activities of flavonoids extracted from the radix of *Scutellaria baicalensis* Georgi. *Biochima et Biophysica Acta.* 1472(3):643–650.

Hui KM, et al. (2000). Interaction of flavones from the roots of *Scutellaria baicalensis* with the benzodiazepine site. *Planta Medica.* 66(1):91–93.

Smolianinov ES, et al. (1997). Effect of *Scutellaria baicalensis* extract on the immunologic status of patients with lung cancer receiving antineoplastic chemotherapy. *Eksperimentalna Klinika Farmakologiia.* 60(6):49–51.

Tang W, Eisenbrand G. (1992). *Chinese Drugs of Plant Origin*. Berlin: Springer-Verlag.

You-ping Z. (1998). *Chinese Materia Medica: Chemistry Pharmacology and Applications*. Amsterdam: Harwood.

NAME: Hyssop (*Hyssopus officinalis*)

Common Name: Hysope (French)

Family: *Lamiaceae*

Description of Plant
- Aromatic perennial member of the mint family, originally from Mediterranean, now cultivated throughout the United States, Britain, and Canada
- Tubular blue-purple flowers bloom July to October, grows 2 feet tall, similar to other members of the mint family in appearance

Medicinal Part: Dried leaves

Constituents and Action (if known)
- Tannins: antiviral activity against herpes simplex when applied topically (Gollapudi et al., 1995)
- Volatile oils (pinocamphone, isopinocamphone, alpha- and beta-pinene, camphene, alpha-terpenene): make up 70% of the essential oil
- Glucosides (hyssopin)
- Rosmarinic acid: antioxidant
- Marubin
- Flavonoids (diosmin and hesperidin)
- Polysaccharides (MR-10) have anti-HIV activity.

Nutritional Ingredients: Used as a flavoring for liqueurs (Chartreuse, Benedictine), puddings, and candies

Traditional Use
- Antibacterial, antiviral, carminative, diaphoretic, expectorant, emmenagogue, antispasmodic
- Antibacterial/antiviral for colds, influenza, sore throats, bronchitis, and pneumonia
- Expectorant for damp coughs
- Emmenagogue for delayed menses
- Antispasmodic for petit mal seizures
- Carminative for digestive upset, gas, and intestinal viruses
- Essential oil used as an insect repellent, insecticide, and pediculicide; used in perfumery

Current Use

- Gargle for sore throats; mix with thyme, sage, or Chinese coptis
- Expectorant and antiviral for bronchitis, viral pneumonia, bronchial catarrh, colds and flu
- Demonstrates antiviral activity (extracts of dried leaves); use topically for herpes infections (oral or genital), mix with lemon balm
- Promotes menstrual flow: for delayed menses (due to stress, travel) or menses with a scanty, clotty flow

Available Forms, Dosage, and Administration Guidelines

Preparations: Dried herb, cut and sifted or powdered; capsules, tinctures, combination products

Typical Dosage

- *Capsules:* Up to six 400- to 500-mg capsules per day
- *Tea:* Steep 1 tsp dried herb in 1 cup hot water (covered) for 10 to 15 minutes; take three times a day for cough, colds.
- *Tincture* (1:5, 40% alcohol): 40 to 60 gtt (2–3 mL) up to four times a day. Or follow manufacturer's or practitioner's recommendations.

Pharmacokinetics—If Available (form or route when known): Unknown

Toxicity: Safe for short-term use at recommended doses

Contraindications: None known

Side Effects: Stomach upset, nausea, diarrhea

Long-Term Safety: Generally recognized as safe by the FDA

Use in Pregnancy/Lactation/Children: Emmenagogue: do not use

Drug/Herb Interactions and Rationale (if known): None known

Special Notes: The essential oil, like all essential oils, is highly concentrated and can be toxic if used internally in excess dosage. Topically it is nonirritating and nonsensitizing to human skin.

BIBLIOGRAPHY

Bartram T. (1995). *Encyclopedia of Herbal Medicine.* Dorset: Grace Publishers.

Gollapudi S, et al. (1995). Isolation of a previously unidentified polysaccharide (MAR-10) from *Hyssop officinalis* that exhibits strong activity against human immunodeficiency virus type 1. *Biochemistry and Biophysics Research Communications.* 210(1):145.

Gruenwald J, et al. (Eds.). (1998). *PDR for Herbal Medicine.* Montvale, NJ: Medical Economics.

Kreis W, et al. (1990). Inhibition of HIV replication by *Hyssop officinalis* extracts. *Antiviral Research.* 14(6):323–338.

Lawrence Review of Natural Products. (1996). St. Louis: Facts and Comparisons.

K

 NAME: Kava Kava (*Piper methysticum*)

Common Names: Ava, awa, kawa, kava, yagana

Family: *Piperaceae*

Description of Plant
- Sprawling shrub in the black pepper family
- Cultivated throughout the South Pacific
- More than 20 varieties have been identified

Medicinal Part: 4- to 6-year-old dried root

Constituents and Action (if known)
- Resins: kava lactones (kava pyrones; 5%–9%)—sedative activity (Lehmann, 1996; Singh et al. 1998) induces sleep; local anesthetic activity through nonopiate pathways
  ○ Methysticin: local anesthetic activity, skeletal muscle relaxant (Lindenburg, 1990; Munte, 1993)
  ○ Kavain: mild sedative, analgesic, and muscle-relaxing effects, similar to lidocaine
- Flavonoids (flavokavains)
- Kava modifies GABA receptors in brain, reduces anxiety (Bone, 1993/4; Lehmann, 1996; Singh et al. 1998; Voltz & Kieser, 1997)

- May act directly on the limbic system
- Suppresses emotional excitability (Munte, 1993) and enhances mood, possibly by binding with GABA receptors; blocks norepinephrine uptake; fungistatic activity.

Nutritional Ingredients: None known

Traditional Use

- Antispasmodic, anxiolytic, diuretic, topical and urinary anodyne, sedative
- Used for hundreds of years by natives of the South Pacific islands as a ceremonial and celebratory nonalcoholic, calming drink
- Also used by South Pacific islanders to treat gonorrhea, urinary conditions, bronchitis, rheumatism, headaches, colds, and sore throats and to enhance wound healing
- Eclectic physicians used kava for urinary tract pain, renal colic, chronic urethritis, neuralgias (optic, trigeminal), mouth and throat pain, and dyspepsia.

Current Use

- Relieves anxiety, nervousness, and tension without affecting alertness. German studies have shown that kava is as effective a treatment for anxiety disorders as tricyclic antidepressants and benzodiazepines, without the side effects and tolerance issues.
- Relieves tension headaches and muscle spasms: restless leg syndrome, back pain, torticollis, temporomandibular joint pain
- Relieves insomnia, enhances rapid eye movement sleep without morning grogginess
- Relieves menopausal anxiety and sleep disorders; may also help other menopausal symptoms, including hot flashes
- May be used for pain control (analgesia through nonopiate pathways): urinary tract pain, muscle pain, mouth and throat pain, fibromyalgia (with black cohosh)
- In Europe, combined with pumpkin seeds to treat irritable bladder syndrome
- May have some antiseizure activity through the GABA receptors

Available Forms, Dosage, and Administration Guidelines

Preparations: Dried root, capsules, tablets, tinctures
Typical Dosage
Absorption may be enhanced if taken with food. Do not use more than 3 to 4 months continuously for self-diagnosed anxiety and sleep disorders.

- *Dried root:* 1.5 to 3 g per day
- *Capsules:* Up to six 400- to 500-mg capsules a day (100–200 mg kava lactones per day)
- *Tea:* 1 to 2 tsp of the dried, cut, sifted root to 8 oz boiling water, decoct 10 to 15 minutes, steep 30 minutes; take 4 oz two or three times per day.
- *Tincture* (1:3, 60% alcohol): 30 to 60 gtt (1.5–3 mL) in water up to three times a day
- Or follow manufacturer's or practitioner's recommendations

Pharmacokinetics—If Available (form or route when known): Metabolism of kava lactones is more rapid and three to five times higher when ingesting whole root extracts rather than isolated lactone extracts.

Toxicity

- Skin discoloration (yellowing of skin, hair, nails), or "kava dermopathy," occurs with abuse only. It may be caused by disruption of cholesterol metabolism (Mills & Bone, 1999).
- Chronic ingestion in large excessive doses may lead to kawaism: dry, flaking, discolored skin, blood count abnormalities (increased red blood cells, decreased platelets, decreased lymphocytes), some pulmonary hypertension, and reddened eyes (also possibly related to interference with cholesterol metabolism). All symptoms are reversible when kava intake is stopped.
- Some authors believe alcohol may increase toxicity, but Herberg's 1993 study showed no synergistic effects or increased toxicity when combining kava with moderate levels of alcohol.

Contraindications: Parkinson's disease: tremors may increase

Side Effects: Changes in motor reflexes and judgment (Spillane et al., 1997), visual disturbances. With chronic, heavy use, low platelet and white blood cell counts; dry, flaky, yellow skin; increased patellar reflexes; shortness of breath; pulmonary hypertension; reduced plasma proteins.

Long-Term Safety: Safe in moderate doses and short term. Kava abuse is a possibility. Withdrawal symptoms have occurred on discontinuation.

Use in Pregnancy/Lactation/Children: Do not use during pregnancy and while breast-feeding; safety is unknown in children.

Drug/Herb Interactions and Rationale (if known)

- Do not use with antiparkinsonian drugs: may increase tremors and make medications less effective.
- May potentiate action of alcohol (Herberg, 1993), tranquilizers (barbiturates), and antidepressants. In one case a patient taking kava and alprazolam was admitted to the hospital in a lethargic and disoriented state; may have been a drug/herb interaction (Almeida et al., 1996).

Special Notes: Research demonstrates that Kava can be an alternative to benzodiazepines and tricyclic antidepressants in anxiety disorders. Take care when operating machinery or driving a vehicle. Do not take kava if depression is present.

BIBLIOGRAPHY

Almeida J, et al. (1996). Coma from health food store: interaction between kava and alprazolam. *Annals of Internal Medicine.* 125:940.

Blumenthal M, et al. (2000). *Herbal Medicine: Expanded Commission E Monographs.* Austin, TX: American Botanical Council.

Bone K. (1993/4). Kava: a safe herbal treatment for anxiety. *British Journal of Phytotherapy.* 3(4):147–153.

Cantor C: Kava and alcohol. *Medical Journal of Australia.* 167:560, 1997.

Herberg KW. (1993). Effect of kava special extract WS 1490 combined with ethyl alcohol on safety relevant performance parameters. *Blutalkohol.* 30:96–105.

Jussogie A, et al. (1994). Kavapyrone extract enriched from *Piper methysticum* as modulator of the GABA binding site in different regions of the rat brain. *Psychopharmacology* (Berlin). 116:469-74.

Lehmann E. (1996). Efficacy of a special kava extract (*Piper methysticum*) in patients with states of anxiety, tension and excitedness of non-mental origin: a double-blind placebo-controlled study of four weeks of treatment. *Phytomedicine.* 3:113–119.

Lindenburg DL. (1990). Kavain in comparison with oxazepam in anxiety disorders. A double-blind study of clinical effectiveness. *Fortschritte fur Medizin.* 108:49–50.

Mills S, Bone K. (1999). *Principles and Practice of Phytotherapy.* Edinburgh: Churchill Livingstone.

Munte TF. (1993). Effects of oxazepam and an extract of kava roots on event-related potentials in a word recognition task. *Neuropsychobiology.* 27:46–53.

Norton S, Ruze P. (1994). Kava dermopathy. *Journal of the American Academy of Dermatology.* 31(1):89–97.

Pittler MH, Ernst E. (2000). Efficacy of kava extract for treating anxiety: systematic review and meta-analysis. *Journal of Clinical Psychopharmacology.* 20(1):84–89.

Ruze P. (1990). Kava-induced dermopathy: a niacin deficiency? *Lancet.* 335(8703):1442–1445.

Singh NN, et al. (1998). A double-blind, placebo controlled study of the effects of kava (Kavatrol) on daily stress and anxiety in adults. *Alternative Therapies.* 4(2):97–98.

Spillane PK, et al. (1997). Neurological manifestations of kava intoxication. *Medical Journal of Australia.* 167:172–173.

Voltz HP, Kieser M. (1997). Kava-kava extract WS 1490 versus placebo in anxiety disorders: a randomized placebo-controlled 25-week outpatient trial. *Pharmacopsychiatry.* 30(1):1–5.

NAME: Kudzu (*Pueraria lobata, P. thomsonii*)

Common Names: Kuzu, ge gen (Chinese), *Pueraria montana* (synonym)

Family: *Fabaceae*

Description of Plant

- A fast-growing perennial vine native to China, Korea, Japan, Burma, and Thailand
- Introduced into the southeastern United States to control erosion, it has now become an aggressive weed.

Medicinal Part: Dried root (usually with the outer bark removed)

Constituents and Action (if known)
- Isoflavones and isoflavone glycosides (average 7.6%)
  - Puerarin: inhibits platelet aggregation and is a beta-adrenergic blocking agent in vitro
  - Daidzein: immunostimulant
  - Daidzein-4, 7-diglucoside, formononetin, genistin: antioxidant, anticancer, antihepatoxic, spasmolytic
- Coumestan derivative (puerarol)
- Aromatic glycosides (puerosides A and B)
- Sapogenins (kudzusapogenols A, B, C, sophoradiol): anti-inflammatory
- Starch (up to 27%): demulcent
- Root extracts (20 g) for 14 days modestly reduced elevated blood pressure in renal hypertensive dogs. The root is a vasodilator, reducing peripheral vascular resistance (You-Ping, 1998).

Nutritional Ingredients: Used in Japanese cooking as a thickening agent. The root is used in Chinese cuisine in soups and stir-fries.

Traditional Use
- Antipyretic, antispasmodic, decongestant, demulcent, cardiotonic, hypotensive, vasodilator
- Flowers (gehua) are used to treat alcohol poisoning (hangovers).
- In traditional Chinese medicine, kudzu root is used to reduce fevers and associated headaches, stiff neck, and muscle pain. It is also indicated to treat diarrhea, dysentery, and constant thirst and to promote the eruption of measles.

Current Use
- Useful for treating irritable bowel syndrome, diarrhea, dysentery, and mucous colitis. Combine with sarsaparilla, yarrow, wild yam, and chamomile.
- One hundred ten patients were given an extract (6:1) of pueraria and hawthorn for angina pain. Ninety percent experienced pain relief, and 43% had improved electrocardiograms. This combination can also be used for mild congestive heart failure.

- Torticollis: this root is very useful for treating stiff neck caused by fevers and hypertension. In hypertensive patients, it also improves other symptoms, including headaches, tinnitus, vertigo, and numbness of the extremities (You-ping, 1998).
- In laboratory studies, alcoholic Syrian golden hamsters voluntarily and significantly reduced their alcohol consumption when given a water extract of kudzu. In clinical practice, some patients have reduced (not stopped) their alcohol consumption; others have seen no benefits from this herb. Additional research would be appropriate.
- A mild decongestant, pueraria can be effective for allergic rhinitis, sinus headaches, and painful otitis media.

Available Forms, Dosage, and Administration Guidelines
- Dried root, tea, capsules, and tincture

Typical Dosage
- *Dried root:* 9 to 15 g
- *Tea:* 1 to 2 tsp dried root in 8 oz water, decoct 20 minutes, steep 30 minutes; take two or three cups per day
- *Capsules* (4:1 extract): Two 500-mg capsules three times a day
- *Tincture* (1:5, 40% alcohol): 40 to 80 gtt (2–4 mL) four times a day

Pharmacokinetics—If Available (form or route when known): Peurarin is quickly but only partially absorbed: 37% was recovered from rat feces in 24 hours.

Toxicity: Safe: long history of use as a food and medicine. Large doses in animals produced no toxic effects.

Contraindications: Do not use kudzu tincture to reduce alcohol cravings.

Side Effects: None known

Long-Term Safety: Safe

Use in Pregnancy/Lactation/Children: Safe

Drug/Herb Interactions and Rationale (if known): None known

Special Notes: Kudzu is an amazing plant. It has taken over the southeastern United States and is considered a noxious and invasive weed. At the same time, the plant can provide medicine (root, flower), food (root starch, root, and young leaves), animal fodder (leaves), and basketry materials (vines) and can provide a source of pulp for paper.

BIBLIOGRAPHY

Chang HM, But P. (1987). *Pharmacology and Applications of Chinese Materia Medica.* Singapore: World Scientific.

de Padua LS, et al. (1999). *Plant Resources of Southeast Asia—Medicinal and Poisonous Plants.* Leiden, Germany: Backhuys Publishing.

Kueng W, et al. (1998). Kudzu root: an ancient Chinese source of modern antidipsotropic agents. *Phytochemistry.* 47(4):499–506.

Leung A, Foster S. (1996). *Encyclopedia of Common Natural Ingredients.* New York: John Wiley & Son.

Tang W, Eisenbrand G. (1992). *Chinese Drugs of Plant Origin.* Berlin: Springer-Verlag.

Winston D. (2000). *Herbal Therapeutics, Specific Indications for Herbs and Herbal Formulas* (7th ed.). Washington, NJ: Herbal Therapeutics Research Library.

Xie C, et al. (1994). Daidzein, an antioxidant isoflavonoid, decreases blood alcohol levels and shortens sleep time induced by ethanol intoxication. *Alcohol Clinical & Experimental Research.* 18(6):1443-1447.

You-ping Z. (1998). *Chinese Materia Medica, Chemistry, Pharmacology, and Applications.* Amsterdam: Harwood.

L

 NAME: Lavender (*Lavendula angustifolia*)

Common Names: English lavender, True lavender

Family: *Lamiaceae*

Description of Plant
- A strongly aromatic, shrubby member of the mint family with blue flowers
- Native to the low mountains of the Mediterranean

Medicinal Part: Dried flowers and essential oil (EO)

Constituents and Action (if known)

- Volatile oils (1%–5%): linalool (25%–38%), linalyl acetate (25%–45%), antispasmodic, inhibited caffeine stimulation by 50%, relaxant, camphor, B-ocimene, and cineole
- Hydroxycoumarins (umbelliferone, herniarin, coumarin)
- Caffeic acid derivatives (rosmarinic acid): antioxidant, anti-inflammatory, antiallergic
- Flavonoids (luteolin): antimutagenic
- Tannins (up to 12%)

Nutritional Ingredients: Flowers are occasionally used in baking cookies and tea cakes. The essential oil is used in tooth powders.

Traditional Use

- Antibacterial, antidepressant, carminative, cholagogue, nervine, rubefacient
- Used for digestive disturbances including gas, nausea, vomiting, biliousness, poor fat digestion, intestinal colic, and nervous stomach
- Used with St. John's wort and lemon balm for "stagnant" depression
- The tea has a long history of use for irritability, insomnia, headaches, and seizures.
- The essential oil has been used topically (diluted) for muscle pain, arthralgias, neuralgia, and Bell's palsy.

Current Use

- Effective treatment for flatulence, borborygmus, nervous stomach, and abdominal bloating. Mix with fennel or chamomile.
- Essential oil (1–2 gtt) in a sitz bath is antibacterial and anti-inflammatory; promotes healing for episiotomy incisions. Essential oil can also be used topically for first- and small second-degree burns, athlete's foot, cuts, and muscle pain. Essential oil, used in aromatherapy, has been effective for anxiety, restlessness, and insomnia of old age and menopause.
- Lavender baths are calming and mildly sedating for occasional insomnia, irritability, premenstrual anger, and stress-induced headaches.

Available Forms, Dosage, and Administration Guidelines

- *Tea:* 1 tsp dried flowers in 8 oz hot water, steep covered for 20 to 30 minutes; take 4 oz three times a day
- *Tincture:* (1:5, 70% alcohol) 30–40 gtt (1.5–2 mL) three to four times a day
- *Essential oil:* 1 to 2 gtt two or three times a day

Pharmacokinetics—If Available (form or route when known): Not known

Toxicity: Herb: none known; essential oil in overdose can be toxic

Contraindications: None known

Side Effects: Herb: none known; essential oil rarely causes skin irritation

Long-Term Safety: Safe

Use in Pregnancy/Lactation/Children: No adverse effects expected from the herb. Avoid using the essential oil internally during pregnancy.

Drug/Herb Interactions and Rationale (if known): None known

Special Notes: Lavender's enduring popularity as a medicine and its use in cosmetics and perfumes has a great deal to do with its odor's ability to alter mood via the olfactory receptors.

BIBLIOGRAPHY
Bisset NG, Wichtl M. (1994). *Herbal Drugs and Phytopharmaceuticals.* Stuttgart: Medpharm.
Blumenthal M, et al. (2000). *Herbal Medicine: Expanded Commission E Monographs.* Austin, TX: American Botanical Council.
Bruneton J. (1999). *Pharmacognosy, Phytochemistry, Medicinal Plants* (2nd ed.). Paris: Lavoisier.
Cornwall S, Dale A. (1995). Lavender oil and perineal repair. *Modern Midwife.* 5(3):31–33.
Fisher C, Painter G. (1996). *Materia Medica of Western Herbs for the Southern Hemisphere.* Auckland, NZ: Authors..
Integrative Medicine Access. (2000). *Lavender.* Newton, MA: Integrative Medicine Communications.

Schulz V, et al. (1998). *Rational Phytotherapy* (3d ed.). Berlin: Springer-Verlag.

Tisserand R, Balics T. (1995). *Essential Oil Safety.* Edinburgh: Churchill Livingstone.

Weiss RF. (1988). *Herbal Medicine.* Beaconsfield, England: Beaconsfield Publishing.

NAME: Lemon balm (*Melissa officinalis*)

Common Names: Balm, melissa, sweet balm

Family: *Lamiaceae*

Description of Plant
- Low perennial herb in the mint family with ovate or heart-shaped leaves
- Has a lemon odor when leaves are rubbed
- Indigenous to Mediterranean but is cultured world-wide

Medicinal Part: Fresh or dried leaves harvested before flowers bloom

Constituents and Action (if known)
- Essential oil (0.2%–0.5%), monoterpenoids, citronellal: sedative and antispasmodic properties (Hener et al., 1995), geranial, neral
  - Sesqueterpenes (beta-caryophyllene, germacrene D)
  - Essential oil is antibacterial, antiviral, and antifungal (Bruneton, 1999).
- Flavonoids (quercitrin, rhamnocitrin, the 7-glucosides of apigenin, and luteolin)
- Phenolic acids (rosmarinic acid, caffeic acid—up to 4.0%): antioxidant effects (may have an effect 10 times greater than vitamin C and E); antiviral activity against herpes simplex cold sores (Hausen & Schulze, 1986; Wobling et al., 1994)
- Freeze-dried extracts bind thyroid-stimulating immunoglobulin and may reduce circulating thyroid hormone.
- Inhibits C3 and C5 in complement cascade, thus reducing inflammation (Peake et al., 1991)

Nutritional Ingredients: Used as a beverage tea

Traditional Use
- Carminative for gas, nausea, and digestive disturbances of children and adults
- Diaphoretic: useful for children's fevers, mixes well with elder flower and peppermint
- Steeped in wine, the ancient Greeks used it as a surgical dressing for wounds and to treat venomous bites and stings.

Current Use
- Headache relief (stress-induced)
- Relieves nervousness, has a mild sedative effect, improves sleep, reduces restlessness and overexcitability (children with attention deficit disorder)
- Antiviral: relieves symptoms and improves healing of herpes simplex cold sores (topically)
- Shown to interfere with cholinesterase, which breaks down acetylcholine; thus, may be helpful in lowering the incidence or slowing the progression of Alzheimer's disease (Perry et al., 1996). In ancient Greece, lemon balm was thought to strengthen the mind, and students wore sprigs of lemon balm in their hair as they studied.
- Mild antidepressant: can be useful for seasonal affective disorder when mixed with St. John's wort
- Thyroxin antagonist: used for hyperthyroidism and Graves' disease; use with buglewood and motherwort
- Gastrointestinal disturbances: epigastric bloating, flatulence, eructations

Available Forms, Dosage, and Administration Guidelines
- *Cream:* Apply as directed at early stages of cold sores and genital herpes
- *Capsules:* 300- to 400-mg capsules up to nine times a day
- *Tea:* steep 1 to 2 tsp dried herb in 1 cup hot water for 10 to 15 minutes; take two to four cups a day
- *Tincture* (1:5, 30% alcohol): 60 to 90 gtt (3–5 mL), three to four times a day

Pharmacokinetics—If Available (form or route when known): None known

Toxicity: None known

Contraindications: None known

Side Effects: None known

Long-Term Safety: Safe

Use in Pregnancy/Lactation/Children: Safe

Drug/Herb Interactions and Rationale (if known): Avoid use with thyroid drugs. Large doses may act as a thyroxin antagonist and affect the action of medications such as levothyroxine.

Special Notes: The essential oil, used in aromatherapy, may be beneficial for mild depression.

BIBLIOGRAPHY

Aufmkolk M, et al. (1985a). Extracts and auto-oxidized constituents of certain plants inhibit the receptor-binding and biological activity of Graves' immunoglobulins. *Endocrinology.* 116(5):1687.

Aufmkolk M, et al. (1985b). The active principles of plant extracts with antithyrotropic activity: oxidation products of derivatives of 3,4-dihydroxycinnamic acid. *Endocrinology.* 116(5):1677.

Blumenthal M. (2000). *Herbal Medicine: Expanded Commission E Monographs.* Austin, TX: American Botanical Council.

Bruneton J. (1999). *Pharmacognosy, Phytochemistry, Medicinal Plants* (2nd ed.). Paris: Lavoisier.

Hener U, et al. (1995). Evaluation of authenticity of balm oil (*Melissa officinalis* L). *Pharmazie.* 50(1):60.

Peake PW, et al. (1991). The inhibitory effect of rosmarinic acid on complement involves the C5 convertase. *International Journal of Immunopharmacology.* 13(7):853.

Perry N, et al. (1996). European herbs with cholinergic activities: potential in dementia therapy. *International Journal of Geriatric Psychiatry.* 11(12):1063–1069.

Review of Natural Products. (1999). St. Louis: Facts and Comparisons.

Wichtl M, Bisset NG. (Eds.). (1994). *Herbal Drugs and Phytopharmaceuticals.* Stuttgart: Medpharm.

 NAME: Licorice (*Glycyrrhiza glabra*)

Common Names: Sweet root, Persian licorice, Spanish licorice, Chinese licorice (*G. uralensis*)

Family: *Fabiaceae*

Description of Plant

- Shrub 4 to 5 feet tall, cultivated in Turkey, Spain, Pakistan, and China
- Glycyrrhiza means "sweet root;" the yellow rhizome is intensely sweet.
- Spanish licorice has pealike blue flowers; Chinese licorice has pale yellow flowers.

Medicinal Part: Rhizome

Constituents and Action (if known)

- Triterpenoid: glycyrrhizin (glycyrrhizic acid)—content varies (2%–6%) depending on growing season and soil
  - Demulcent, expectorant properties
  - Pseudoaldosterone effects (sodium retention, hypertension, and edema) may be seen with doses of 700 to 1,400 mg licorice per day (Bernardi et al., 1994).
  - Suppresses scalp sebum secretion (10% glycyrrhizin shampoo) for an additional 24 hours compared with citric acid shampoo (Snow, 1996).
  - Binds to mineralocorticoid and glucocorticoid receptors in vitro (Farese et al., 1991; MacKenzie et al., 1990)
  - Reduces mucosal injury associated with aspirin administration; may increase gastric mucosal blood flow (Johnston & McIssac, 1981; Van Marle et al., 1981)
  - Inhibits production of oxygen free radicals by neutrophils (Akamatsu et al., 1991)
  - Mild anti-inflammatory and antiarthritic activity
  - May enhance clearance of immune complexes, so may benefit autoimmune disease (Matsumoto, 1996)
  - Stimulates gastric mucosa repair (LaBrooy et al., 1979; Maxton et al., 1990)
- Flavonoids (1%–1.5%; liquiritin, isoliquiritin, glabrol)
- Isoflavones (formononetin, glabrone)
- Coumarins

Nutritional Ingredients: Used as a sweetening and flavoring agent. Licorice is 50 times sweeter than sugar and is used in candies and liqueurs. Contains starches and sugars (glucose, mannose, sucrose).

Traditional Use

- Adaptogen, carminative, expectorant, antispasmodic, anti-inflammatory, immune amphoteric, antiviral, antihepatotoxin
- Used by ancient Greek and Roman physicians such as Hippocrates and Pliny the Elder (23 AD) as an expectorant for asthma and dry coughs and as a carminative
- In China, licorice is one of the most frequently prescribed herbs. It is used to treat sore throats and sticky, hard-to-expectorate mucus; to tonify the stomach, spleen, and lungs, to control abdominal spasms; and as an antidote for poisonous substances.

Current Use

- Expectorant, antitussive (similar to codeine): useful for bronchial congestion, spastic coughs, pertussis, bronchitis, and allergies
- Mild systemic anti-inflammatory: similar in action to cortisone
- Soothes irritated mucous membranes (gastritis, gastric and duodenal ulcer, irritable bowel syndrome, and sore throat)
- Heals herpetic lesions and shingles (topical use)
- Antihepatotoxin and antiviral activity (intravenous): has shown benefits in Japanese studies with patients with active hepatitis C (Arase et al., 1997)
- Used to support adrenal exhaustion and mild cases of Addison's disease (Mills & Bone, 1999)
- Immune amphoteric and adaptogen: studies have shown that licorice is beneficial for autoimmune conditions such as lupus and possibly immune deficiency conditions such as chronic fatigue syndrome (Baschetti, 1995) and HIV/AIDS (Mills & Bone, 1999)
- Inhibits low-density lipoprotein cholesterol peroxidation
- Postural hypertension because of its pseudoaldosterone activity
- Polycystic ovarian disease: licorice, along with white peony, was given to eight women in an uncontrolled study. After 8 weeks, serum testosterone levels had become normal in seven patients and six of the women were ovulating regularly (Mills & Bone, 1999).

- Peptic ulcer: shown in clinical studies to be as effective as cimetidine for treating ulcers, and has a superior ability to prevent recurrence
- Improves vasovagal syncope

Available Forms, Dosage, and Administration Guidelines

Preparations: Dried root whole, sliced, cut and sifted; capsules; extracts; tablets; tinctures; standardized products. European products are formulated to deliver 5 to 15 g (1–2 tsp) root, which contains 200 to 600 mg glycyrrhizin. Several studies have assessed the efficacy of deglycyrrhizinated licorice (DGL), in which all the glycyrrhizin is removed, with inconclusive results. DGL products show none of the serious side effects associated with licorice.

Typical Dosage:

- *Capsules:* Up to six 400- to 500-mg capsules a day for no more than 4 to 6 weeks
- *Tincture* (1:5, 30% alcohol): 30 to 60 gtt (1.5–3 mL) up to three times a day
- *Powdered root:* 1 to 2 g one to three times a day
- *Solid (dry powder) extract* (4:1): 250 to 500 mg (adverse effects may occur with 100 mg/day)
- *DGL extract:* 380 to 760 mg three times a day
- Or follow manufacturer's or practitioner's recommendations

Pharmacokinetics—If Available (form or route when known): Studies have shown that glycyrrhizin is less bioavailable and has less toxicity when given in a whole extract rather than as an isolated substance (Cantelli-Forti et al., 1994).

Toxicity: A mineralocorticoid-like effect can occur that can cause lethargy, headache, hypertension, hypokalemia, sodium retention and edema, weight gain, and pulmonary hypertension; in rare cases, it may contribute to congestive heart failure.

Contraindications: Hypersensitivity to licorice; pre-existing renal, hepatic (cirrhosis and cholestatic liver disorders), and cardiovascular disease (congestive heart failure) because of risk of side effects; hypertension; low potassium level (hypokalemia). Elderly patients may be more sensitive to licorice.

Side Effects: Hyperaldosteronism, hypertension, edema, hypokalemia, sodium retention. The DGL form will not cause any of these side effects.

Long-Term Safety: Long history of human use as a food and medicine. Safe when used in small quantities or for limited periods of time.

Use in Pregnancy/Lactation/Children: Cautious use is advised. Use low doses in children. Avoid using for more than 2 weeks during pregnancy because it may increase blood pressure.

Drug/Herb Interactions and Rationale (if known)

- Do not use with diuretics: inhibits fluid loss and increases potassium loss.
- Do not use with digitalis: decreases effectiveness and increases side effects related to K+ and Na+.
- Use cautiously with antihypertensives: may inhibit activity.
- Use cautiously with corticosteroids: can potentiate effects. Dosage of medication may need to be adjusted.
- Use cautiously with laxatives: may increase potassium loss and cause hypokalemia.

Special Notes: Licorice preparations can be deglycyrrhizinated. This removes the side effects of pseudoaldosteronism but may reduce some of the herb's activity. Much of the licorice candy in the United States is flavored with anise oil and does not really contain licorice. Do not overconsume licorice. Eat a diet high in K+ and low in sodium when taking licorice. Monitor patient's blood pressure regularly. Most cases of hyperaldosteronism have occurred with overconsumption of real licorice candies; there are fewer reports of adverse reactions in patients who take recommended therapeutic doses of whole licorice extracts.

BIBLIOGRAPHY

Akamatsu H, et al. (1991). Mechanism of anti-inflammatory action of glycyrrhizin: effect on neutrophil functions including reactive oxygen species generation. *Planta Medica.* 57:119–121.

Arase Y, et al. (1997). The long-term efficacy of glycyrrhizin in chronic hepatitis C patients. *Cancer.* 79:1494–1500.

Baschetti R. (April 25, 1995). Chronic fatigue syndrome and liquorice [letter]. *New Zealand Medical Journal.* pp. 156–157.

Bernardi M, et al. (1994). Effects of prolonged ingestion of graded doses of licorice by healthy volunteers. *Life Sciences.* 55:863–872.

Blythe SL. (1999). Use of licorice root to treat vasovagal syncope. *HerbalGram.* 46:24.

Bruneton J. (1999). *Pharmacognosy, Phytochemistry, Medicinal Plants* (2nd ed.). Paris: Lavoisier Publishing.

Cantelli-Forti G, et al. (1994). Interaction of licorice on glycyrrhizin pharmacokinetics. *Environmental Health Perspectives.* 102(suppl. 9): 65–68.

Chamberlain J, Abolnik I. (1997). Pulmonary edema following a licorice binge [letter]. *Western Journal of Medicine.* 167(3):184–185.

Farese RV, et al. (1991). Licorice-induced hypermineralocorticoidism. *New England Journal of Medicine.* 325:1223–1227.

Johnston BJ, McIssac RL. (1981). The effect of some anti-ulcer agents on basal gastric mucosal blood flow and transmucosal flux of hydrogen and sodium ions in the conscious dog. *British Journal of Pharmacology.* 73:308P.

LaBrooy SJ, et al. (1979). Controlled comparison of cimetidine and carbenoxolone sodium in gastric ulcer. *British Medical Journal.* 1:1308–1309.

Lawrence Review of Natural Products. (1998). St. Louis: Facts and Comparisons.

MacKenzie MA, et al. (1990). The influence of glycyrrhetinic acid on plasma cortisol and cortisone in healthy young volunteers. *Journal of Clinical Endocrinology and Metabolism.* 70:1637–1643.

Matsumoto T, et al. (1996). Licorice may fight lupus. *Journal of Ethnopharmacology.* 53:1–4.

Maxton DG, et al. (1990). Controlled trial of pyrogastrone and cimetidine in the treatment of reflux oesophagitis. *Gut.* 31:351–354.

Mills S, Bone K. (1999). *Principles and Practice of Phytotherapy.* Edinburgh: Churchill Livingstone.

Snow JM. (Winter 1996). *Glycyrrhiza glabra* L. (Leguminaceae). *Protocol Journal of Botanical Medicine.* pp. 9–14.

Van Marle J, et al. (1981). Deglycyrrhizinated liquorice (DGL) and the renewal of rat stomach epithelium. *European Journal of Pharmacology.* 72:219–225.

NAME: Lobelia (*Lobelia inflata*)

Common Names: Asthma weed, pukeweed, Indian tobacco

Family: *Campanulaceae*

Description of Plant
- Small, hardy annual or biennial herb with pale blue flowers and inflated calyxes
- Native to eastern North America

Medicinal Part: Dried leaves and tops, seeds

Constituents and Action (if known)
- Lobeline (0.26%–0.40%): primary alkaloid, but at least 14 different piperidine alkaloids have been identified, including lobelanine and lobelanidine
  - Acts on nicotine receptors in body, crosses blood and placental barriers but is less potent than nicotine; because it binds to nicotine receptors, it decreases cravings for nicotine
  - Respiratory effect: in low doses, stimulation; in high doses, depression by inhibiting respiratory center in brain stem (Damaj et al., 1997)
  - Increases gastric acid secretion, gastrointestinal tone, and mobility (Westfall & Meldrum, 1986)
- Beta-amyrin palmitate: may possess sedative activity (Subarnas et al., 1993)

Nutritional Ingredients: None known

Traditional Use
- Antispasmodic, antiasthmatic, anodyne, bronchodilator, sedative, expectorant, emetic
- Important herbal medicine for the Thomsonians, physiomedicalists, and eclectic physicians (1822–1930). It was used to treat asthma, bronchitis (cough with a sense of oppression and a feeling of fullness in the chest, mucous rales), pertussis, pleurisy, angina, petit mal seizures, and muscle spasms.
- Topically, used for bruises, sprains, insect bites, and muscle spasms

- Lobelia and lobeline sulphate have been used as a smoking deterrent because of their nicotine-like effects. The FDA has banned its use as an antismoking aid not because of toxicity but because proof of efficacy is lacking. No companies were willing to spend the money to do sufficient research, because the product could not be patented.

Current Use: Spasmodic, asthma, and chronic obstructive pulmonary disease. Lobelia, along with ma huang, thyme, and khella (*Amni visnaga*), can be an effective treatment for mild asthma. Lobelia seed oil is a very effective topical treatment for muscle spasms, sore muscles, strains, and bruises.

Available Forms, Dosage, and Administration Guidelines
Preparations: Capsules, tinctures, tea; lobeline sulphate tablets or lozenges
Typical Dosage
- *Capsule* (usually no more than 15% of a formula): Two or three capsules per day
- *Tea:* 0.5 tsp dried herb in 8 oz hot water, steep half-hour; take 2 oz three times a day. Always mixed with milder, less acrid herbs.
- *Tincture:* (1:2, 40% alcohol, 10% acetic acid) 2 to 10 gtt three times a day; (1:5, 40% alcohol, 10% acetic acid) 5 to 20 gtt three times a day

Pharmacokinetics—If Available (form or route when known): Absorbed well by mucous membranes (mouth, gastrointestinal, and respiratory tract); metabolized in liver, kidney, and lungs; excreted in kidneys (Westfall & Meldrum 1986). Lobeline is rapidly metabolized and its effects are rather transitory when taken orally (Bradley, 1992).

Toxicity: At high doses, respiratory depression and tachycardia. The isolated alkaloid lobeline sulphate is substantially more toxic than the herb or whole herb extract.

Contraindications: Nausea, dyspnea, hypotension

Side Effects: Nausea, vomiting, dizziness, dyspnea, changes in heart rate, blood pressure (hypotension), diaphoresis, palpitations

Long-Term Safety: Unknown

Use in Pregnancy/Lactation/Children: Contraindicated, except as an aid during childbirth (helps to relax and dilate the cervix) by trained midwives or obstetricians

Drug/Herb Interactions and Rationale (if known): Do not use with smoking cessation products: may potentiate side effects.

Special Notes: There is much confusion about the toxicity of this herb. Recent analysis of the literature suggests that the acute dangers of this herb have been exaggerated (Bergner, 1998). Because of the strong potential for adverse effects with this herb (especially nausea, dizziness, and dyspnea), do not use for self-medication; it should be prescribed by a knowledgeable clinician. Patients should be warned that safer methods of smoking cessation are FDA-approved; it should be used for 6 weeks only and with behavior modification.

BIBLIOGRAPHY

Bartram T. (1995). *Encyclopedia of Herbal Medicine.* Dorset: Grace Publishers.

Bergner P. (1998). Lobelia toxicity: a literature review. *Medical Herbalism.* 10(1-2):15–34.

Bradley PR. (Ed.). (1992). *British Herbal Compendium.* Dorset: British Herbal Medicine Association.

Damaj MI, et al. (1997). Pharmacology of lobeline, a nicotine receptor ligand. *Journal of Pharmacology & Experimental Therapy.* 282:410–419.

Leung A, Foster S. (1996). *Encyclopedia of Common Natural Ingredients* (2nd ed.). New York: John Wiley & Sons.

Subarnas A, et al. (1993). Pharmacological properties of beta-amyrin palmitate, a novel centrally acting compound, isolated from *Lobelia inflata* leaves. *Journal of Pharmacy & Pharmacology.* 45(6):545–550.

Westfall TC, Meldrum MJ. (1986). Ganglionic blocking agents. In: Craig CR, Stizel RE. *Modern Pharmacology* (2d ed.). Boston: Little, Brown & Co.

NAME: Ma Huang (*Ephedra sinica, E. equisetina, E. intermedia*)

Common Names: Ephedra, Chinese ephedra

Family: *Ephedraceae*

Description of Plant: A small perennial evergreen shrub native to China, Japan, Tibet, India, Pakistan, and southern Siberia

Medicinal Part: Dried twigs (stem)

Constituents and Action (if known)

- Phenylproamine alkaloids(0.487%–2.436%)
  - Ephedrine (12%–75%): sympathomimetic agent acting on alpha- and beta-adrenergic receptors. Increases heart rate, blood pressure; bronchodilator; relaxes bronchi; anti-inflammatory; inhibits inflammatory PGE_2 prostaglandins and other proinflammatory substances (histamine, serotonin, bradykinin, PGE_1) (You Ping, 1998)
  - Pseudoephedrine (12%–75%): bronchodilating effects; increases heart rate, blood pressure; diuretic; anti-inflammatory; inhibits inflammatory PGE_2 prostaglandins and other proinflammatory substances (histamine, serotonin, bradykinin, PGE_1) (You Ping, 1998)
  - Methylephedrine
  - Methylpseudoephedrine
  - Norephedrine
  - Norpseudoephedrine
  - Ephedroxane: anti-inflammatory (You Ping, 1998)
  - Tannins: inhibit angiotensin II production
- Research suggests:
  - Volatile oils (tetramethylpyrazine, L-alpha-terpineol): antiasthmatic (AHPA, 1999)
  - Whole ephedra has fewer side effects than isolated ephedrine hydrochloride because of the balancing effect of its two major alkaloids.

- ○ Ephedra decoction has in vitro antibacterial activity against *Staphylococcus aureus, Bacillus anthracis, B. diphtheriae, B. dysenteriae, B. typhosus*, and *Pseudomonas aeruginosa*.
- Each species of ephedra has a different alkaloidal profile:

Nutritional Ingredients: None

Traditional Use: Antiallergic, bronchodilator, decongestant, central nervous system stimulant, diaphoretic, diuretic. In traditional Chinese medicine, ma huang is used in formulas for treating bronchial asthma, nasal congestion, head colds, fevers without perspiration, and headache and as a diuretic for edema.

Current Use

- Decongestant for allergies and hay fever: isolated ephedrine sulfate is found in over-the-counter medicines used to treat allergic rhinitis, allergic sinusitis, and head colds. The herb, in combination with herbs such as eyebright, osha root, and bayberry root, works very well with little or no adverse reactions (Winston, 2000).
- Asthma: ephedrine sulfate is used as an over-the-counter medication in some inhalers. The herb ephedra can be a useful part of an herbal protocol for mild asthma. It can be combined with other herbs such as lobelia), thyme, and khella (*Amni visnaga*).
- Weight loss: the benefits of thermogenic formulas for weight loss in patients with a sluggish metabolism seem to outweigh the potential risks, as long as the patient has no contraindications. The obvious health risks of obesity and the potential dangers of approved antiobesity medications make ma huang and various thermogenic formulas (usually including some form of caffeine and acetylsalicylic acid) a reasonable therapeutic protocol, if used in the recommended dosage and monitored by a physician (along with healthy diet, exercise, and behavior modification).
- Recent studies in China found that ma huang could be used to treat chronic bedwetting in children. Dosage was based on age; therapy lasted 1 month. In one study, 50 children were given a ma huang decoction every night before bed; 42

were cured with no recurrence after 6 months, 5 stopped bedwetting but resumed after the herb was discontinued, and 3 did not respond (AHPA, 1999).

Available Forms, Dosage, and Administration Guidelines

Preparations: Dried herb, tea, tincture, tablets, capsules, standardized extract. The American Herb Products Association (AHPA) has established upper limits for ephedra use of 25 mg ephedra alkaloids per dose and 100 mg ephedra alkaloids per day.

Typical Dosage

- *Dried herb:* 1 to 2 g per dose (approximately 13 mg total alkaloids) two or three times a day
- *Capsules* (ground whole herb): 500 to 1,000 mg two or three times a day
- *Standardized extract:* 12 to 25 mg total alkaloids two or three times a day
- *Tea:* 0.5 tsp dried herb in 8 oz hot water, decoct 15 minutes, steep 30 minutes; take 4 oz three times a day
- *Tincture* (1:5, 40% alcohol): 15 to 30 gtt (0.75–1.5 mL) up to three times a day

Pharmacokinetics—If Available (form or route when known):
With oral administration of ephedrine, peak effect occurs in 1 hour and activity lasts up to 6 hours. Whole ephedra is absorbed more slowly; the effects are less dramatic but more sustained (AHPA, 1999).

Toxicity: Overdose associated with hypertension, tachycardia, cardiac arrhythmia, myocardial infarction, and stroke (Blumenthal & King, 1995; Morton, 1977; Weiss, 1988)

Contraindications: Hypertension, insomnia, heart disease, glaucoma, benign prostatic hypertrophy, thyrotoxicosis, pheochromocytoma

Side Effects: Dry mouth, nervousness, anxiety, increased blood pressure, insomnia, palpitations, adrenal exhaustion, headache, nausea

Long-Term Safety: Unknown, not appropriate for long-term use except as prescribed by a physician

Use in Pregnancy/Lactation/Children: Use only if prescribed by a knowledgeable clinician. Inappropriate for self-medication by pregnant or nursing women or children.

Drug/Herb Interactions and Rationale (if known)

- Caffeine and other xanthine alkaloids: increased effects and potential toxicity
- Monoamine oxidase inhibitors: increased sympathomimetic effects
- Cardiac glycosides (digoxin): can cause arrhythmia
- Guanethidine: increased sympathomimetic effect
- Halothane: can cause arrhythmia
- Oxytocin: can increase hypertensive effects

Special Notes: Ephedra is being used inappropriately as an "herbal amphetamine" and energy aid and for sports training. It should not be used for any of these purposes. It may be of some value for sluggish metabolism obesity but should be used only under a physician's supervision in otherwise relatively healthy patients.

BIBLIOGRAPHY

(1999). AHPA Ephedra International Symposium, American Herb Products Association, Silver Spring, MD.

Blumenthal M, et al. (2000). *Herbal Medicine: Expanded Commission E Monographs*. Austin, TX: American Botanical Council.

Blumenthal M, King P. (1995). Ma huang: ancient herb, modern medicine regulatory dilemma. *HerbalGram*. 34:22.

McCaleb R, et al. (2000). *Encyclopedia of Popular Herbs*. Roseville, CA: Prima Publishing.

Morton JF. (1977). *Major Medicinal Plants: Botany, Culture and Uses*. Springfield, IL: Charles C. Thomas.

Schulz V, et al. (1998). *Rational Phytotherapy, A Physician's Guide to Herbal Medicine*. Berlin: Springer-Verlag.

Weiss RF. (1988). *Herbal Medicine*. Gothenburg, Sweden: AB Arcanum.

Winston D. (2000). *Herbal Therapeutics—Specific Indications*. (7th ed.). Washington, NJ: Herbal Therapeutics Research Library.

You-Ping Z. (1998). *Chinese Materia Medica*. Amsterdam: Harwood Academic Publishers.

NAME: Meadowsweet (*Filipendula ulmaria*)

Common Names: Queen of the meadow, bridewort, lady of the meadow

Family: *Rosaceae*

Description of Plant
- Perennial herb growing up to 3 to 5 feet tall, with panicles of small white flowers
- Native to Europe but grows well in North America
- Prefers damp, moist soil

Medicinal Part: Dried herb and flowers

Constituents and Action (if known)
- Phenolic glycosides (spiraein, monotropin, isosalicin): anti-inflammatory, antipyretic, analgesic activity (Bisset, 1994; Schultz et al., 1998)
- Flavonoids (rutin, hyperoside, spiraeoside) (Bisset, 1994)
- Polyphenols (tannins) (10%–15%): rugosin-D has astringent properties and may help with diarrhea (Duke, 1989; Newall et al., 1996)
- A heparin-like compound; may be responsible for anticoagulant activity (Kudriashov et al., 1990)
- Volatile oils (0.2%): mostly salicylaldehyde

Nutritional Ingredients: Used as a flavoring in alcoholic beverages in the United Kingdom

History: Considered a sacred herb by the Druids. Salicylic acid was first isolated from *Filipendula* (spirae) flowers. The pure salicylic acid caused acute GI distress, so researchers found a related compound, acetylsalicylic acid, that had the benefits of the salicylic acid without as much of the adverse reactions. The word aspirin comes from A (acetyl) + spirae (old name for meadowsweet).

Traditional Use
- Antacid, astringent, antipyretic, analgesic, anti-inflammatory, astringent, diuretic, stomachic
- To settle the stomach and treat indigestion, heartburn, irritable bowel syndrome, and diarrhea

- To treat arthritis, bursitis, muscle pain, and rheumatic pain
- To treat headaches, fevers, and abdominal cramps
- Nonirritating antiseptic diuretic for cystitis, urinary calculi, and gout

Current Use

- Supportive therapy for colds because of its anti-inflammatory, analgesic, antipyretic activity
- Digestive remedy for acid indigestion (dyspepsia), gastritis, and peptic ulcers
- Used to treat rheumatic and arthritic pains (orally and topically)
- Intravaginal administration of meadowsweet ointment in 48 patients with cervical dysplasia resulted in an improvement in 32 women and a complete remission in 25.

Available Forms, Dosage, and Administration Guidelines

- *Dried flowers/herb:* 2 to 6 g
- *Tea:* 1 to 2 tsp dried herb/flowers in 8 oz hot water, steep 30 minutes; take two or three cups per day
- *Tincture* (1:5, 30% alcohol): 40 to 80 gtt (2–4 mL) up to three times a day

Pharmacokinetics—If Available (form or route when known): Not known

Toxicity: None known

Contraindications: Salicylate sensitivity

Side Effects: None known

Long-Term Safety: Not known

Use in Pregnancy/Lactation/Children: No research available; no restrictions known (McGuffin et al, 1997)

Drug/Herb Interactions and Rationale (if known):
Possible interaction with anticoagulants. Use cautiously together, especially if using other herb or supplement products that could cause a cumulative effect (fish oils, vitamin E, ginkgo, garlic). Obtain prothrombin time and

International Normalized Ratio (INR) to rule out possible interactions.

BIBLIOGRAPHY

Bisset N. (1994). *Herbal Drugs and Phytopharmaceuticals.* Stuttgart, Germany: CRC Press.

Blumenthal M, ed. (1998). *The Complete German Commission E Monographs.* Boston: American Botanical Council.

Bradley PR. (1992). *British Herbal Compendium.* Dorset: British Herbal Medicine Association.

Duke J. (1989). *CRC Handbook of Medicinal Herbs.* Boca Raton, FL: CRC Press Inc.

Kudriashov B, et al. (1990). The content of a heparin-like anticoagulant in the flowers of the meadowsweet. *Farmakology Toksikologia.* 53(4):39–41.

Liapina LA, Kovalchuk GA. (1993). A comparative study of the action on the hemostatic system of extracts from the flowers and seeds of the meadowsweet. *Izv Akad Nauk Ser Biol.* 4:625–628.

McGuffin M, et al. (1997). *American Herbal Product Association's Botanical Safety Handbook.* Boca Raton, FL: CRC Press.

Mills S, Bone K. (1999). *Principles and Practice of Phytotherapy.* Edinburgh: Churchill Livingstone.

Newall C, et al. (1996). *Herbal Medicines.* London: Pharmaceutical Press.

Review of Natural Products. (1999). St. Louis: Facts and Comparisons.

Schultz V, et al. (1998). *Rational Phytotherapy.* Berlin: Springer-Verlag.

 NAME: Milk Thistle (*Silybum marianum*)

Common Names: Lady's thistle, Marion thistle, Mary's thistle, *Cardii marianus*

Family: *Asteraceae*

Description of Plant

- Annual/biennial weedy plant found in rocky soils in southern and western Europe and North Africa; naturalized in some parts of the United States
- Grows 2 to 4 feet high. Has dark shiny green leaves with white veins.

- The spiny flower heads are purple and bloom from June to August.

Medicinal Part: Seeds

Constituents and Action (if known)

- Silymarin (1.5%–3%) consists of several flavonolignans: silybin (antioxidant and hepatoprotection), silychristin, silydianin, and isosilybin.
  - Binds with hepatocellular membranes and protects against damaging chemicals and toxins (Albrecht, 1992; Awang, 1993)
  - Prevents lysoperoxidative hepatic damage from alcohol and drugs (Buzzelli, 1993, Flora et al., 1998; Hobbs, 1992)
  - Prevents hepatocyte damage (Flora et al., 1998)
  - Powerful oxygen free radical scavenger activity (Bisset, 1994)
  - Increases level of glutathione in liver
  - Reduces blood cholesterol (Skottova & Kreeman, 1998)
  - Increases superoxide dismutase levels in red blood cells of chronic alcoholics (Muzes et al., 1991)
  - Increases protein synthesis in hepatocytes, thereby increasing liver cell regeneration (Grossman, 1995; Mascarella, 1993)
  - Prevents toxins from entering liver cells by preventing binding (Foster, 1991, Morazzoni & Bombardelli, 1995)
  - Prevents liver damage from alcohol, tetracycline, acetaminophen, thallium, erythromycin, amitriptyline, long-term phenothiazine use, carbon tetrachloride, lorazepam, and anesthesia (Morazzoni & Bombardelli, 1995; Palasciancio et al., 1994; von Schonfeld et al., 1997)
- Flavonoids (quercitin, taxifolin, eriodyctiol, chrysoeriol)
- Fixed oil (20%–30%)

Additional Actions

- Antioxidant: inhibits lipid peroxidation of hepatic microsomes
- May have anti-inflammatory activity (studies in vitro)
- May enhance immune function (polymorphonuclear neutrophils, T lymphocytes)

- Increases motility of neutrophils and leukocytes
- Lowers biliary cholesterol and phospholipid concentrations without affecting bile flow (Morazzoni & Bombardelli, 1995)
- Increases bile secretion
- May reduce diabetic complications: studies showed less diabetic neuropathy resulting from prevention of inhibition of protein mono-adenosine diphosphate ribosylation
- Decreases prostaglandin synthesis

Nutritional Ingredients: Once grown in Europe as a vegetable: the despined leaves were used as a spinach substitute and the flower was eaten like an artichoke. The roasted seeds were used as a coffee substitute.

Traditional Use

- Used for more than 2,000 years as a liver herb and protectant
- Used in England to remove obstructions of the liver and spleen and to treat jaundice, constipation, hemorrhoids, and insufficient bile flow with clay-colored stools
- In the 19th and 20th century, the seed was used to treat hepatomegaly, splenomegaly, dry, scaly skin, pancreatitis (with ceanothus), and gallstones
- Leaves have been used to stimulate milk production in lactating women, as a bitter digestive tonic, and as a mild liver tonic.

Current Use

- The best-researched hepatoprotective herb
- Improves survival in patients with cirrhosis: slows liver disease and may reverse liver damage. Patient must stop drinking to maximize effectiveness.
- Improves immune function and appetite and reduces nausea in patients with cirrhosis
- Improves both acute progressive and chronic persistent hepatitis (A, B, and possibly C)
- Reduces liver damage and helps to restore hepatic function in nonviral hepatitis (drug-induced or of unknown origin)

- Reduces side effects in patients undergoing chemotherapy for cancer
- May prevent or treat gallstones
- Persons exposed to hepatotoxins (farmers, chemical workers) use it to protect the liver from damage.
- Used in Europe for *Amanita* (death cap) mushroom poisoning: inhibits hepatic uptake of the phallotoxins and renal uptake of alpha-amanitine, thus preventing liver and kidney damage and death (primarily used as an injection)

Available Forms, Dosage, and Administration Guidelines

Preparations: Whole or powdered seed, capsules, tablets, tinctures. Most products are standardized to 70% to 80% silymarin. The product researched most widely and available in Europe is Legalon. Another product, Thisilyn, also widely researched in Europe, is available in the United States through Nature's Way. Alcohol-based extracts should be used cautiously in patients with liver damage because of the need to administer relatively high amounts of alcohol to obtain an adequate dose of silymarin.

Typical Dosage

- *Capsules* (standardized to 70% silymarin): 140 mg silymarin three times a day. After 6 weeks, reduce to 90 mg three times a day.
- *Tea:* Steep 2 to 3 tsp dried, powered seed in 1 cup hot water for 10 to 15 minutes. Silymarin is poorly soluble in water, so aqueous preparations such as teas are only marginally effective, if at all.
- *Tincture* (1:5, 70% alcohol): 60 to 100 gtt (3–5 mL) up to three times a day
- Or follow manufacturer's or practitioner's recommendations

Pharmacokinetics—If Available (form or route when known): Absorbs readily: 20% to 50% of silymarin is absorbed by oral administration. Peak action occurs in 1 hour. Excretion: 80% of silymarin is excreted in the bile. Functional onset: 5 to 8 days. Reversal of liver damage occurs in 1 to 2 months, remission of chronic hepatitis in 6 months to 1 year.

Toxicity: Considered completely safe

Contraindications: None known

Side Effects: Mostly devoid of side effects; mild laxative effect and GI symptoms, usually subside in 2 to 3 days; mild allergic reactions

Long-Term Safety: Completely safe and nontoxic

Use in Pregnancy/Lactation/Children: Safe

Drug/Herb Interactions and Rationale (if known): None known

BIBLIOGRAPHY

Albrecht M. (1992). Therapy of toxic liver pathologies with Legalon. *Z Klin Med.* 47(2):87–92.

Awang D. (1993). Milk thistle. *Canadian Pharmaceutical Journal.* 422,403,404.

Bisset N. (1994). *Herbal Drugs and Phytopharmaceuticals.* London: CRC Press.

Bruneton J. (1999). *Pharmacognosy, Phytochemistry, Medicinal Plants.* Paris: Lavoisier.

Buzzelli G. (1993). A pilot study on the liver protective effect of silybin-phosphatidylcholine complex (IdB1016) in chronic active hepatitis. *International Journal of Clinical Pharmacology Therapy & Toxicology.* 31:456–460.

Flora K, et al. (1998). Milk thistle (*Silybum marianum*) for the therapy of liver disease. *American Journal of Gastroenterology.* 93(2):139–143.

Foster S. (1991). Milk thistle (*Silybum marianum*). *Botanical Series #305.* Austin, TX: American Botanical Council.

Grossman M. (1995). Spontaneous regression of hepatocellular carcinoma. *American Journal of Gastroenterology.* 90(9):1500–1503.

Hobbs C. (1992). *Milk Thistle: The Liver Herb.* Capitola, CA: Botanica Press.

Mascarella S. (1993). Therapeutic and antilipoperoxidant effects of silybin-phosphatidylcholine complex in chronic liver disease: preliminary result. *Current Therapeutic Research.* 53(1):98–102.

Morazzoni P, Bombardelli E. (1995). *Silybum marianum (Carduus marianus).* Fitoterapia. 66(1):3–42.

Muzes G, et al. (1991). Effect of the bioflavonoid silymarin on the in vitro activity and expression of superoxide dismutase enzyme. *Acta Physiologica Hungarica.* 78:3–9.

Palasciancio G, et al. (1994). The effect of silymarin on plasma levels of malondialdehyde in patients receiving long-term treatment with psychotropic drugs. *Current Therapeutic Research.* 55(5):537–545.

Review of Natural Products. (1998). St. Louis: Facts and Comparisons.

Schulz V. (1998). *Rational Phytotherapy: A Physician's Guide to Herbal Medicine.* Berlin: Springer-Verlag.

Skottova N, Kreeman V. (1998). Silymarin as a potential hypocholesterolaemic drug. *Physiology Research.* 47(1):1–7.

von Schonfeld J, et al. (1997). Silibinin, a plant extract with antioxidant and membrane stabilizing properties, protects exocrine pancreas from cyclosporin A toxicity. *Cellular Molecular Life Sciences.* 53(11-12):917–920.

 NAME: Motherwort (*Leonurus cardiaca*)

Common Names: The Chinese species *L. heterophyllyus* (yi mu cao) is similar in activity.

Family: *Lamiaceae*

Description of Plant
- A nonaromatic perennial member of the mint family.
- Naturalized in the United States and Canada, it grows 2 to 4 feet tall, with pink flowers and sharp, thorny calyxes.

Medicinal Part: Dried leaves

Constituents and Action (if known)
- Triterpenes
  - Ursolic acid: tumor-inhibiting for leukemia, lung, mammary, and colon cancers (Nagasawa et al., 1992)
  - Antiviral (Epstein-Barr virus) (Tokuda, 1986)
  - Cardioactive: stimulates alpha- and beta-adrenoreceptors and inhibits calcium chloride (Newall et al., 1996)
  - Cytotoxic
- Iridoid glycosides (leonuride)
- Alkaloids
- Leonurine: produces transient central nervous system depression and hypotensive effects when given intravenously

(Bradley, 1992); uterine stimulant (You-Ping, 1998), L-stachydrine
- Tannins (5%–9%)

Traditional Use
- Antispasmodic, anxiolytic, cardiotonic, emmenagogue, hypotensive, nervine/sedative
- Cardiovascular conditions such as palpitations and mild hypertension
- Reduces the pain of menstrual cramps and other smooth muscle, parasympathetic cramps, including vaginismus
- Increases or stimulates menstrual flow for women with amenorrhea or a clotty, scanty flow with cramps

Current Use
- Stress-induced cardiac disorders: palpitations and mild hypertension. For hypertension use with hawthorn, olive leaf, linden flower, and black haw.
- Nervine: sedative, antispasmodic, useful for general anxiety, including premenstrual and menopausal anxiety. Use with blue vervain, scullcap, or fresh oat extract. Motherwort is also useful for pelvic and lumbar pain, including mild to moderate dysmenorrhea.
- Use for hyperthyroidism with bugleweed and lemon balm, especially if nervousness and palpitations are part of the patient's symptoms.

Available Forms, Dosage, and Administration Guidelines
Preparations: Infusion, dried herb, capsules, tincture
Typical Dosage
- Unless otherwise prescribed, 3 to 6 g per day of dried herb
- *Infusion:* 2 tsp dried herb in 8 oz hot water, steep 30 minutes; take two or three cups a day
- *Capsules:* Two or three 500-mg capsules three times a day
- *Tincture* (1:5, 30% alcohol): 60 to 100 gtt (3–5 mL) three times a day

Pharmacokinetics—If Available (form or route when known): Not known

Toxicity: None known

Contraindications: None known

Side Effects: May increase menstrual bleeding

Long-Term Safety: Safe when used in normal therapeutic doses

Use in Pregnancy/Lactation/Children: Not recommended in pregnancy because it is an emmenagogue; no restrictions in lactation

Drug/Herb Interactions and Rationale (if known): None known

Special Notes: The *Botanical Safety Handbook* notes, "A dose in excess of 3.0 grams of a powdered extract may cause diarrhea, uterine bleeding, and stomach irritation" (McGuffin et al, 1997). There is no mention in the original literature of what type of extract was used or the concentration. This warning is not repeated anywhere else in the literature and does not apply to the crude herb or tincture.

BIBLIOGRAPHY

Bradley PR. (Ed.). (1992). *British Herbal Compendium, Vol. 1.* Bournemouth: British Herbal Medicine Association.

McGuffin M, et al. (1997). *American Herbal Product Association's Botanical Safety Handbook.* Boca Raton, FL: CRC Press.

Moore M. (1979). *Medicinal Plants of the Mountain West.* Museum of New Mexico Press.

Nagasawa H, et al. (1992). Further study on the effects of motherwort (*Leonurus sibiricus* L.) preneoplastic and neoplastic mammary gland growth in multiparous GR/A mice. *Anticancer Research.* 12(1):141–143.

Newall CA, et al. (1996). *Herbal Medicines: A Guide for Health Care Professionals.* London: Pharmaceutical Press.

Sherman JA. (1993). *Complete Botanical Prescriber* (3rd ed.). Portland, OR: Author.

Tokuda H, et al.(1986). Inhibitory effects of ursolic and oleanolic acid on skin tumor promotion by 12-0-tetradecanoylphorbol-13-acetate. *Cancer Letters.* 33(3):279–285.

Weiss R. (1988). *Herbal Medicine* (6th ed.). Beaconsfield: Beaconsfield Publishing.

You-Ping Z. (1998). *Chinese Materia Medica-Chemistry, Pharmacology, and Applications*. Amsterdam: Harwood Academic Publishers.

Zou QZ, et al. (1989). Effect of motherwort on blood hyperviscosity. *American Journal of Chinese Medicine*. 17(1-2):65–70.

NAME: Myrrh (*Commiphora myrrha, C. molmol, C. madagascariensis*)

Common Names: African myrrh, Somali myrrh, Yemen myrrh, Gum myrrh

Family: *Burseraceae*

Description of Plant

- A shrub or small tree that grows to 30 feet; native to Egypt, Sudan, Somalia, Yemen, and Ethiopia
- The gum resin exudes from natural fractures in the bark and from man-made incisions, then hardens into red-brown or yellowish-red tears.

Medicinal Part: Air-hardened gum resin

Constituents and Action (if known)

- Volatile oils (limonene, dipentene, alpha coprene, elemene, lindestrene, boubonene)
- Resins: alpha, beta, and gamma commiphoric acids (25%–40%), alpha and beta heerabomyrrols, heeraboresene, burseracin
- Gum (30%–60%) contains proteoglycans
- Sesquiterpenes/lactones/terpenes (commiferin): smooth muscle relaxant (Andersson et al., 1997)

Other Actions

- Antitumor activity
- Analgesic activity (Dolara et al., 1996)
- Cytoprotective effect: antiulcer effect against numerous necrotizing agents

Nutritional Ingredients: Used as flavor for beverages, liqueurs, and foods

History: Used since ancient times as an incense, a medicine, and for embalming mummies in Egypt

Traditional Use

- Astringent, antibacterial, anti-inflammatory, antiulcer, carminative, analgesic, antispasmodic
- Used for sore throats, gum disease, bronchial infections, topically for sores, infections, and muscle pain
- Long tradition of therapeutic use in traditional Chinese medicine and Tibetan and Unani medical traditions to treat mouth ulcers, poorly healing sores, boils, bruises, abdominal pains, and amenorrhea

Current Use

- Useful therapy with echinacea and sage for tonsillitis or pharyngitis
- Astringent and antibacterial in mouthwashes for gingivitis, aphthous ulcers, and pyorrhea
- Improves granulation and is used topically as a salve or as dusting powder to treat wounds, hemorrhoids, oozing skin conditions, and bedsores

Available Forms, Dosage, and Administration Guidelines

Preparations: Unless otherwise prescribed, powdered gum resin, myrrh tincture, and other galenical preparations for topical use. Dental powders contain 10% powdered gum resin.

Typical Dosage

- *Tincture* (1:5, 90% alcohol): For use in gargles, mouthwashes, and rinses; dilute with water or it may irritate mucous membranes
- *Mouthwash or gargle solution:* Add 30 to 60 gtt tincture to a glass of warm water

Pharmacokinetics—If Available (form or route when known): Not known

Toxicity: None known

Contraindications: None known

Side Effects: Dermatitis from local contact (Gallo et al., 1999)

Long-Term Safety: Although no formal clinical studies have been reported, it is clear from ethnopharmacologic evidence that myrrh has been extensively used both internally and externally without apparent adverse effects (ESCOP, 1999).

Use in Pregnancy/Lactation/Children: Avoid internal use during pregnancy; topical use is fine. No known restrictions for breast-feeding and with children.

Drug/Herb Interactions and Rationale (if known): None known

BIBLIOGRAPHY

Al-Harbi MM, et al. (1994). Anticarcinogenic effect of *Commiphora molmol* on solid tumors induced by Ehrlich carcinoma cells in mice. *Chemotherapy.* 40:337–347.

Al-Harbi MM, et al. (1997). Gastric antiulcer and cytoprotective effect of *Commiphora molmol* in rats. *Journal of Ethnopharmacology.* 55:141–150.

Andersson M, et al. (1997). Minor components with smooth muscle relaxing properties from scented myrrh (*Commiphora guidotti*). *Planta Medica.* 63(3):251–254.

Blumenthal M, et al. (2000). *Herbal Medicine: Expanded Commission E Monographs.* Austin, TX: American Botanical Council.

Bradley P. (1992). *British Herbal Compendium, Vol. 1.* Bournemouth: British Herbal Medicine Association.

Dolara P, et al. (1996). Analgesic effects of myrrh. *Nature.* 379(6560):29.

ESCOP Monographs on the Medicinal Uses of Plant Drugs. (1999). Exeter: ESCOP.

Gallo R, et al. (1999). Allergic contact dermatitis from myrrh. *Contact Dermatitis.* 41(4):230–231.

Lawrence Review of Natural Products. (1994). St. Louis: Facts and Comparisons.

Leung A, Foster S. (1996). *Encyclopedia of Common Natural Ingredients.* New York: John Wiley & Sons.

NAME: Nettles (*Urtica dioica*)

Common Names: Common nettles, greater nettles, stinging nettles

Family: *Urticaceae*

Description of Plant
- Common weedy perennial found throughout the United States, Europe, and most temperate climates. Can grow 3 to 4 feet tall.
- Hairs on stem and leaves release formic acid when touched and can sting for hours.

Medicinal Part: Root, leaf, seed

Constituents and Action (if known)
- Roots and flowers: scopoletin (coumarin): anti-inflammatory activity (Chrubasik et al., 1997)
- Roots: steroids: inhibit membrane Na+/K+ ATPase activity of the prostate (Hirano et al., 1994)
  - Phenylpropanes
  - Lignans (secoisolariciresinol, enterodiol, enterolactone): reduced binding affinity of human sex hormone-binding globulin in vitro. Lignans may also inhibit the sex hormone-binding globulin and 5-dihydrotestosterone interaction (Mills & Bone, 1999).
- A single-chain lectin, UDA, inhibits the sex hormone-binding globulin to the receptor, thus decreasing the symptoms of benign prostatic hypertrophy (Gansser, 1995; Hartmann et al., 1996); suppresses prostate cell metabolism (Krzeski et al., 1993); inhibits cytomegalovirus and HIV (Balzarini et al., 1992)
- Leaf: flavonal glycosides: vitamins C, B complex, K, carotenoids, minerals
- Stinging hairs contain amines (histamine, serotonin, acetylcholine, formic acid).

Nutritional Ingredients: As a food, nettles contain 25% to 42% protein and are rich in Ca++, Mg++, zinc, K+, selenium, silicon, and vitamins B, C, D, K, and carotenoids. Steamed nettles taste like spinach. Collect the plants when they are young, tender, light green, and no more than 6 to 10 inches tall. Use gloves when gathering nettles!

Traditional Use

- High iron content used to treat low hemoglobin/hematocrit and iron deficiency anemia
- Used to stop excessive menstrual flow, hematuria, hemoptysis; applied topically to stop bleeding (nose bleeds, cuts)
- Used to reduce pain of arthritis
- Tea was applied to the head to increase hair growth.
- Used for skin conditions where the skin looks and feels papery and tears easily
- Nonirritating diuretic used for low-grade kidney infections with low back pain

Current Use

- Reduces inflammation (especially arthralgias) and may reduce the need for nonsteroidal anti-inflammatories by as much as 50%
- Freeze-dried product has a moderate ability to reduce allergic reaction and reduce symptoms of seasonal allergies.
- Leaf has a mild diuretic effect (potassium-sparing) and therefore may benefit persons with hypertension, heart failure, and kidney disorders.
- Root improves urinary output and inhibits cellular proliferation in benign prostatic hyperplasia; use for stage 1 and 2 benign prostatic hyperplasia. Usually mixed with saw palmetto and pygeum bark.
- Root weakly inhibits interaction between 5-alpha-reductase and dihydrotestosterone. Root also inhibits aromatase, which converts testosterone into estradiol (Winston, 1999).
- Seed is used as a kidney trophorestorative in experimental protocols for glomerulonephritis and chronic nephritis with degeneration. The results have been promising (Winston, 2000).

Available Forms, Dosage, and Administration Guidelines

Preparations: Dried leaf, dried root (may be combined with saw palmetto); capsules, tablets, tea, tincture. Studies conflict as to whether the aqueous or alcoholic extract of the root is more effective (Hryb et al., 1995; Mills & Bone, 1999). The freeze-dried herb in capsules is the most effective form for antihistamine activity.

Typical Dosage

- *Dried leaf:* 6 to 10 g per day
- *Capsules (root)* (5:1 extract): 600 to 1,200 mg a day
- *Tea (root):* Steep 1 to 2 tsp dried root in a cup of hot water; take one or two cups daily
- *Tea (leaf):* Steep 1 to 2 tsp dried herb in a cup of hot water; take two to four cups daily
- *Tincture (root)* (1:5, 30% alcohol): 40 to 60 gtt (2–3 mL) three times a day
- *Tincture (leaf)* (1:5, 30% alcohol): 60 to 100 gtt (3–5 mL) three times a day
- Or follow manufacturer's or practitioner's recommendations

Pharmacokinetics—If Available (form or route when known): The lectin UDA is primarily excreted via the intestines (30%–50%) and to a minor degree by the kidneys (less than 1%).

Toxicity: None known

Contraindications: Hemochromatosis

Side Effects: Contact dermatitis: the rash and blisters from nettles can last up to 12 hours. Nettle root rarely causes nausea or vomiting; take with food. May raise glucose serum levels (Roman et al., 1992).

Long-Term Safety: Safe; has been eaten as a food for millennia

Use in Pregnancy/Lactation/Children: Herb is safe; long history of use as a food; no data for the root

Drug/Herb Interactions and Rationale (if known): Use cautiously with diuretics: may potentiate action

Special Notes: Alert patients not to self-diagnose benign prostatic hyperplasia. Recommend that they seek medical attention before beginning any prostate protocol to rule out a serious medical condition. For nettle rash, apply a compress of plantain leaf, chickweed, or jewelweed juice.

BIBLIOGRAPHY

Balzarini J, et al. (1992). The mannose-specific plant lectins from *Cymbidium hybrid* and *Epipactis helleborine* and the (N-acetylglucosamine) n-specific plant lectin from *Urtica dioica* are potent and selective inhibitors of human immunodeficiency virus and cytomegalovirus replication in vitro. *Antiviral Research.* 18(2):191–207.

Bisset N, Wictl M. (Eds.). (1994). *Herbal Drugs and Phytopharmaceuticals.* Stuttgart: CRC Press.

Chrubasik S, et al. (1997). Evidence for antirheumatic effectiveness of Herba *Urtica dioica* in acute arthritis: a pilot study. *Phytomedicine.* 4(2):105–108.

Davidov M, et al. (1995). Phytoperfusion of the bladder after adenectomy. *Urologiia I Nefrologiia.* (5):19-20.

Gansser D. (1995). Plant constituents interfering with human sex hormone-binding globulin. Evaluation of a test method and its application to Urtica dioica root extracts. *A Naturforsch [C]* 50:98-104.

Hartmann RW, et al. (1996). Inhibition of 5 a-reductase and aromatase by PHL-00801 (Prostatonin), a combination of PY 102 (*Pygeum africanum*) and UR 102 (*Urtica dioica*) extracts. *Phytomedicine.* 3(2):121–128.

Hirano T, et al. (1994). Effects of stinging nettle root extracts and their steroidal components on the Na+, K+-ATPase of the benign prostatic hyperplasia. *Planta Medica.* 60(1):30–33.

Hryb D, et al. (1995). The effect of extracts of the roots of the stinging nettle (*Urtica dioica*) on the interaction of SHBG with its receptor on human prostatic membranes. *Planta Medica.* 61(1):31–32.

Krzeski T, et al. (1993). Combined extracts of *Urtica dioica* and *Pygeum africanum* in the treatment of benign prostatic hyperplasia: double-blind comparison of two doses. *Clinical Therapeutics.* 15(6):1011–1020.

Mills S, Bone K. (1999). *Principles and Practice of Phytotherapy.* Edinburgh, UK: Churchill-Livingstone.

Mittman P. (1990). Randomized, double-blind study of freeze-dried *Urtica dioica* in the treatment of allergic rhinitis. *Planta Medica.* 56:44–47.

Roman R, et al. (1992). Hypoglycemic effect of plants used in Mexico as antidiabetics. *Archives of Medical Research.* 23(1):59–64.

Wagner H, et al. (1994). Search for the antiprostatic principle of stinging nettle (*Urtica dioica*) roots. *Phytomedicine.* 1(3):213–224.

White A. (1995). Stinging nettles for osteoarthritis pain of the hip. *British Journal of General Practice.* 45(392):162.

Winston D. (1999). *Saw Palmetto for Men and Women.* Pownal, CT: Storey Publishing.

Winston D. (2000). *Herbal Therapeutics: Specific Indications for Herbs and Herbal Formulas* (7th ed.). Washington, NJ: Herbal Therapeutics Research Library.

🌿 NAME: Noni (*Morinda citrifolia*)

Common Names: Hog apple, Indian mulberry, nonu

Family: *Rubiaceae*

Description of Plant

- An evergreen shrub or small tree native to Southeast Asia; has become naturalized in Polynesia, Australia, Mexico, the Caribbean, and Central America.
- Has white flowers and yellow fruit about the size of a potato with a bumpy surface. Ripe fruit has cheeselike, offensive odor.

Medicinal Part: Fruit, leaves, bark

Constituents and Action (if known)

- Anthraquinones: laxative, antibacterial
- Fatty acids: linoleic, oleic, caproic, caprylic acids, octanic acid: insecticidal activity (Dixon et al., 1999)
- Root extracts show central analgesic activity and possible sedative properties (Younos et al., 1990).
- Alcohol extracts of leaves display anthelmintic activity against human *Ascaris lumbricoides*.
- Immunodulatory polysaccharide: noni PPT (Hirazumi & Furusawa, 1999)
- A researcher has claimed to have identified an "alkaloid/xeronine;" it is theorized to work at the molecular level to repair damaged cells to regulate their function (digestive, respiratory, bone, and skin can all benefit) (Hirazumi & Furusawa, 1999; U.S. Patent #5,288,491, 1994). No other researchers have validated this claim; in fact, they have dismissed this research as seriously flawed.

- Other actions: may have anticancer activity (studied in Lewis lung carcinoma in mice) by enhancing immune system activity (Hirazumi et al., 1994; Hirazumi & Furusawa, 1999)

Nutritional Ingredients: Contains vitamin A; edible fruit is usually layered in sugar; leaves are consumed raw or cooked

Traditional Use
- Traditional ethnobotanical use by Hawaiians and other Polynesian peoples was primarily as a topical application for boils, ringworm, rheumatic pain, neuralgia, bruises, gout, and infections.
- Seeds were used as a purgative and anthelmintic in the Philippines.
- In Hawaii, by the 1930s, noni had become a popular ingredient in many compound formulas (usually mixed with ginger, coconut milk, or sugar cane juice); it was taken orally for tuberculosis, intestinal worms, and sexually transmitted diseases and for "purifying the blood."

Current Use
- Promoted as a panacea for a wide range of diseases, including cancer, atherosclerosis, AIDS, obesity, hypertension, and diabetes. There is currently no research on the effectiveness of this herb for these conditions. The product seems to have a low potential for toxicity, but it is unclear whether noni has any real health benefits.
- Based on a long history of use for topical complaints, noni may be useful as a local application for skin infections, abscesses, boils, carbuncles, abrasions, blemishes, wounds, bruises, and arthritic pain.

Available Forms, Dosage, and Administration Guidelines
Preparations: Noni juice (10%–97% noni mixed with fruit juices), dried fruit leather, dry extract, tincture
Typical Dosage: The juice product should be taken on an empty stomach 30 minutes before meals. Take 1 to 2 oz twice a day.

Pharmacokinetics—If Available (form or route when known): Not known

Toxicity: Not known

Contraindications: Hyperkalemia: the juice products contain fruit juices that often have substantial potassium content (Mueller et al., 2000)

Side Effects: None known

Long-Term Safety: Has been used for thousands of years as a healing plant and food; would appear to be safe

Use in Pregnancy/Lactation/Children: According to one manufacturer of noni juice, it is safe in pregnant and lactating women and children 7 months and older.

Drug/Herb Interactions and Rationale (if known): None known

Special Notes: Most research has been done by companies with commercial interests in the product.

BIBLIOGRAPHY

Dittmar A. (1993). *Morinda citrifolia* L.: use in indigenous Samoan medicine. *Journal of Herbs, Spices and Medicinal Plants.* 1(3):77–92.

Dixon AR, et al. (1999). Ferment this: the transformation of noni, a traditional Polynesian medicine (*Morinda citrifolia*, Rubiaceae). *Economic Botany.* 53(1):51–68.

Hirazumi A, et al. (1994). Anticancer activity of *Morinda citrifolia* (noni) on intraperitoneally implanted Lewis lung carcinoma in syngeneic mice. *Proceedings of the Western Pharmacologic Society.* 37:145–146.

Hirazumi A, et al. (1996). Immunomodulation contributes to the anticancer activity of *Morinda citrifolia* (noni) fruit juice. *Proceedings of the Western Pharmacologic Society.* 39:7–9.

Hirazumi A, Furusawa E. (1999). An immunomodulatory polysaccharide-rich substance from the fruit juice of *Morinda citrifolia* (noni) with antitumor activity. *Phytotherapy Research.* 13(5):380–387.

Morton J. (1981). *Atlas of Medicinal Plants of Middle America.* Springfield, IL: Charles Thomas.

Morton J. (1992). The ocean-going noni, or Indian mulberry (*Morinda citrifolia*, Rubiaceae) and some of its "colorful" relatives. *Economic Botany.* 46(3):241–256.

Mueller BA, et al. (2000). Noni juice (*Morinda citrifolia*): hidden potential for hyperkalemia? *American Journal of Kidney Disease.* 35(2):310–312.

Review of Natural Products. (1997). St. Louis: Facts and Comparisons.

Srivastava M, et al. (1993). *International Journal of Pharmacognosy.* 31(3):182–184.

U.S. Patent #5,288,491; date of patent Feb. 22, 1994.

Younos CR, et al. (1990). Analgesic and behavioral effects of *Morinda citrifolia*. *Planta Medica.* 56:430–434.

 NAME: Olive Leaf (*Olea europaea*)

Common Names: Olive leaf

Family: *Oleaceae*

Description of Plant

- Evergreen tree, grows to 25 to 30 feet tall, source of olives and olive oil
- Native to Mediterranean but cultivated in the Americas.
- Leaves can be gathered throughout the year.

Medicinal Part: Leaves

Constituents and Action (if known)

- Secoiridoid glycosides
  - Oleuropein (oleouropeoside): antibacterial: *Staphylococcus*, *Bacillus cereus*, antiviral, antifungal properties, reduces blood pressure (in animal studies) through vasodilation, antiarrhythmic, mild calcium antagonist (Weiss & Fintelmann, 2000), inhibits oxidation of low-density lipoprotein (Zheng, 1999)
  - Antioxidant properties (Bruneton, 1999), inhibits oxidation of low-density lipoprotein (Zheng, 1999), antispasmodic, coronary vasodilator (Zarzuelo et al., 1991)
  - Antidiabetic activity by increasing peripheral uptake of glucose and potentiates glucose-induced insulin release (Gonzalez et al., 1992)

- Calcium elenolate, a hydrolyzed form of oleuropein, shows antiviral activity (Zheng, 1999)
- Ligustroside, oleuroside, oleacein: inhibits vasoconstriction by blocking production of angiotensin II (Zheng, 1999)
- Flavonoids (rutin, glycosides of apigenin and leuteolin) (Bruneton, 1999)
- Phenols: caffeic acid, antioxidant; 2-(3,4 dihydroxyphenyl) ethanol, inhibits platelet aggregation and production of thromboxane A_2 (Zheng, 1999)
- Triterpenes (oleanolic acid, maslinic acid, erythrodiol)

Nutritional Ingredients: None known

Traditional Use
- Hypoglycemic agent, hypotensive, diuretic, astringent, febrifuge
- Used in Europe for mild hypertension
- Used to treat malaria
- Astringent and antiseptic for skin
- Used to treat diabetes in Trinidad and Tobago as well as in European folk medicine

Current Use: To lower blood pressure: useful for mild hypertension, usually combined with other herbs such as hawthorn, motherwort, black haw, and dandelion leaf; may be useful for borderline type II diabetes and insulin resistance (syndrome X), but more research is needed

Available Forms, Dosage, and Administration Guidelines
Preparations: Dried leaf; extracts containing 6% to 15% oleuropein, tincture, pills, capsules. Take with meals to avoid gastrointestinal upset.
Typical Dosage
- *Tea:* Steep 1 tsp dried leaves in 1 cup hot water for 20 minutes; take a half-cup two or three times a day.
- *Tincture* (1:5, 60% alcohol): 30 to 40 gtt (1.5–2 mL) three times a day
- *Capsules:* One or two capsules twice a day with meals to avoid GI upset or follow manufacturer's recommendations

Pharmacokinetics—If Available (form or route when known): None known

Toxicity: None known

Contraindications: May lower blood sugar in patients with diabetes (Gonzalez et al., 1992)

Side Effects: GI upset occasionally has been reported.

Long-Term Safety: Not known

Use in Pregnancy/Lactation/Children: No research; do not use

Drug/Herb Interactions and Rationale (if known): None known

Special Notes: A current testimonial claims that this herb should be used for chronic fatigue syndrome, herpes and other viral infections, arthritis, yeast infections, and skin conditions. No real research exists to support these claims.

BIBLIOGRAPHY

Bruneton J. (1999). *Pharmacognosy, Phytochemistry, Medicinal Plants.* Paris: Lavoisier.

Chevallier A. (1996). *Encyclopedia of Medicinal Plants.* New York: DK Publishing.

Gonzalez M, et al. (1992). Hypoglycemic activity of olive leaf. *Planta Medica.* 58(6):513–515.

Hansen K, et al. (1996). Isolation of an angiotensin-converting enzyme (ACE) inhibitor from *Olea europaea* and *Olea lancea*. *Phytomedicine.* 2(4):319–325.

Review of Natural Products. (1999). St. Louis: Facts and Comparisons.

Tranter HS, et al. (1993). The effect of the olive phenolic compound, Oleuropein, on growth and enterotoxin B production by *Staphylococcus aureus. Journal of Applied Bacteriology.* 74:253–259.

Vioque B, et al. (1989). Peroxidases and ethylene formation in olive tree leaves. *Revista Espanolade Fisiologie.* 45(1):47–52.

Weiss R, Fintelmann V. (2000). *Herbal Medicine.* (2nd ed.). Stuttgart: Thieme.

Zarzuelo A, et al. (1991). Vasodilator effect of olive leaf. *Planta Medica.* 57(5):417–419.

Zheng QY, et al. (1999). *Review of Pharmacology and Chemistry of Olive Leaf (Olea europaea L.).* [Unpublished manuscript.]

NAME: Passion flower (*Passiflora incarnata*)

Common Names: Apricot vine, passionfruit, water lemon, maypop

Family: *Passifloraceae*

Description of Plant

- Most plants in this family are vines. There are more than 400 different species. Some have edible fruit, and many have showy flowers.
- Different species are native to tropical and subtropical areas of the Americas; *P. incarnata* is a creeping vine native to the southeastern United States.

Medicinal Part: Dried above-ground herb and flower

Constituents and Action (if known)

- Flavonoids (2.5%) (shaftoside, isoshaftoside, isovitexin, isoorientin, lucenin-2, vicenin-2): may account for sedative activity (Bokstaller et al., 1997; Bourin et al., 1997; Rehwald et al., 1994)
- Maltol (0.05%): relaxes skeletal muscle (Yaniv et al., 1995), reduces corneal reflexes, reduces spontaneous activity, induces sleep (Bourin et al., 1997)
- Cyanogenic glycosides (0.01%): gynocardin
- Indole alkaloids (trace amounts only) (harmine, harman, harmol): have sedative effects through monoamine oxidase inhibition; not enough present to have any activity

Other Actions

- In vitro, has antimicrobial activity against a hemolytic streptococci, *Staphylococcus* aureus, and *Candida*
- Antibacterial (Bokstaller et al., 1997; Nicolis et al., 1973)
- No single constituent or group of constituents has been found to be responsible for passion flower's activity. Recent research suggests that two unidentified compounds that are not alkaloids or flavonoids may have significant activity (Bruneton, 1999).

Nutritional Ingredients: Fruit used for juices and jellies

History: Folklore suggests the flower resembles the crucifixion: the three styles are the nails, the five stamens are the five wounds, the ovary resembles a hammer, the corona resembles the crown of thorns, the petals represent the 10 true apostles, the white color symbolizes purity, and the purple color heaven.

Traditional Use
- Sedative, nervine, antispasmodic
- The eclectic indications for this herb are insomnia with circular thinking: the patient can't seem to turn off his or her mind.
- Used for insomnia, anxiety, nervous tachycardia, neuralgias

Current Use
- GI disturbance caused by stress; combine with catnip, valerian, or chamomile
- Reduces menopausal anxiety and sleeplessness; use with motherwort and black cohosh
- Minor sleeplessness associated with stress; combine with hawthorn, valerian, lemon balm, or linden flower

Available Forms, Dosage, and Administration Guidelines
Preparations: Dried herb, fluid extract, tea, tincture, combination products with other nervine herbs
Typical Dosage
- *Dried herb:* 1 to 2 g three times a day
- *Tea:* Steep 1 tsp dried herb in 1 cup hot water for 15 to 20 minutes; take two cups per day
- *Tincture* (1:5, 40% alcohol): 40 to 80 gtt (2–4 mL) up to four times a day
- *Fluid extracts* (1:1 in 25% alcohol): 0.5 to 2 mL three times a day
- Or follow manufacturer's or practitioner's recommendation

Pharmacokinetics—If Available (form or route when known): None known

Toxicity: None known

Contraindications: None known

Side Effects: Slight CNS depression

Long-Term Safety: Unknown

Use in Pregnancy/Lactation/Children: No restrictions known

Drug/Herb Interactions and Rationale (if known):
Possible additive effect with CNS depressants; theoretical concern

BIBLIOGRAPHY

Birner J, et al. (1973). Passicol, an antibacterial and antifungal agent produced by *Passiflora* plant species: preparation and physicochemical characteristics. *Antimicrobial Agents & Chemotherapy.* 3(1):105–109.

Bokstaller S, et al. (1997). Comparative study on the content of passionflower flavonoids and sesquiterpenes from valerian root extracts in pharmaceutical preparations by HPLC. *Pharmazie.* 52:552–557.

Bourin M, et al. (1997). A combination of plant extracts in the treatment of outpatients with adjustment disorder with anxious mood: controlled study vs. placebo. *Fundamentals of Clinical Pharmacology.* 11(2):127–132.

Bradley P. (1992). *British Herbal Compendium,* Vol. 1. Dorset: British Herbal Medicine Association.

Bruneton J. (1999). *Pharmacognosy, Phytochemistry, Medicinal Plants.* Paris: Lavoisier.

Israel D, et al. (1997). Herbal therapies for perimenopausal and menopausal complaints. *Pharmacotherapy.* 17(5):970–984.

Lawrence Review of Natural Products. (1999). St. Louis: Facts and Comparisons.

Nicolis J, et al. (1973). Passicol, an antibacterial and antifungal agent produced by *Passiflora* plant species: qualitative and quantitative range of activity. *Antimicrobial Agents & Chemotherapy.* 3:110–117.

Rehwald A, et al. (1994). Qualitative and quantitative reversed-phase high-performance liquid chromatography of flavonoids in *Passiflora incarnata* L. *Pharmaceutica Acta Helvetiae.* 69(3):153–158.

Schulz V, et al. (1998). *Rational Phytotherapy,* 3rd ed. Berlin: Springer-Verlag. 1998.

Yaniv R, et al. (1995). Natural premedication for mast cell proliferative disorders. *Journal of Ethnopharmacology.* 46(1):71–72.

NAME: Pau d'arco (*Tabebuia impetiginosa, T. ipe*)

Common Names: Ipe roxo, lapacho colorado, lapacho morado, purple lapacho, red lapacho, taheebo

Family: *Bignoniaceae*

Description of Plant
- Evergreen flowering trees with red, violet, and pink flowers. Species that have yellow flowers are considered to be inferior as a medicine.
- Native to South America, especially Brazil and Argentina

Medicinal Part: Inner bark or heart wood

Constituents and Action (if known)
- Quinone compounds (naphthoquinones)
  ○ Lapachol and beta-lapachone: antimicrobial activity against primarily gram-positive organisms (Guiraud et al., 1994), antitumor activity, antimalarial, antischistosomal, antifungal, antiviral, anticoagulant (Mills & Bone, 1999)
  ○ Xyloidone, deoxylapachol
- Anthroquinone: tabebuin
- Furonaphthoquinones

Nutritional Ingredients: None known

Traditional Use
- Anticancer, antibacterial, antiviral, and antifungal agent
- Used for a broad spectrum of diseases, including dysentery, gastric ulcers, snake bites, fevers, and malaria
- Skin diseases: topically and orally for fungal infections, skin cancers, eczema, psoriasis, and wounds
- Cancer cure for a wide range of carcinomas, including leukemia

Current Use
- In Brazil, used to treat cancer; effectiveness is unproven; may be useful as an adjunctive immune stimulant
- Adjunctive therapy to treat viral infections such as herpes, flu, and colds
- Used to treat fungal and bacterial infections (candidiasis overgrowth)

- Possible use for treating malaria and schistosomiasis; additional research needed

Available Forms, Dosage, and Administration Guidelines
Preparations: Dried bark, capsules, tincture, tea
Typical Dosage
- No therapeutic dosage has been established.
- *Capsules:* Up to four 500- to 600-mg capsules or nine 300-mg capsules a day
- *Tea:* Simmer 2 to 3 tsp inner bark in 2 cups water for 15 minutes; divide into two or three daily doses
- *Tincture* (1:5, 40% alcohol): 20 to 50 gtt (1–2.5 mL) up to four times a day
- Or follow manufacturer's or practitioner's recommendations

Pharmacokinetics—If Available (form or route when known): None known

Toxicity: Very low

Contraindications: Blood clotting disorders

Side Effects: Nausea, vomiting, intestinal discomfort (isolated lapachol); pink urine; anticoagulant effects with high doses

Long-Term Safety: Unknown

Use in Pregnancy/Lactation/Children: The isolated phytochemical lapachol has abortive and teratogenic effects. The whole herb, which contains very small amounts of lapachol, should be used very cautiously if at all during pregnancy and only under clinical supervision.

Drug/Herb Interactions and Rationale (if known): Use cautiously with anticoagulants; may potentiate effects. Obtain prothrombin time and INR to rule out possible interactions.

Special Notes: Research has primarily been done in the laboratory and not on living organisms. National Cancer Institute researchers isolated lapachol in the 1960s and 1970s, with no significant findings. The anticancer activity might come from the whole bark rather than one isolated constituent.

More research is necessary. Most products in the North American marketplace have very low levels of lapachol; Brazilian products have much higher levels of this therapeutically active phytochemical (Awang, 1988).

BIBLIOGRAPHY

Awang DVC. (1988). Commercial taheebo lacks active ingredient. *Canadian Pharmacy Journal.* 5:323–326.

Block JB, et al. (1974). Early clinical studies with lapachol (NSC-11905). *Cancer Chemotherapy Reports.* 4:27–28.

Dinnen RD, Ebisuzaki K. (1997). Search for novel anticancer agents: a differentiation-based assay and analysis of a folklore product. *Anticancer Research.* 17:1027–1034.

Guiraud P, et al. (1994). Comparison of antibacterial and antifungal activities of lapachol and beta-lapachone. *Planta Medica.* 60:373–374.

Mills S, Bone K. (1999). *Principles and Practice of Phytotherapy.* Edinburgh: Churchill Livingstone.

Schutes RE, Raffauf, RF. (1990). *The Healing Forest, Medicinal and Toxic Plants of the Northwest Amazonia.* Portland, OR: Dioscorides Press.

NAME: Pennyroyal (*Hedeoma pulegioides, Mentha pulegium*)

Common Names: American pennyroyal (*H. pulegioides*), European pennyroyal (*M. pulegium*), squaw mint

Family: *Lamiaceae*

Description of Plant
- Both plants are small members of the mint family with a very strong mint odor.
- American pennyroyal is a small, upright annual herb; European pennyroyal is a creeping perennial

Medicinal Part: Herb, EO (very toxic)

Constituents and Action (if known): Volatile oils (monoterpene ketones): pulegone (hepatotoxic; Khojasteh-Bakht et al., 1999), isomenthone, menthone, piperitenone

Nutritional Ingredients: None

Traditional Use

- Abortifacient, carminative, diaphoretic, emmenagogue
- Used to induce "herbal" abortions: this is a very dangerous procedure with the EO and not a very effective one with the herb or tea
- Used as a carminative for gas, nausea, and vomiting

Current Use: The tea can be useful for scanty menstruation with a clotty flow and cramps. Use mixed with ginger, chamomile, and motherwort. Short-term use only.

Available Forms, Dosage, and Administration Guidelines

Preparations: Tea, tincture, EO

Typical Dosage

- *Tea:* 0.5 tsp dried herb in 8 oz hot water, steep 15 minutes (covered); take 4 oz twice daily. Take for no more than a few days per month.
- *Tincture* (1:5, 35% alcohol): avoid
- *EO:* Toxic; do not use

Pharmacokinetics—If Available (form or route when known): Metabolized by the liver, where pulegone is converted by cytochrome P450 enzymes into menthofuran, a proximate hepatotoxic metabolite of pulegone

Toxicity: Causes uterine contractions. The EO is associated with seizures, respiratory depression, liver failure, and death.

Contraindications: Pregnancy, menorrhagia, liver disease, kidney disease, seizure disorders

Side Effects: Some pregnant women become nauseated just from smelling pennyroyal.

Long-Term Safety: Use only the tea in healthy adults and on a short-term basis. Not recommended for regular use (Bruneton, 1999).

Use in Pregnancy/Lactation/Children: Avoid in all.

Drug/Herb Interactions and Rationale (if known): None known

Special Notes: Do not use the EO topically or orally. Pet owners who have heard that the oil repels mosquitoes and ticks have applied it to pets who, on licking it off, have experienced liver and kidney failure and death. N-acetylcysteine has been successfully used to treat poisoning caused by ingestion of pennyroyal EO.

BIBLIOGRAPHY

Anderson IB, et al. (1996). Pennyroyal toxicity: measurement of toxic metabolite levels in two cases and review of the literature. *Annals of Internal Medicine.* 124(8):726–734.

Bakerink JA, et al. (1996). Multiple organ failure after ingestion of pennyroyal oil from herbal tea in two infants. *Pediatrics.* 98(5):944–947.

Bruneton J. (1999). *Pharmacognosy, Phytochemistry, Medicinal Plants.* Paris: Lavoisier.

Duke J. (1989). *Hedeoma pulegioides.* In: *CRC Handbook of Medicinal Herbs.* Boca Raton, FL: CRC Press.

Khojasteh-Bakht S, et al. (1999). Metabolism of (R)-(+)-pulegone and (R)-(+)-menthofuran by human liver cytochrome P-450s: evidence for formation of a furan epoxide. *Drug Metabolism & Disposition.* 28(5):574–580.

Lawless J. (1995). Pennyroyal. In: *The Illustrated Encyclopedia of Essential Oils.* Rockport, MA: Element Books, Inc.

Newall C, et al. (1996). Pennyroyal. In: *Herbal Medicines.* London: Pharmaceutical Press.

Sudekum M, et al. (1992). Pennyroyal oil toxicosis in a dog. *Journal of the American Veterinary Medical Association.* 200(6):817–818.

Sullivan JB Jr, et al. (1979). Pennyroyal oil poisoning and hepatotoxicity. *Journal of the American Medical Association.* 242(26):2873–2874.

NAME: Peppermint *(Mentha × piperita)* (hybrid of spearmint [*M. spicata*] and water mint [*M. aquatica*])

Common Names: Peppermint

Family: *Lamiaceae*

Description of Plant

- Aromatic perennial member of the mint family with square purple-green stems and leaves and small, lilac-colored flowers

- Plant is sterile and spreads through rhizomes underground
- Many varieties of peppermint exist and are cultivated worldwide.

Medicinal Part: Dried herb, essential oil

Constituents and Action (if known)

- More than 100 components have been identified.
- Volatile oils
  - Menthol (35%–55%): antispasmodic in the colon, calcium antagonist effect, reduces abdominal pain, smooth muscle relaxant (Taylor et al., 1985), decongestant, topical analgesic (ESCOP, 1997)
  - Mentone (10%–35%), isomenthone (1.5%–10%), menthyl acetate (2.8%–10%), limonene (1%–5%)
- Flavonoids (luteolin, rutin, hesperidin, erioeitrin): bile-stimulating activity in doses of 0.1 to 50 mg/kg (dogs and guinea pigs) but 25 to 50 mg/kg constricted the sphincter
- Phenolic acids

Other Actions

- Peppermint EO stimulated bile secretion.
- EO and menthol have antibacterial activity.

Nutritional Ingredients: Flavoring for mouthwashes, teas, candies; fresh leaves are used in Middle Eastern cuisine

Traditional Use

- Carminative, GI antispasmodic, choleretic, antipruritic (menthol), nervine, topical analgesic
- Used with elderflower for fevers in small children
- Used to treat digestive upsets, including flatulence, nausea, borborygmus, and intestinal cramps
- Used to relieve colic in infants in combination with chamomile; often given to breast-feeding mothers: the oils pass into the breast milk, relieving gas in the infant

Current Use

- EO is used as a smooth muscle relaxant for irritable bowel syndrome.
- Used as part of decongestant formulas for cough and colds, usually combined with eucalyptus, thyme, or tea tree

- Digestive disturbances: dyspepsia, flatulence, nausea, biliousness, stress-induced GI disturbance (combined with valerian, catnip, or chamomile)
- Used as a counterirritant in topical analgesics (EO) for rheumatic pain, toothache, and headache
- Antipruritic in topical creams (EO or menthol) for symptomatic relief of itching caused by poison ivy, insect bites, dry skin, and so forth
- A tea of peppermint leaf mixed with linden flower, chamomile, or lemon balm is flavorful and relaxing for minor stress, insomnia, or tension headaches.

Available Forms, Dosage, and Administration Guidelines

Preparations: Dried herb, tea, capsules, tincture, EO, ointment (semisolid preparation containing 5%–20% EO in base of beeswax and olive oil)

Typical Dosage

- *Leaf:* 3 to 6 g per day of dried cut leaf for infusions or in capsules, unless otherwise prescribed
- *Infusion:* 2 tsp dried herb in 8 oz. of hot water, steep covered 15 to 20 minutes; take two to four cups per day
- *Tincture* (1:5, 30% alcohol): 100–160 gtt (5 to 8 mL), two or three times daily
- *EO:* 6 to 12 gtt per day for internal and external use, unless otherwise prescribed. Average single dose for internal use is 0.2 to 0.4 mL of EO diluted in carrier oils. Average daily dose is 0.6 mL of EO in the enteric-coated form (for irritable bowel syndrome).
- *Inhalant:* Add 3 to 4 gtt EO to hot water; deeply inhale the steam vapor
- *External use:* Rub a few drops of EO into the affected skin areas. Should be diluted with a carrier such as apricot, olive, or sesame oil.
- *Ointment or unguent:* Apply locally by massage

Pharmacokinetics—If Available (form or route when known): Menthol and other terpenes are fat-soluble and rapidly absorbed by the small intestine. Excretion by the kidney peaks in 3 hours.

Toxicity: None known

Contraindications: Hiatal hernia and GRD, because it relaxes the GI smooth muscle and may worsen symptoms. Do not use EO on the face or mucous membranes (conjunctiva, vagina).

Side Effects: Menthol component may cause allergic reaction and contact dermatitis.

Long-Term Safety: Safe

Use in Pregnancy/Lactation/Children: No restrictions for pregnant or breast-feeding women. Do not give to or apply directly to the nasal or chest area of infants and small children because there is a risk of laryngeal or bronchial spasms. Give to the mother, and the oils will pass through the breast milk.

Drug/Herb Interactions and Rationale (if known): None known

Special Notes: Studies (Freise & Kohler, 1999; Madisch et al., 1999) using peppermint oil and caraway oil for functional dyspepsia found results comparable to those of cisapride. Peppermint EO has low toxicity compared with many other EOs; however, it is still a highly concentrated substance and should be diluted before use and used with caution.

BIBLIOGRAPHY

Briggs C. (1993). Peppermint: medicinal herb and flavoring agent. *Canadian Pharmacy Journal.* 129:89–92.

ESCOP Monographs on the Medicinal Uses of Plant Drugs. (1997). Exeter: ESCOP.

Freise J, Kohler S. (199). Peppermint oil–caraway oil fixed combination in non-ulcer dyspepsia: comparison of the effects of enteric preparations. *Pharmazie.* 54(3):210–215.

Gershenzon J, et al. (2000). Regulation of monoterpene accumulation in leaves of peppermint. *Plant Physiology.* 122(1):205–214.

Hills JM, Aaronson PI. (1991). The mechanism of action of peppermint oil in gastrointestinal smooth muscle. *Gastroenterology.* 101:55–65.

Kingham JGC. (1995). Commentary: peppermint oil and colon spasm. *Lancet.* 346:986.

Lawrence Review of Natural Products. (1990). St. Louis: Facts and Comparisons.

Leung AY, Foster R. (1996). *Encyclopedia of Common Natural Ingredients Used in Food, Drugs, and Cosmetics* (2nd ed.). New York: Wiley Interscience.

Madisch A, et al. (1999). Treatment of functional dyspepsia with a fixed peppermint oil and caraway oil combination preparation as compared to cisapride. A multicenter, reference-controlled double-blind equivalence study. *Arzneimittelforschung.* 49(11):925–932.

Pittler MH, Ernst E. (1998). Peppermint oil for irritable bowel syndrome: a critical review and meta-analysis. *American Journal of Gastroenterology.* 93(7):1131–1135.

Tate S. (1997). Peppermint oil: a treatment for postoperative nausea. *Journal of Advanced Nursing.* 26(3):543–549.

Taylor BA, et al. (April 1985). *Proceedings of the British Pharmacologic Society.*

Weiss RF, Fintelmann V. (2000). *Herbal Medicine* (2nd ed.). Stuttgart: Thieme.

 NAME: Picrorrhiza (*Picrorrhiza kurroa*)

Common Names: Katuka

Family: *Scrophulariaceae*

Description of Plant: A small perennial herb native to the northwestern Himalayas, from Kashmir to Sikkim.

Medicinal Part: Root

Constituents and Action (if known)
- Iridoid glycosides (picoside I, II, III, kutkoside): hepatoprotective (Bone, 1994)
- Triterpenes (cucurbitacin glycosides)
- Bitter substances (apocynin, androsin)

Nutritional Ingredients: None

Traditional Use: Antihepatotoxin, anti-inflammatory, bitter tonic, choleretic, laxative; used in Ayurvedic medicine as a liver and bowel stimulant, for constipation, and for periodic fevers (malaria), to treat hepatitis A with jaundice, and used topically for snake bites and scorpion stings

Current Use

- Hepatoprotective agent: used to prevent and treat liver damage caused by hepatitis A, B, or C, industrial solvents, and pharmaceutical drugs by inhibiting lipid peroxidation of liver microsomes, increasing free radical scavenging activity, and increasing nucleic acid and protein synthesis in rat livers. Reduces elevated liver enzymes, reduces nausea, vomiting, and anorexia, and has shown superior activity to the well-researched herb milk thistle.
- Useful for treating asthma: stabilizes mast cells and inhibits allergen and PAF-induced bronchial obstruction by a nonspecific anti-inflammatory effect (Bone, 1991)
- Immune potentiation and modulator: an ethanotic extract of this herb increased T-cell, B-cell, and phagocytic function. Oral administration of the standardized Picroliv at 10 mg/kg for 7 days stimulated antigen-specific and nonspecific immune response; there was a 10-fold increase in antibody production and a 77.5% increase in activated lymphocytes (Bone, 1991).
- In a 7-year study, picrorrhiza combined with psoralens and light therapy dramatically decreased the number and size of depigmented skin patches in vitiligo.
- Vitiligo and other autoimmune diseases (rheumatoid arthritis, ankylosing spondylitis, and psoriasis) have shown improvement with picrorrhiza treatment.

Available Forms, Dosage, and Administration Guidelines

Preparations: Dried root, tea, tincture, standardized extract (60% picroside I and kutkoside)

Typical Dosage

- *Dried root:* 300 to 500 mg, up to 2 g per day
- *Tea:* 0.5 tsp dried root in 8 oz hot water, decoct 15 to 20 minutes, steep 15 minutes; take 4 oz three times a day. Use with other herbs; the intensely bitter taste will reduce compliance significantly.
- *Tincture* (1:5, 30% alcohol): 10 to 40 gtt (0.5–2 mL) three times a day
- *Standardized extract* (Picroliv): Follow manufacturer's recommended dosage.

Pharmacokinetics—If Available (form or route when known): Not known

Toxicity: Low potential for toxicity

Contraindications: Pregnancy

Side Effects: Nausea, diarrhea and intestinal cramping (at higher doses), skin rash

Long-Term Safety: Safe when used in recommended doses. Animal studies have found no chronic toxicity.

Use in Pregnancy/Lactation/Children: Avoid in all.

Drug/Herb Interactions and Rationale (if known): None known

Special Notes: An important ingredient in many Ayurvedic preparations

BIBLIOGRAPHY
Bone K. (1996). *Clinical Applications of Ayurvedic and Chinese Herbs.* Queensland, Australia: Phytotherapy Press
Bone K. (1994). Picrorrhiza: important modulator of immune function. *Mediherb Professional Newsletter.* #40-41.
Doshi VB, et al. (1983). *Picrorrhiza kurroa* in bronchial asthma. *Journal of Postgraduate Medicine.* 28(2):89–95.
Joy KL, et al. (2000). Effect of *Picrorrhiza kurroa* extract on transplanted tumours and chemical carcinogenesis in mice. *Journal of Ethnopharmacology.* 71(1-2):261–266.
Joy KL, Kuttan R. (1999). Antidiabetic activity of *Picrorrhiza kurroa* extract. *Journal of Ethnopharmacology.* 67(2):143–148.
Kapoor CD. (1990). *CRC Handbook of Ayurvedic Medicinal Plants.* Boca Raton, FL: CRC Press.
Mehrotra R, et al. (1990). In vitro studies on the effect of certain natural products against hepatitis B virus. *Indian Journal of Medical Research.* 92:133–138.
Saraswat B, et al. (1999). Ex vivo and in vivo investigations of picroliv from *Picrorrhiza kurroa* in an alcohol intoxication model in rats. *Journal of Ethnopharmacology.* 66(3):263–270.
(1992). *Selected Medicinal Plants of India.* Bombay: Chemexcil.

NAME: Plantain (*Plantago lanceolata, P. major*)

Common Names: English plantain, broadleaf plantain, buckhorn, common plantain, greater plantain, white man's foot, lanceleaf plantain

Family: *Plantaginaceae*

Description of Plant

- Small perennial weedy plant with a rosette of basal leaves and inconspicuous flowers in heads or spikes
- The genus contains up to 270 species throughout the world.

Medicinal Part: Leaves and root

Constituents and Action (if known)

Leaves

- Iridoid glycosides
  - Aucubin: anti-inflammatory, spasmolytic, antihepatotoxin, antibacterial (Samuelson, 2000)
  - Catapol, gardoside, geniposidic acid, mayoroside, melittoside
- Terpenoids: loliolid, ursolic acid (anti-inflammatory), oleanolic acid (antihyperlipidemic, tumor inhibitor, antihepatotoxic activity) (Samuelson, 2000)
- Caffeic acid derivatives: caffeic acid, chlorogenic acid, plantamajoside R (anti-inflammatory, antioxidant), aceteoside R (antibacterial, antioxidant, inhibits lipid peroxidation, immunosuppressant, analgesic) (Samuelson, 2000)
- Polysaccharides: plantaglucide, glucomannon, PMII, PMIa (activates human monocytes in vitro for increased production of tumor necrosis factor)
- Alkaloids: indicain, plantagonin
- Polyholozide: gastroprotective, laxative (Hriscu et al., 1990)
- Flavonoids and flavone glucosides: luteolin-7 glucoside, hispidulin 7-glucuronide, apigenin, balcalein, scutallarin, plantaginin: antioxidant, free radical scavengers, inhibit lipid peroxidation, anti-inflammatory, antiallergic (Samuelson, 2000)

Seeds

- Tannins

- *P. major* seeds contain polysaccharides but are much less mucilaginous than its relative psyllium.
- Fatty acids

Nutritional Ingredients: Young leaves can be cooked and eaten as greens. They contain vitamin C, K, carotenoids, zinc, and potassium.

Traditional Use

- Astringent, vulnerary, anti-inflammatory, expectorant, topical anodyne, antibacterial, styptic
- The tea of the leaf and root was used for hemoptysis, hematuria, sore throats, coughs, diarrhea, and dysentery.
- Local application for hemorrhoids (baths), cervicitis (vaginal douche), rectal fissures (suppository)
- Vulnerary for insect bites, snake bites, cuts, bruises, and boils

Current Use

Oral Use

- Gastroprotective: heals gastric and intestinal inflammation (gastritis, gastric and duodenal ulcers, mild colitis)
- Bronchial irritation and coughs: reduces upper respiratory tract irritation and bronchitis
- UTI (interstitial cystitis, hematuria, cystitis)

Topical Use

- Astringent and vulnerary for burns, cuts, wounds, cervical erosion, rectal fissures, hemorrhoids, and episiotomy incisions
- Reduces inflammation and pain of insect bites and stings (bee, wasp, spider, scorpion, ants) and poison ivy

Available Forms, Dosage, and Administration Guidelines

Preparations: Dried herb, tea, capsules, tincture

Typical Dosage

- *Tea:* Steep 2 tsp dried herb in 1 cup hot water for 10 to 15 minutes; take 8 oz three or four times a day as needed
- *Tincture* (1:2, 30% alcohol): 60 to 120 gtt (3–6 mL) three times a day
- Or follow manufacturer's or practitioner's recommendations

Pharmacokinetics—If Available (form or route when known): None known

Toxicity: None known

Contraindications: None known

Side Effects: None

Long-Term Safety: Safe. Long-term human use as a food and medicine and animal studies show no toxicity.

Use in Pregnancy/Lactation/Children: Safe

Drug/Herb Interactions and Rationale (if known): None known

Special Notes: Be sure the suppliers of the dried herb use guaranteed botanical identification. In the past few years, plantain was accidentally adulterated with foxglove (digitalis), with one known death.

BIBLIOGRAPHY

Hriscu A, et al. (1990). A pharmacodynamic investigation of the effect of polyholozidic substances extracted from *Plantago* sp. on the digestive tract. *Rev Med Chir Soc Med Nat Iasi.* 94(1):165–170.

Matev M, et al. (1982). Clinical trial of a *Plantago major* preparation in the treatment of chronic bronchitis. *Vutreshni Bolesti.* 21(2):133–137.

Mauri M, et al. (1995). Phenylethanoids in the herb of *Plantago lanceolata* and inhibitory effect on arachidonic acid-induced mouse ear edema. *Planta Medica.* 61(5):479–480.

Ringbom T, et al. (1998). Ursolic acid from *Plantago major*, a selective inhibitor of cyclooxygenase-2 catalyzed prostaglandin biosynthesis. *Journal of Natural Products.* 61(10):1212–1215.

Samuelson AB. (2000). The traditional uses, chemical constituents, and biological activities of *Plantago major*: a review. *Journal of Ethnopharmacology.* 71(1-2):1–22.

Wegener T, Kraft K. (1999). Plantain (*Plantago lanceolata* L.): anti-inflammatory action in upper respiratory tract infections. *Wien Medizinische Wochenschrift.* 149(8-10):211–216.

Wichtl M, Bisset NG. (1994). *Herbal Drugs and Phytopharmaceuticals.* Boca Raton, FL: CRC Press.

NAME: Psyllium Seed (*Plantago psyllium, P. ovata*)

Common Names: Black psyllium (*P. psyllium*), blonde psyllium (*P. ovata*), ispaghula

Family: *Plantaginaceae*

Description of Plant
- Black psyllium is native to the Mediterranean.
- Blonde psyllium is native to the Mediterranean, North Africa, and Western Asia.

Medicinal Part: Seeds and husks

Constituents and Action (if known)
- Soluble fiber (47%), mucilage (10%–30%): when soaked in water, increases greatly in volume, adding bulk to the stool (ESCOP, 1997; McRorie et al., 1998)
  - May be able to reduce diarrhea in patients receiving enteral feedings (Belknap et al., 1997; Brown et al., 1999; Olson et al., 1997)
  - Lowers cholesterol (Anderson et al., 2000; ESCOP, 1997); reduces the ratio of LDL to HDL (Jenkins et al., 1997)
  - Reduces glucose absorption, improving postprandial glucose in persons with type 1 and 2 diabetes (Anderson et al. 1999; Frati Munari et al., 1998; Rodriguez-Moran M et al., 1998)
- Insoluble fiber (53%)
- Fixed oils and unsaturated fatty acids
- Trisaccharide (planteose)

Nutritional Ingredients: Protein (15%–20%)

Traditional Use
- Tea (mucilage) used for sore throats, dry coughs, and gastric irritation
- Bulk laxative
- Topically used as a poultice for styes, boils, and sores

Current Use
- Increases fiber in stool
- Short-term (3–4 days) treatment of nonspecific diarrhea

- Reduces cholesterol (Larkin, 2000); binds bile acids and increases their fecal excretion, which in turn stimulates further bile salt synthesis from cholesterol (ESCOP, 1997)
- Bulk laxative and stool softener for habitual constipation, especially in patients with anal fissures, hemorrhoids, after rectal surgery, and during pregnancy (ESCOP, 1997)
- Reduces symptoms of irritable bowel syndrome; psyllium decreases B-glucuronidase activity of intestinal bacteria, inhibiting cleavage of toxic compounds from their liver conjugates
- Short-chain fatty acids (acetate, proprionate, butyrate) that are released from the digestible part of the fiber by bacterial fermentation have a normalizing effect on mucosal cells (ESCOP, 1997). Psyllium is superior to bran in maintaining stool frequency without producing flatulence (Blumenthal et al., 2000)
- May reduce blood sugar by slowing glucose absorption in gut

Available Forms, Dosage, and Administration Guidelines
- A single dose usually contains 1.7 g soluble fiber. Unless otherwise prescribed, take 10 to 30 g/day whole or ground seeds or other galenical preparations for oral use.
- *Seed:* 5 to 10 g seed, two or three times daily. Presoak seeds in 100 to 200 mL warm water for several hours. Follow each dose by drinking at least another 200 mL water. WHO recommends an average dose of 7.5 g dissolved in 240 mL water or juice, one to three times daily. Children 6 to 12 years should take half the adult dosage.

Pharmacokinetics—If Available (form or route when known): Not known

Toxicity: None known

Contraindications: Psyllium allergies, bowel obstruction, stenosis of the esophagus or GI tract

Side Effects: Allergic reactions may occur.

Long-Term Safety: Safe

Use in Pregnancy/Lactation/Children: Safe

Drug/Herb Interactions and Rationale (if known):
Separate by 2 hours from all other drugs. If taken with diabetic drugs, may need to reduce dose because blood sugar can be reduced.

Special Notes: Always take with sufficient fluids to ensure the seeds do not cause bowel obstruction.

BIBLIOGRAPHY

Anderson JW, et al. (2000). Cholesterol-lowering effects of psyllium intake adjunctive to diet therapy in men and women with hypercholesterolemia: meta-analysis of 8 controlled trials. *American Journal of Clinical Nutrition.* 71(2):472–479.

Anderson JW, et al. (1999). Effects of psyllium on glucose and serum lipid responses in men with type 2 diabetes and hypercholesterolemia. *American Journal of Clinical Nutrition.* 70(4):466–473.

Belknap D, et al. (1997). The effects of psyllium hydrophilic mucilloid on diarrhea in enterally fed patients. *Heart & Lung.* 26(3):229–237.

Blumenthal M, et al. (2000). *Herbal Medicine Expanded Commission E Monographs.* Austin, TX: American Botanical Council.

Bradley PR. (Ed.). (1992). *British Herbal Compendium,* Vol. I. Dorset: British Herbal Medicine Association.

Brown L, et al. (1999). Cholesterol-lowering effects of dietary fiber: a meta-analysis. *American Journal of Clinical Nutrition.* 69(1):30–42.

Bruneton J. (1999). *Pharmacognosy, Phytochemistry, Medicinal Plants.* Paris: Lavoisier.

ESCOP Monographs on the Medicinal Uses of Plant Drugs. (1997). Exeter: ESCOP.

Frati Munari AC, et al. (1998). Lowering glycemic index of food by acarbodse and *Plantago psyllium* mucilage. *Archives of Medical Research.* 29(2):137–141.

Jenkins DJ, et al. (1997). Effect of psyllium in hypercholesterolemia at two monounsaturated fatty acid intakes. *American Journal of Clinical Nutrition.* 65(5):1524–1533.

Larkin M. (2000). Functional foods nibble away at serum cholesterol concentrations. *Lancet.* 355(9203):555.

McRorie JW, et al. (1998). Psyllium is superior to docusate sodium for treatment of chronic constipation. *Alimentary Pharmacology and Therapeutics.* 12(5):491–497.

Olson BH, et al. (1997). Psyllium-enriched cereals lower blood total cholesterol and LDL cholesterol, but not HDL cholesterol, in hypercholesterolemic adult: results of a meta-analysis. *Journal of Nutrition.* 127(10):1973–1980.

Rodriguez-Moran M, et al. (1998). Lipid and glucose-lowering efficacy of *Plantago psyllium* in type I diabetes. *Journal of Diabetes Complications.* 12(5):273–278.

NAME: Pygeum (*Prunus africana*)

Common Names: African plum

Family: *Rosaceae*

Description of Plant
- A tall evergreen tree native to southern and central Africa
- Grows in highland mountain forests above 2500 feet. Much of its natural habitat has been lost to clear-cutting.

Medicinal Part: Bark

Constituents and Action (if known)
- Fatty acids
  - Decrease inflammation in prostate by antagonizing 5-lipoxygenase (Bruneton, 1999; Krzeski et al., 1993; Levin et al., 1997)
  - Reduce hormonal level in prostate (Chevallier, 1996)
  - Increase bladder elasticity (Levin et al., 1997)
  - Histologically modify glandular cells (Levin et al., 1997)
  - Increase prostatic secretions (Mathe et al., 1995; Paubert-Barquet et al., 1994; Yablonski et al., 1997)
- Phytosterols (beta-sitosterol, beta-sitosterone, campesterol)
  - Reduce inflammation and edema in and near prostate (Bassi et al., 1987; Dagues et al., 1995; Krzeski et al., 1993)
  - Inhibit prostaglandin biosynthesis (Schulz et al., 1998)
  - Inhibit 5-alpha-reductase, an enzyme that increases the production of DHT (Bruneton, 1999; Paubert-Barquet et al., 1994)
  - Inhibits biosynthesis (Schulz et al., 1998)

- Triterpenoid pentacyclic acids (ursolic, oleanolic): anti-inflammatory (Schulz et al., 1998)
  - Ferulic acid esters (n-docosanol and n-tetracosanol): lower testosterone and prolactin levels
- Organic acids (hydrocyanic acid)

Nutritional Ingredients: None

Traditional Use: Used to treat intercostal pain, improve kidney function, improve difficult urination; taken in milk for dysuria, stomach ache

Current Use
- Relieves symptoms of BPH, including dysuria, nocturia, pollakiuria, and volume of residual urine
- Commonly used in Italy and France for BPH along with saw palmetto, nettle root, and rye pollen
- May reduce prostate gland size
- May reverse impotence and sterility associated with a reduction in prostatic secretions and improve seminal fluid composition
- Also used to treat prostatitis

Available Forms, Dosage, and Administration Guidelines
Preparations: Dried bark, capsules, tablets, tinctures. Some products are standardized to 14% beta-sitosterol and/or 12% to 13% phytosterols and 0.5% n-docosanol.
Typical Dosage: For standardized products, take 100 to 200 mg/day, or follow manufacturer's or practitioner's recommendations. Take with meals. Take in 6- to 8-week cycles with at least 1 week in between. May be started at half the therapeutic dose to prevent gland enlargement. Men should start therapy in their early 40s.

Pharmacokinetics—If Available (form or route when known): Not known

Toxicity: None known

Contraindications: None known

Side Effects: Nausea, stomach pain

Long-Term Safety: Safe

Use in Pregnancy/Lactation/Children: Do not use.

Drug/Herb Interactions and Rationale (if known): None known

Special Notes: In comparative studies, pygeum was less effective than saw palmetto and less well tolerated by patients (Winston, 1999). Pygeum is often combined with saw palmetto, nettle root, or pumpkin seed oil to treat BPH, because each herb has a slightly different mechanism of action and the combinations have a synergistic effect superior to any one single treatment. Patients should be seen by a medical practitioner first for baseline studies, including prostatic-specific antigen. Use only cultivated bark; pygeum has been drastically overharvested.

BIBLIOGRAPHY

Barlet A, et al. (1990). Efficacy of *Pygeum africanum* extract in the treatment of micturitional disorders due to benign prostatic hyperplasia. *Wien Klinische Wochenschrift.* 22:667–673.

Bassi P, et al. (1987). Standardized *Pygeum africanum* extract in the treatment of benign prostatic hypertrophy. *Minerva Urologica e Nefrologica.* 39:45–50.

Bruneton J. (1999). *Pharmacognosy, Phytochemistry, Medicinal Plants.* Paris: Lavoisier.

Chatelain C, et al. (1999). Comparison of once- and twice-daily dosage forms of *Pygeum africanum* extract in patients with benign prostatic hyperplasia: a randomized, double-blind study, with long-term open label extension. *Urology.* 54(3):473–478.

Chevallier A. (1996). *Encyclopedia of Medicinal Plants.* New York: DK Publishing.

Dagues F, et al. (1995). Medical treatment of disorders of the bladder sphincter. *Review du Praticien.* 45(3):337–341.

Hutchings A, et al. (1996). *Zulu Medicinal Plants: An Inventory.* Scottsville, South Africa: University of Natal Press.

Krzeski T, et al. (1993). Combined extracts of *Urtica dioica* and *Pygeum africanum* in the treatment of benign prostatic hyperplasia: double-blind comparison of two doses. *Clinical Therapeutics.* 15(6):1011–1020.

Levin R, et al. (1997). Cellular and molecular aspects of bladder hypertrophy. *European Urology.* 32(Suppl. 1):15–21.

Mathe G, et al. (1995). The so-called phyto-estrogenic aciton of *Pygeum africanum* extract. *Biomedical Pharmacotherapeutics.* 49(7-8):339–343.

Murray MT. (1995). *The Healing Power of Herbs.* Rocklin, CA: Prima Publishing.

Paubert-Barquet M, et al. (1994). Effect of *Pygeum africanum* extract on A23187-stimulated production of lipoxygenase metabolites from human polymorphonuclear cells. *Lipid Mediated Cell Signals.* 9(3):285–290.

Review of Natural Products. (1998). St. Louis: Facts & Comparisons.

Schulz V, et al. (1998). *Rational Phytotherapy.* Berlin: Springer-Verlag.

Winston D. (1999). *Saw Palmetto for Men and Women.* Pownal, VT: Storey Publishing.

 NAME: Raspberry (*Rubus idaeus, R. stryosus*)

Common Names: Red raspberry, raspberry leaf

Family: *Rosaceae*

Description of Plant
- Cultivated throughout the world as a food plant for its berries
- Plant has thorny canes with three- to five-toothed leaflets
- Fruit is usually red but can also be yellow

Medicinal Part: Leaves, fruit

Constituents and Action (if known)
- Gallo- and elligitannins: astringent properties for diarrhea or as mouthwash (Haslam et al., 1989), antiviral activity
- Flavonoids (rutin, kaemferol, quercitin): antioxidants, anti-inflammatory
- Volatile oils (monoterpenes): geraniol, linolool
- Raspberry leaf may lower blood glucose (Briggs & Briggs, 1997).

Nutritional Ingredients: The fruit is a source of vitamin C, flavonoids, pectin, and fructose. The leaves contain calcium, magnesium, and flavonoids.

Traditional Use
- Astringent, uterine tonic, styptic, mild antispasmodic
- As an astringent to treat diarrhea, hematuria, and enuresis
- Pregnancy tonic, as a tea, to strengthen the uterus, reduce morning sickness, and prevent miscarriage
- As a uterine tonic for a boggy atonic uterus, uterine prolapse, and menorrhagia
- As an astringent gargle for inflammation of the mouth, gums, and throat
- Dried raspberry fruit (*fu pen zi*) is used in TCM for frequent urination, bedwetting, and impotence.

Current Use
- Pregnancy tonic (see use in pregnancy section)
- Astringent tea to treat mild diarrhea and mouth sores
- Mild uterine tonic for women in their 40s and 50s with uterine prolapse, menorrhagia, worsening dysmenorrhea, and pelvic congestion. Preliminary studies suggest the leaves may have antispasmodic activity (Wren, 1988).

Available Forms, Dosage, and Administration Guidelines
- *Dried herb:* 4 to 8 g
- *Tea:* 1 to 2 tsp herb in 8 oz hot water, steep half-hour; take one to three cups per day
- *Tincture* (1:5, 30% alcohol): 60 to 100 gtt (3–5 mL) three times a day

Pharmacokinetics—If Available (form or route when known): Not known

Toxicity: None known

Contraindications: None known

Side Effects: None known

Long-Term Safety: Safe

Use in Pregnancy/Lactation/Children: Used for millennia as a pregnancy tonic; empirical use as well as as clinical use by midwives suggests it is not only safe but that it improves the pregnancy and makes the labor easier

Drug/Herb Interactions and Rationale (if known): None known

Special Notes: There is little scientific information on this herb because of a lack of studies. Ethnobotanical and empirical use suggests numerous benefits, and studies of related species suggest that this herb may have anti-inflammatory, antiviral, and antioxidant activity.

BIBLIOGRAPHY
Bisset NG, Wichtl M. (1994). *Herbal Drugs and Phytopharmaceuticals*. Stuttgart: Medpharm.
Briggs CJ, Briggs K. (1997). Raspberry. *Canadian Pharmaceutical Journal*. 130:41–43.
Haslam E, et al. (1989). Traditional herbal medicines: the role of polyphenols. *Planta Medica*. 55:1.
Hobbs C, Keville K. (1998). *Women's Herbs, Women's Health*. Loveland, CO: Interweave Press.
McIntyre A. (1995). *The Complete Woman's Herbal*. New York: Henry Holt Co.
Review of Natural Products. (1999). St. Louis: Facts and Comparisons.
Wren RC. (1988). *Potter's New Cyclopaedia of Botanical Drugs and Preparations*. Saffron Waldon, England: CW Daniel Co. Ltd.

 NAME: Red Clover (*Trifolium pratense*)

Common Names: Meadow clover, purple clover, wild clover, beebread

Family: Fabiaceae

Description of Plant
- Native to Europe but naturalized in the United States
- Low-growing perennial with trifoliate leaves and purplish flowers

Medicinal Part: Flowering tops

Constituents and Action (if known)
- More than 125 phytochemicals have been isolated from red clover.

- Flavone glycosides, including genistein, diadzen, biochanin A, formononetin, and calycosin, are responsible for weak estrogen-like actions (Kelly et al., 1979).
  - Anticancer activity: inhibit cancers in vitro and breast cancer in rats, inhibit angiogenesis and cancer cell adhesion (Kelly et al., 1998)
  - Increase follicle-stimulating hormone and alter luteinizing hormone, therefore helping to decrease many menopausal signs and changes (Wilcox et al., 1990; Zava et al., 1998); inhibit oxidation of steroid hormones and increase production of sex hormone-binding globulin (Kelly et al., 1998)
  - Increase arterial compliance, which may assist with blood pressure control (no effect on lipids) (Nestel et al., 1999)
  - Promote calcium storage and maintain bone density (Kelly et al., 1998)
- Coumarins (warfarin, medicagol) may affect platelet activity; antioxidant, lipid-reducing, and antitumor activity (McCaleb et al., 2000)
- Saponins
- Minerals: calcium, iron, magnesium, manganese, potassium, copper
- May have antitumor activity; is part of the controversial Hoxsey formula used to treat cancer in Mexico (Cassady et al., 1988). Used in more than 30 countries to treat cancer (McCaleb et al., 2000).

Nutritional Ingredients: Florets can be added to salads and used as edible garnishes. They are rich in minerals (potassium, iron, magnesium, calcium, manganese). Widely grown as animal fodder.

Traditional Use
- Alterative, anticancer remedy, expectorant
- Used as an "alterative or blood cleanser" for cancer, especially breast, lymph, and lung cancers
- Topical use: chronic skin conditions including skin cancer (Samuel Thomson's Cancer Salve), eczema, and dermatitis

- Used as a tea and cough syrup to suppress coughs, useful for colds, bronchitis, and pertussis
- Lymph tonic for chronic lymphatic congestion associated with skin problems, mastitis, and arthritis

Current Use
- Standardized product is a source of isoflavones. It is used as a "natural hormone replacement" therapy to control menopausal symptoms and changes (hot flashes, night sweats) and as a means of maintaining prostate health.
- 5-alpha-reductase and aromatase inhibition, estrogen receptor antagonist, increases uridine diphosphate-glucuronyltransferase
- Further research should be done to assess this plant's possible activity for treating human cancers.

Available Forms, Dosage, and Administration Guidelines
Preparations: Dried flowering tops, tea, tincture, capsules. Promensil is a widely used standardized product for control of menopausal symptoms.

Typical Dosage
- *Standardized tablets:* Two per day, each containing 40 mg isoflavones
- *Capsules:* Up to five 500-mg capsules a day
- *Tea:* 1 to 2 tsp dried flowering tops in 8 oz hot water, steep half-hour; take two or three cups per day
- *Tincture* (1:5, 30% alcohol): 60 to 100 gtt (3–5 mL) up to three times a day
- Or follow manufacturer's or practitioner's recommendations

Pharmacokinetics—If Available (form or route when known): None known

Toxicity: None

Contraindications: Use cautiously in patients with bleeding disorders. Use of phytoestrogens is controversial in patients with estrogen-positive cancers. Some researchers speculate that these substances may stimulate estrogen-sensitive tumor growth. Studies show that genistein and biochanin prevent the

growth of cancer cell lines (prostate, stomach) in vitro and inhibit breast cancer in rats.

Side Effects: Theoretical possibility of decreased clotting; infertility in animals (cows, sheep) who eat large quantities of this plant and are much more sensitive to isoflavones than humans

Long-Term Safety: Safe; FDA GRAS list

Use in Pregnancy/Lactation/Children: Avoid using the standardized isoflavone products during pregnancy. Long history of use with children; no adverse effects expected.

Drug/Herb Interactions and Rationale (if known)

• Use cautiously with anticoagulants (coumarin, warfarin) and antiplatelet agents (ASA, ticlopidine): theoretical possibility of effects on platelets and an increase of bleeding. Obtain prothrombin time and INR to assess possible interactions.

• Use cautiously with oral contraceptives: theoretical concern that concurrent use of the isolated isoflavone may enhance effects

Special Notes: There is a major difference between red clover as a herb or crude extract and the standardized preparations, which are highly concentrated for isoflavones. Epidemiologists believe cultures that eat food rich in isoflavones have a lower incidence of cancer. Population studies clearly show that in Asian cultures where daily consumption of isoflavones is usually 40 mg (vs. 2–5 mg in the United States), there is a lower incidence of prostate cancer in men and breast cancer in women.

BIBLIOGRAPHY

Bradley PR. (Ed.). (1992). *British Herbal Compendium,* Vol. I. Bournemouth, UK: British Herbal Medicine Association.

Cassady JM, et al. (1988). Use of a mammalian cell culture benzo(a)pyrene metabolism assay for the detection of potential anticarcinogens from natural products: inhibition of metabolism by biochanin A, an isoflavone from *Trifolium pratense* L. *Cancer Research.* 48:6257–6261.

Kelly G, et al. (1998). *Standardized Red Clover Extract Clinical Monograph.* Seattle: Natural Products Research Consultants, Inc.

Kelly RW, et al. (1979). Formononentin content of grasslands pawera red clover and its estrogenic activity in sheep. *New Zealand Journal of Experimental Agriculture.* 7:131–134.

McCaleb R, et al. (2000). *Encyclopedia of Popular Herbs.* Roseville, CA: Prima Publishers.

Nachtigall L, et al. (1999). *The effects of isoflavone derived from red clover on vasomotor symptoms, endometrial thickness, and reproductive hormone concentrations in menopausal women.* Endocrine Society 81st annual meeting, June 12–15, 1999.

Nestel PJ, et al. (1999). Isoflavones from red clover improve systemic arterial compliance but not plasma lipids in menopausal women. *Journal of Clinical Endocrinology & Metabolism.* 84(3):895–899.

Wilcox G, et al. (1990). Estrogenic effects of plant foods in postmenopausal women. *British Medical Journal.* 301:905–906.

Yanagihara K, et al. (1993). Antiproliferative effects of isoflavones on human cancer cell lines established from the gastrointestinal tract. *Cancer Research.* 53:5815–5821.

Zava DT, et al. (1998). Estrogen and progestin bioactivity of foods, herbs and spices. *Proceedings of the Society for Experimental Biology & Medicine.* 217:369–378.

 NAME: Reishi (*Ganoderma lucidum*)

Common Names: Varnish shelf fungus, *ling zhi* and *ling chih* (Chinese)

Family: *Polyporaceae*

Description of Plant
- A woody shelf fungus (polypore) with a shiny red or reddish-brown upper surface
- The mushroom grows on oak trees in China, Japan, Russia, and the eastern United States.

Medicinal Part: Fruiting body and mycelium

Constituents and Action (if known)
- Polysaccharides
  - Beta-D-glucans: enhance protein synthesis and nucleic acid metabolism
  - Ganoderans A, B, and C: hypoglycemic

- ○ GL-1: antitumor, immunostimulating
- ○ FA, F1, F1-1a: antitumor, immunostimulating
- ○ Other polysaccharides have shown cardiotonic activity.
- Triterpenes
  - ○ Ganoderic acids A, B, C, D: inhibit histamine release
  - ○ Ganoderic acids R and S: antihepatotoxin
  - ○ Ganoderic acids B, D, F, H, K, S, Y: antihypertensive, inhibit angiotensin-converting enzyme
  - ○ Ganoderic acids B and M: inhibit cholesterol synthesis
  - ○ Ganodermadiol: antihypertensive, inhibit angiotensin-converting enzyme
- Protein (ling-zhi-8): antiallergic, immunomodulator
- Steroid (ganodosterone): antihepatotoxin
- Whole ganoderma extracts have also shown anti-inflammatory, antioxidant, expectorant, adrenal stimulant, radiation protective, antiulcer, and antitumor activity (Hobbs, 1995).
- Protects against ultraviolet and x-ray radiation in mice (Kim & Kim, 1999)

Nutritional Ingredients: Black ganoderma (*G. sinensis*) has been used for millennia to make a stock for soups.

Traditional Use
- Adaptogen, immune amphoteric, antihepatotoxin, nervine, cardiotonic
- The Chinese considered *ling zhi* a profoundly powerful tonic remedy; it was rare and reserved for the emperor and his court.
- In TCM, *ling zhi* is used to tonify the blood and vital energy. It is also used to calm disturbed *shen* and as an antitussive for coughs. Ganoderma is used in formulas for insomnia, palpitations, anxiety, impaired memory, general weakness and debility, heart disease, cancer, allergies, and hypertension.

Current Use
- Immune amphoteric: normalizes immune response and can be used for immune deficiency and hyperimmune response (autoimmune conditions [rheumatoid arthritis, lupus,

scleroderma, ankylosing spondylitis, multiple sclerosis] and allergies)
- Immunostimulant: enhances NK cells, interleukin 1 and 2, and interferon production in vitro and in vivo. Has been used clinically for HIV/AIDS, herpes virus, hepatitis B and C, CFS, fibromyalgia, acute myeloid leukemia, and recurrent nasopharyngeal carcinomas.
- Use is sanctioned by the Japanese Health Ministry as an adjunct treatment for cancer. Increases the activity of chemotherapeutic agents and reduces adverse effects such as nausea, decreased white blood cell counts, and cachexia.
- Antihepatotoxin: used to protect the liver against damage caused by viral, drug, or environmental liver toxins. Used with vitamin C for treating hepatitis B and C; also effective for treating toxipathic hepatitis caused by ingestion of poisonous mushrooms, hepatodynia, and hyperlipidemia
- Useful as a cardiotonic; enhances myocardial metabolism and improves coronary artery hemodynamics. Symptoms that showed improvement include palpitations, dyspnea, arrhythmias, elevated cholesterol, and high blood pressure (Hobbs, 1995)
- In Chinese clinical trials, tablets were given to more than 2,000 patients with chronic bronchitis. In 2 weeks, 60% to 90% of the patients had improvement of symptoms and increased appetite. Also beneficial for allergic asthma and allergic rhinitis because of its ability to inhibit histamine release.
- Prevention and possibly treatment of atherosclerosis
- Treatment of altitude sickness: use with schisandra, ginkgo, or Siberian ginseng
- Effective for treating the symptoms of a rare genetic disease, myotonia dystrophica (Hobbs, 1995)
- Useful as an adaptogen for reducing the effects of chronic stress. Improves adrenal function, sleep quality, appetite; acts as an antioxidant; reduces anxiety and inflammation.

Available Forms, Dosage, and Administration Guidelines
Preparations: Dried mushroom, tea, tincture, spray dried extract

Typical Dosage
- *Dried mushroom (finely ground):* 3 to 10 g per day
- *Tea:* 2 tsp ground mushroom in 16 oz water, decoct slowly until the water is reduced by half (8 oz); take two or three cups per day
- *Tincture* (1:5, 30% alcohol): 80 to 160 gtt (4–8 mL) three times a day
- *Spray dried extract* (5:1): Three 300-mg capsules three times a day

Pharmacokinetics—If Available (form or route when known): Not known

Toxicity: None

Contraindications: Mushroom allergies

Side Effects: Diarrhea (large doses)

Long-Term Safety: Safe

Use in Pregnancy/Lactation/Children: Safe

Drug/Herb Interactions and Rationale (if known): None known

Special Notes: Various species (*G. sinensis, G. tsugae, G. applanatum, G. tenue, G. capense, G. japonicum*) have shown medicinal activity.

BIBLIOGRAPHY

el-Mekkawy S, et al. (1998). Anti-HIV-1 and Anti-HIV-1-protease substances from *Ganoderma lucidum*. *Phytochemistry.* 49(6):1651–1657.

Hijikata Y, Yamada S. (1998). Effect of *Ganoderma lucidum* on postherpetic neuralgia. *American Journal of Chinese Medicine.* 26(3-4):375–381.

Hobbs C. (1995). *Medicinal Mushrooms* (2nd ed.). Santa Cruz, CA: Botanica Press.

Jones K. (1996). *Reishi: Ancient Herb for Modern Times.* Seattle: Sylvan Press.

Kim KD, Kim IG. (1999). *Ganoderma lucidum* extract protects DNA from strand breakage caused by hydroxyl radical and UV irradiation. *International Journal of Molecular Medicine.* 4(3):273–277.

Kim DH, et al. (1999). Beta-glucuronidase-inhibitory activity and hepatoprotective effect of *Ganoderma lucidum*. *Biological Pharmacy Bulletin*. 22(2):162–164.

Patocka J. (1999). Anti-inflammatory triterpenoids from mysterious mushroom *Ganoderma lucidum* and their potential possibility in modern medicine. *Acta Medica (Hradec Kralove)*. 42(4):123–125.

Seong-Kug E, et al. (1999). Antiherpetic activities of various protein-bound polysaccharides isolated from *Ganoderma lucidum*. *Journal of Ethnopharmacology*. 68:175–181.

Willard T. (1990). *Reishi Mushroom*. Issaquah, WA: Sylvan Press.

Ying J, et al. (1987). *Icones of Medicinal Fungi from China*. Beijing: Science Press.

Zhu M, et al. (1999). Triterpene antioxidants from *Ganoderma lucidum*. *Phytotherapy Research*. 13(6):529–531.

 NAME: Rosemary *(Rosmarinus officinalis)*

Common Names: Garden rosemary

Family: *Lamiaceae*

Description of Plant

- A highly aromatic member of the mint family with waxy linear leaves and pale blue flowers.
- A small, bushy shrub native to the southern Mediterranean; now commonly cultivated throughout the world.
- Leaves are harvested and can be used fresh or dried.

Medicinal Part: Leaves, flowering tops, EO

Constituents and Action (if known)

- Volatile oils (0.5%–2.5%): monoterpenes: camphor (15%–25%), cineole (15%–50%), alpha-pinene (10%–25%), camphene, and borneol (spasmolytic): antibacterial, antiviral, and antifungal activity
- Flavonoids (diosmin, diosmetin, genkwanin, luteolin, apigenin)
  - May reduce capillary permeability and fragility
  - Antioxidant activity (Okamura et al., 1994)

- May have anti-inflammatory activity (Parnham & Kesselring, 1985)
- Phenolic acids
  - Rosmarinic acid: anti-inflammatory, antioxidant; reduces smooth muscle activity (in vitro); suppresses release of thromboxane A_2, prostacyclin (al-Sereiti et al., 1999; Bult et al., 1985), chlorogenic acid (Bruneton, 1999)
  - Caffeic acid: antioxidant (al-Sereiti et al., 1999)
  - Phenolic compounds inhibit cancers by inhibiting activation of phase I enzymes (cyclic P450) and stimulating phase II enzymes (glutathione S-transferase). In laboratory animals, adding 1% rosemary extract to the diet reduced the incidence of experimentally caused mammary tumors by 47%. Skin tumors were also inhibited by topical application.
- Tricyclic diterpenes
  - Carnosolic (carnosic) and labiatic acids: antioxidant and anticancer properties (Offord et al., 1995); carnosol, rosmanol, rosmariquinone, rosmadial: anti-inflammatory, antioxidant, antiviral (ESCOP, 1997)
  - Inhibitory against HIV-1 protease (Paris et al., 1993)

Other Actions

- Rosemary extracts have a strong antiviral activity.
- Extracts have a topical anti-inflammatory activity.
- May have potential as a chemoprotectant (more studies in humans are needed) (Huang et al., 1994; Offord et al., 1997)

Nutritional Ingredients: A versatile spice that can be used to flavor meat, fish, and fowl; can also be used in rolls and bread

Traditional Use

- Astringent, antioxidant, carminative, antispasmodic, choleretic, circulatory tonic
- Digestive tonic for flatulence, borborygmus, eructations, nausea, and biliousness
- Tea used to stimulate hair growth and prevent baldness
- Used to strengthen the memory and cerebral circulation
- Used in Europe for headaches, hypotension, and impaired circulation

- EO in a carrier oil is used as a massage oil for arthritic pain and muscle spasms.

Current Use
Internal
- Liver/gallbladder tonic for impaired fat digestion, biliousness, nausea, and biliary dyskinesia. Rosemary enhanced the activity of two liver enzymes (GSH-transferase, NAD(P)H-quinone reductase) when included at very low levels in the diet of rats.
- Reduces GI upset, gas, and distention
- Powerful dietary antioxidant that may reduce the risk of cancers, arteriosclerosis, and other oxidative diseases
- A mild circulatory tonic for hypotension, impaired memory

Topical: Topical application of rosemary extract in carrier oils or liniments is useful for muscle pain and arthralgias and may inhibit risk of skin cancers.

Available Forms, Dosage, and Administration Guidelines
Preparations: Dried herb, tincture, capsules, EO, ointment (semisolid preparation containing 6%–10% EO in base of beeswax and vegetable oil)
Typical Dosage
- *Dried herb:* 4 to 6 g per day
- *Infusion:* 1 tsp dried herb in 8 oz hot water, steep covered 15 to 20 minutes; take two cups per day
- *Tincture* (1:5, 40% alcohol): 40 to 80 gtt (2–4 mL) three times a day
- *Capsules:* One or two 500-mg capsules three times a day
- *EO:* 2 gtt two or three times per day
- *Rosemary wine:* macerate 1 oz dried leaf in 1 L wine for 1 to 5 days, stirring occasionally
- *Bath additive:* infuse 2 oz leaf in 1 qt water, let stand covered for 15 to 30 minutes, strain, and add to one full bath
- *Ointment:* massage into affected areas

Pharmacokinetics—If Available (form or route when known): Not known

Toxicity: Herb: none known; EO: overdoses can cause irritation of the stomach and intestines and kidney damage.

Contraindications: Avoid internal use of EO in patients with seizures.

Side Effects: Contact dermatitis with external use (Fernandez et al., 1997); GI disturbances with large internal doses

Long-Term Safety: Safe; long history of human consumption as a spice and medicine

Use in Pregnancy/Lactation/Children: Avoid in pregnancy; may have adverse effects on fetus and uterus. No restrictions during lactation.

Drug/Herb Interactions and Rationale (if known): None known

Special Notes: Rosemary EO, like all EOs, is highly concentrated and should be used internally in very minute amounts. Topically, the EO should be diluted before being applied to the skin.

BIBLIOGRAPHY

Al-Sereiti MR, et al. (1999). Pharmacology of rosemary (*Rosmarinus officinalis* Linn.) and its therapeutic potentials. *Indian Journal of Experimental Biology.* 37(2):124–130.

Blumenthal M, et al. (2000). *Herbal Medicine: Expanded Commission E Monographs.* Austin, TX: American Botanical Council.

Bruneton J. (1999). *Pharmacognosy, Phytochemistry, Medicinal Plants* (2nd ed.). Paris: Lavoisier.

Bult H, et al. (1985). Modification of endotoxin-induced hemodynamic and hematologic changes in the rabbit by methylprednisolone, F(ab')2 fragments and rosmarinic acid. *Biochemistry & Pharmacology.* 35:1397–1400.

Correa Dias P, et al. (2000). Antiulcerogenic activity of crude hydroalcoholic extract of *Rosmarinus officinalis* L. *Journal of Ethnopharmacology.* 69(1):57–62.

ESCOP Monographs on the Medicinal Uses of Plant Drugs. (1997). Exeter: ESCOP.

Fahim FA, et al. (1999). Allied studies on the effect of *Rosmarinus officinalis* L. on experimental hepatotoxicity and mutagenesis. *International Journal of Food Science & Nutrition.* 50(6):413–427.

Fernandez L, et al. (1997). Allergic contact dermatitis from rosemary (*Rosmarinus officinalis* L). *Contact Dermatitis.* 37(5):248–249.

Hjorther AB, et al. (1997). Occupational allergic contact dermatitis from carnoso, a naturally-occurring compound present in rosemary. *Contact Dermatitis.* 37(3):99–100.

Huang MT, et al. (1994). Inhibition of skin tumorigenesis by rosemary and its constituents carnosol and ursolic acid. *Cancer Research.* 54:701–708.

Offord EA, et al. (1995). Rosemary components inhibit benzo (a) pyrene-induced genotoxicity in human bronchial cells. *Carcinogenesis.* 16(9):2057–2062.

Offord EA, et al. (1997). Mechanisms involved in the chemoprotective effects of rosemary extract studied in human liver and bronchial cells. *Cancer Letters.* 114:275–281.

Okamura N, et al. (1994). Flavonoids in *Rosmarinus officinalis* leaves. *Phytochemistry.* 37(5):1463–1466.

Paris A, et al. (1993). Inhibitory effect of carnosic acid on HIV-1 protease in cell-free assays. *Journal of Natural Products.* 56(8):1426–1430.

Parnham MJ, Kesselring K. (1985). Rosmarinic acid. *Drug Future.* 10:756–757.

Review of Natural Products. (2000). St. Louis: Facts and Comparisons.

Tisserand R, Balacs T. (1995). *Essential Oil Safety.* Edinburgh: Churchill Livingstone.

Weiss R, Fintelmann V. (2000). *Herbal Medicine.* (2nd ed.). Stuttgart: Thieme.

S

 NAME: Sarsaparilla (*Smilax* species)

Common Names: Honduras or brown sarsaparilla (*S. regelii*), Mexican or gray sarsaparilla (*S. medica*), Jamaican or red sarsaparilla (*S. ornata*), Ecuadorian sarsaparilla (*S. febrifuga*)

Family: *Liliaceae*

Description of Plant

- Woody, trailing vine that can grow to 150 feet
- Numerous species are used, and many are similar in appearance.
- Cultivated in Mexico, Jamaica, and Central and South America

Medicinal Part: Rhizome

Constituents and Action (if known)
- Steroidal saponins
  - Sarsaponin, sarasapogenin, smilagenin, smilasaponin: have ability to bind endotoxins, so may be beneficial in liver disease, psoriasis, fever, and inflammatory processes; may have antibiotic properties (Murray, 1995; Newall et al., 1996)
  - Diosgenin, tigogenin, and asperagenin (Newall et al., 1996)
- Phytosterols (sitosterol, stigmasterol, pollinastanol) (Newall et al., 1996)
- Other constituents include starch (50%), resin (2.5%), kaempferol, quercetin.
- Minerals: potassium, chromium, magnesium, selenium, calcium, and zinc

Nutritional Ingredients: Root has mild spicy-sweet taste and has been used as a natural flavoring in medicines, foods, and nonalcoholic beverages.

Traditional Use
- Anti-inflammatory, alterative, diuretic, hepatoprotective, antirheumatic
- Used with guaiac to treat syphilis. A Chinese species, *S. glabra,* along with five other herbs, has been reported to be 90% effective in curing acute syphilis and 50% effective in treating chronic cases (confirmed by blood tests).
- For red, hot, and inflamed skin and connective tissue conditions (psoriatic and rheumatoid arthritis and psoriasis); use with gotu cola
- Systemic anti-inflammatory for arthralgias

Current Use
- Reduces inflammation in arthritis, bursitis, rheumatoid arthritis, and gout. Increases uric acid excretion and binds endotoxin, reducing the oxidative load in the bowel. Combine with additional anti-inflammatory herbs, such as turmeric, bupleurum, or boswellia.
- Moderate hepatoprotective activity

- Anti-inflammatory to the large and small intestines; a useful therapy for dysbiosis, leaky gut syndrome, and irritable bowel syndrome. Use with yarrow, chamomile, turmeric, or marshmallow.
- Adjunctive therapy for leprosy

Available Forms, Dosage, and Administration Guidelines

Preparations: Dried root, powdered; capsules, tablets, tincture, combination products

Typical Dosage
- *Dried root:* 6 to 10 g
- *Capsules:* Up to six 500-mg capsules a day
- *Tea:* 2 tsp powdered root, decoct in 10 oz hot water for 10 to 15 minutes, steep half-hour; take two or three cups per day
- *Tincture* (1:5, 30% alcohol): 60 to 100 gtt (3–5 mL) three times a day
- Or follow manufacturer's or practitioner's recommendations

Pharmacokinetics—If Available (form or route when known): None known

Toxicity: None known

Contraindications: None known

Side Effects: GI irritation and nausea in large doses; asthma may occur from exposure to sarsaparilla dust (Vandenplas et al., 1996)

Long-Term Safety: Long history of human use in beverages and as a medicine; no adverse effects expected in normal therapeutic dosage

Use in Pregnancy/Lactation/Children: No known problems, but no research to establish safety

Drug/Herb Interactions and Rationale (if known): Separate from all other oral drugs by 2 hours; saponins may affect absorption.

Special Notes: Advertising claims suggest that sarsaparilla is a natural source of testosterone (this is false) and that it enhances exercise performance (this is unsubstantiated). Few studies are available on the Western species of *Smilax*, but the Chinese species, *S. glabra*, has been well studied and shown to be effective in treating rheumatoid arthritis and leptospirosis.

BIBLIOGRAPHY

Bradley PR. (1992). *British Herbal Compendium,* Vol. I. Bournemouth, UK: British Herbal Medicine Association.

Bernardo RR, et al. (1996). Steroidal saponins from *Smilax officinalis*. *Phytochemistry.* 43(20):465–469.

Leung A, Foster S. (1996). *Encyclopedia of Common Natural Ingredients*. (2nd ed.). New York: John Wiley & Sons.

Murray M. (1995). *The Healing Power of Herbs*. (2nd ed.). Rocklin, CA: Prima Publishing.

Newall C, et al. (1996). *Herbal Medicines*. London: Pharmaceutical Press.

Rafatullah S, et al. (1991). Hepatoprotective and safety evaluation studies on sarsaparilla. *International Journal of Pharmacognosy.* 29(4):296–301.

Review of Natural Products. (1999). St. Louis: Facts and Comparisons.

Vandenplas O, et al. (1996). Occupational asthma caused by sarsaparilla root dust. *Journal of Allergy & Clinical Immunology.* 97(6):1416–1418.

 NAME: Sassafras (*Sassafras albidum*)

Common Names: Ague tree, cinnamon wood, lignum floridium, root bark, lignum sassafras, saloop

Family: *Lauraceae*

Description of Plant
- Common deciduous tree found growing throughout the eastern United States
- Leaves have three distinct forms (entire, mitten, and trident)

Medicinal Part: Root bark

Constituents and Action (if known): Volatile oils (5%–9%): safrole (80%), alpha-pinene, alpha- and beta-phellandrene; tannins

Nutritional Ingredients: Commonly used as a beverage tea throughout the southeastern and south-central United States.

The leaf is dried and powdered and sold as filé, a spice and thickener in Creole cooking.

Traditional Use

- Carminative, diaphoretic, diuretic
- Used for digestive disturbances (gas, nausea, vomiting, and borborygmus)
- Taken as a hot tea to stimulate sweating and break fevers
- A spring tonic or "blood purifier" used to stimulate elimination of wastes by the kidney, liver, and skin

Current Use: Not commonly used, except as a home remedy and beverage tea. The purported toxicity of sassafras as a tea is overstated, and its occasional ingestion in small amounts is not a cause for serious concern. The carcinogen safrole is poorly water-soluble, so very little is consumed in a tea. Avoid the EO, capsules, and tincture because of their high safrole content.

Available Forms, Dosage, and Administration Guidelines

Preparations: Dried root bark, tea
Typical Dosage

- *Tea:* 1 tsp dried root bark in 8 oz water, steep covered 5 minutes
- *Tincture:* Not recommended
- *EO:* Toxic; avoid

Pharmacokinetics—If Available (form or route when known): Safrole is broken down to 1-hydroxysafrole, a potent hepatic carcinogen.

Toxicity: Safrole, a component of the EO, is a potential carcinogen and is banned in the United States, even as a flavoring or fragrance (Duke, 1989; Newall et al., 1996). However, it is still sold and labeled "not for human consumption."

Contraindications: Pregnancy

Side Effects: Nausea or vomiting in large doses. The hot tea may cause excess sweating, especially in obese or menopausal patients.

Long-Term Safety: Avoid regular long-term use.

Use in Pregnancy/Lactation/Children: Avoid in all.

Drug/Herb Interactions and Rationale (if known): None known

Special Notes: Studies in mice clearly show the toxicity of safrole. There are no known cases of human toxicity from consuming the tea.

BIBLIOGRAPHY

Bruneton J. (1999). *Pharmacognosy, Phytochemistry, Medicinal Plants.* (2d ed.). Paris: Lavoisier.

DeSmet PAGM. (1997). *Adverse Effects of Herbal Drugs,* Vol. 3. Berlin: Springer-Verlag.

Duke J. (1989). *Sassafras albidum* (Nutt.). In: *CRC Handbook of Medicinal Herbs.* Boca Raton, FL: CRC Press.

Leung A, Foster S. (1996). *Encyclopedia of Common Natural Ingredients.* (2nd ed.). New York: John Wiley & Son.

Newall C, et al. (1996). *Sassafras.* In: *Herbal Medicine.* London: Pharmaceutical Press.

Review of Natural Products. (1997). St. Louis: Facts and Comparisons.

Tisserand R, Balacs T. (1995). *Essential Oil Safety.* Edinburgh: Churchill Livingstone.

 NAME: Saw Palmetto (*Serenoa repens*)

Common Names: Dwarf palmetto, fan palm

Family: *Palmae*

Description of Plant

- Small palm tree native to the Atlantic and Gulf coasts of North America, from South Carolina to Florida to Alabama
- Grows 6 to 10 feet high, with 2- to 4-foot spiny-toothed leaves that form a circular fan shape
- Berries are blue-black with an oily texture and a pungent, cheesy aroma.

Medicinal Part: Berries (drupes)

Constituents and Action (if known)

- Fatty acids (63%–65%) (lauric, capric, caproic, caprylic, oleic, linoleic, linolenic, myristic, palmitic and stearic acids): reduce the formation of dihydrotestosterone by being a weak inhibitor of 5-alpha-reductase (Dathe & Schmid, 1991; Goepel et al., 1999; Marks & Tyler, 1999; McKinney, 1999); anti-inflammatory for prostatic tissue (Gerber et al., 1998)
- High-molecular-weight alcohols (n-docosanol, n-octacosanol, n-tricosanol, and hexacosanol): inhibit both subtypes of 5-alpha-reductase (Tenover, 1991; Weisser et al., 1996); inhibit prolactin (DiSilverio et al., 1992) and growth-factor-induced prostatic cell proliferation (Champault et al., 1984a, 1984b; Paubert-Braquet et al., 1996)
- Fatty acids (ethyl esters and sterols: beta-sitosterol, stigmasterol): anti-inflammatory, antitumor; lupeol, campesterol: anti-inflammatory
- Diterpenes (geranylgeraniol, phytol)
- Triterpenes (cycloartenal): bactericide, hypocholesterolemic
- Polysaccharides (S1, S2, S3, S4): immunostimulating; found in herb, not in standardized extracts (Winston, 1999)

Nutritional Ingredients: Used by the native people of Florida as a food; used as a flavoring in cognac; in the early part of the 20th century it was used to flavor a soft drink called Metto.

Traditional Use

- Adaptogen, anti-inflammatory, diuretic, demulcent, immune amphoteric, urinary antiseptic
- Used by native people as a food; there is no history of them using the berries as a medicine
- Introduced into Western medical practice in 1877 as a digestive tonic and nutritive and to relieve irritation of the mucous membranes and upper respiratory tract. Was used for anorexia, pertussis, laryngitis, chronic coughs, tuberculosis, bronchitis, asthma, and weakness and deficiency after a serious illness.
- The eclectic physicians popularized *Serenoa* as a urinary tract and reproductive remedy and used it for orchitis,

epididymitis, ovarian pain, prostatic hypertrophy, pelvic congestion, and atrophy of the testes and ovaries.

Current Use

- Improves urine flow rate, relieves nocturia by up to 73%, reduces residual urine volume, decreases dysuric pain and pollakiuria. Reduces prostatic swelling, prevents further progression of the condition (reducing the need for later surgery), and does not affect prostatic-specific antigen levels.
- A valuable upper respiratory herb (capsule, tea, tincture) useful for chronic irritable coughs, laryngitis, chronic bronchitis, and asthma
- The tea or encapsulated herb is an immune tonic and adaptogen and can be used for patients with immune deficiency, frequent colds, cachexia, anorexia, and allergies.
- A mild, nonirritating diuretic, the berries can be beneficial for interstitial cystitis, UTIs, and scalding urine.
- Reduces symptoms of pelvic congestion syndrome (Winston, 1999)
- Useful along with chaste tree for treating polycystic ovarian disease, ovarian pain, and female infertility caused by excessive androgens
- Can be beneficial for deep cystic acne, combined with red alder, Oregon grape root, and chaste tree

Available Forms, Dosage, and Administration Guidelines

Preparations: Dried fruit (whole or ground), capsules, tablets, tinctures. Standardized products are made with fat-soluble carriers containing high levels of free fatty acids.

Typical Dosage
- *Dried herb:* 2 to 6 g per day
- *Standardized preparations* (85%–95% fatty acids and sterols): Once or twice a day for a daily dose of 320 mg
- *Capsules* (nonstandardized): Six to nine 500-mg capsules a day
- *Tincture* (1:3, 70% alcohol): 60 to 100 gtt (3–5 mL) up to four times a day, or follow manufacturer's or practitioner's recommendations

- *Tea:* 1 tsp crushed berries to 8 oz hot water, decoct 15 minutes, steep half-hour; take two or three cups per day. The taste is terrible and will severely limit patient compliance.

Pharmacokinetics—If Available (form or route when known): None known

Toxicity: Completely safe

Contraindications: None known

Side Effects: GI upset (take with meals to minimize), diarrhea, headache (rare)

Long-Term Safety: Very safe

Use in Pregnancy/Lactation/Children: Used as a food by native people so it is probably safe, but because there is no current research, best to avoid. Avoid in breast-feeding women because it inhibits prolactin and may interfere with lactation.

Drug/Herb Interactions and Rationale (if known): None known

Special Notes: A medical diagnosis of BPH before starting treatment with saw palmetto and appropriate medical follow-up are recommended.

BIBLIOGRAPHY

Bach D, Ebeling L. (1996). Long-term drug treatment of benign prostatic hyperplasia: results of a three-year multicenter study, *Phytomedicine.* 3(2):105–111.

Bach D, Schmitt M, Ebeling L. (1997). Phytopharmaceutical and synthetic agents in the treatment of benign prostatic hyperplasia. *Phytomedicine.* 3(4):309–313.

Batchelder H. (Winter 1996). Allopathic specific condition review: BPH. *Protocol Journal of Botanical Medicine.* 19–20.

Bennett BC, Hicklin JR. (1998). Uses of saw palmetto (*Serenoa repens, Arecaceae*) in Florida. *Economic Botany.* 52(4):381–393.

Bombardelli E, Morazzoni P. (1997). *Serenoa repens* (Bartram). *Fitoterapia.* 68(2):99–114.

Braeckman J. (1994). The extract of *Serenoa repens* in the treatment of benign prostatic hyperplasia. *Current Therapeutic Research.* 55:776–785.

Bruneton J. (2000). *Pharmacognosy, Phytochemistry, Medicinal Plants.* (2nd ed.). Paris: Lavoisier.

Champault G, et al. (1984a). Medical treatment of the prostatic adenoma: a controlled test of PA 109 (Permixon): *Serenoa repens* extract) vs. placebo in 100 patients. *Annual Journal of Urology.* 18(6):407–410.

Champault G, et al. (1984b). A double-blind trial of an extract of the plant *Serenoa repens* in benign prostatic hyperplasia. *British Journal of Clinical Pharmacy.* 18:461–462.

Dathe G, Schmid H. (1991). Phytotherapy of benign prostatic hyperplasia (BPH) with extractum *Serenoa repens. Urology.* 31:220–223.

DiSilverio F, et al. (1992). Evidence that *Serenoa repens* extract displays an antiestrogenic activity in prostatic tissue of benign prostatic hypertrophy patients. *European Urology.* 21:309–314.

Gerber GS, et al. (1998). Saw palmetto (*Serenoa repens*) in men with lower urinary tract symptoms: effects on urodynamic parameters and voiding symptoms. *Urology.* 51:1003–1007.

Goepel M, et al. (1999). Saw palmetto extracts potently and noncompetitively inhibit human alpha 1-adrenoceptors in vitro. *Prostate.* 38(3):208–215.

Marandola P, et al. (1997). Main phytoderivatives in the management of benign prostatic hyperplasia. *Fitoterapia.* 68(3):195–204.

Marks LS, et al. (2000). Effects of a saw palmetto herbal blend in men with symptomatic benign prostatic hyperplasia. *Journal of Urology.* 163(5):1451–1456.

Marks LS, Tyler VE. (1999). Saw palmetto extract: newest (and oldest) treatment alternative for men with symptomatic benign prostatic hyperplasia. *Urology.* 53(3):457–461.

McPartland JM, Pruitt PL. (2000). Benign prostatic hyperplasia treated with saw palmetto: a literature search and an experimental case study. *Journal of the American Osteopathic Association.* 100(2):89–96.

McKinney DE. (1999). Saw palmetto for benign prostatic hyperplasia. *Journal of the American Medical Association.* 281(18):1699.

Paubert-Braquet M, et al. (1996). Effect of *Serenoa repens* extract (Permixon) on estradiol/testosterone-induced experimental prostate enlargement in the rat. *Pharmacology Research.* 34:171–179.

Plosker GL, Brogden RN. (1996). *Serenoa repens* (Permixon): a review of its pharmacology and therapeutic efficacy in benign prostatic hyperplasia. *Drugs in Aging.* 9:379–395.

Schneider HJ, et al. (1995). Treatment of benign prostatic hyperplasia. Results of a surveillance study in the practices of urological specialists using a combined plant-based preparation. *Fortschritte der Medizin.* 113:37–40.

Tenover JS. (1991). Prostates, pates, and pimples. The potential medical uses of steroid 5-alpha-reductase inhibitors. *Endocrinology & Metabolism Clinics of North America.* 20:893–903.

Weisser H, et al. (1996). Effects of the *Sabal surrulata* extract IDS 89 and its subfractions on 5-alpha-reductase activity in human benign prostatic hyperplasia. *Prostate.* 28:300–306.

Wilt TJ, et al. (1998). Saw palmetto extracts for treatment of benign prostatic hyperplasia: a systematic view. *Journal of the American Medical Association.* 280(18):1604–1609.

Winston D. (1999). *Saw Palmetto for Men and Women.* Pownal, VT: Storey Publishing.

 NAME: Schisandra (*Schisandra chinensis*)

Common Names: Schizandra, *gomishi* (Japanese), *wu-wei-zi* (Chinese), Chinese magnolia vine

Family: *Schisandraceae*

Description of Plant
- Climbing woody vine with white to pink flowers producing purple-red globular fruits with kidney-shaped seeds
- Native to China, Russia, Korea, and Japan
- Fruit is harvested in autumn.

Medicinal Part: Dried fruit

Constituents and Action (if known)
- Dibenzo[a,c] cycloactadiene lignans (18% of seeds): approximately 40 have been identified
  - Gomisins D, E, F, G, H, J, N, schizandrol A, B, schisandrin A, b, Schisantherin A, B, C, gomisins wu-wei-zi-su C
  - PAF antagonist activity (Lee et al., 1999)
  - May have cardioprotective activity (in rats) and protect from hypoxia (Li et al., 1996), antioxidants (Bone, 1996)
  - Enhance glutathione protection in liver (Ko et al., 1995), stimulate liver glycogen and protein synthesis, inhibit lipid

peroxidation; enhanced survival in experimental fulminant hepatitis from 7.5% to 80% and prevented liver cell necrosis (Bone, 1996)
  ○ Gomisin N, schisandrin B, schizandrol B protect the liver against halothane-induced hepatitis, carbon tetrachloride, hepatic failure induced by bacteria (Ip et al., 1996; Ko et al., 1995; Upton, 1999)
- Gomisin A (schizandrol B)
  ○ May improve bile acid metabolism
  ○ Improves liver regeneration and hepatic blood flow (in rats)
  ○ May decrease amphetamine-induced motor activity
  ○ Antitussive activity (in pigs)
  ○ Inhibits hepatocarcinogenesis in rats, improves excretion of carcinogens
  ○ Anti-inflammatory
- N granoic acid may inhibit HIV-1 reverse transcriptase replication (Sun et al., 1996)
- Volatile oils: monoterpenes (borneal, 1,8-cineol, citral) and sesquiterpenes (sesquicarene, ylangene, chamigrenol)
- Vitamins A, C, E (Chevallier, 1996; Upton, 1999)
- Organic acids (10% by weight): malic, citric, tartaric
- Fixed oils (38%): linoleic, oleic, linolenic, lauric, and palmitic acids

Other Actions
- Nervous system stimulant; enhances memory in humans (Chevallier, 1996; Nishiyama et al., 1995); antidepressant (Bone, 1996); anticonvulsant
- May enhance neuron growth and prevent neuron atrophy
- Used to treat insomnia (Chevallier, 1996)

Nutritional Ingredients: Fresh berry juice with sugar and water has been used as a beverage ("sandra berry" juice).

Traditional Use
- Adaptogen, anti-inflammatory, astringent, hepatoprotective, antiasthmatic
- Commonly used in TCM; the berries are used in formulas to calm *shen* (insomnia, palpitations, impaired memory) and to astringe the *jing* (frequent urination, spermatorrhea, leukorrhea, night sweats, and early morning diarrhea)
- Relieves dry coughs, dyspnea, asthma

Current Use

- Tonic and restorative herb (adaptogen); effective for deficiency conditions such as neurasthenia, CFS, insomnia, impaired memory, fatigue, chronic stress, and depression
- Human athletes and race horses improved performance, displayed accelerated recovery after exercise, and had greater stamina after taking schisandra for 2 weeks.
- Hepatoprotective; use with milk thistle, turmeric, or picrorrhiza to prevent or treat liver damage caused by alcohol, industrial solvents, viruses, or pharmaceutical medications. In one controlled study of 189 patients with hepatitis B and elevated SGPT levels, levels returned to normal in 68% of patients after 4 weeks of taking schisandra (Upton, 1999).
- To treat respiratory conditions such as allergic asthma with wheezing, dyspnea, and chronic coughs
- Cardiac antioxidant: in animal studies, the berries reduced ischemic myocardial damage. Reduces stress-induced palpitations.

Available Forms, Dosage, and Administration Guidelines

Preparations: Dried fruit, tea, capsules, tinctures

Typical Dosage

- *Dried berry:* 1.5 to 6 g per day
- *Capsules:* Up to six 500-mg capsules a day
- *Tea:* Steep 1 tsp dried fruit in 1 cup hot water, decoct for 10 to 15 minutes, steep 15 minutes; take 4 oz three times a day
- *Tincture* (1:5, 35% alcohol): 40 to 80 gtt (2–4 mL) three times a day, or follow manufacturer's or practitioner's recommendations

Pharmacokinetics—If Available (form or route when known): Not known

Toxicity: Experimental overdose in mice caused decreased activity, apathy, and increased body weight.

Contraindications: Epilepsy, pregnancy

Side Effects: Acid indigestion and GI upset, urticaria

Long-Term Safety: Safe. Very low toxicity when used in normal therapeutic doses.

Use in Pregnancy/Lactation/Children: Avoid during pregnancy; may stimulate uterine contractions (Bone, 1996). No adverse reactions expected during lactation (Upton, 1999).

Drug/Herb Interactions and Rationale (if known): Use cautiously with pentobarbitol and barbitol; may potentiate action. May antagonize the CNS-stimulatory effect of caffeine and amphetamines.

Special Notes: Lignan content has been well studied, and it seems to be responsible for schisandra's hepatoprotective effects.

BIBLIOGRAPHY

Bone K. (1996). *Clinical Applications of Ayurvedic and Chinese Herbs.* Queensland, Australia: Phytotherapy Press.

Chevallier A. (1996). *Encyclopedia of Medicinal Plants.* New York: DK Publishing.

Hancke J, et al. (1996). Reduction of serum hepatic transaminases and CPK in sports horses with poor performance treated with a standardized *Schisandra chinensis* fruit extract. *Phytomedicine.* 3(3):237–240.

Ip SP, et al. (1996). Effect of a lignan-enriched extract of *Schisandra chinensis* on aflatoxin B1 and cadmium chloride-induced hepatotoxicity in rats. *Pharmacology & Toxicology.* 78(6):413–416.

Jung KY, et al. (1997). Lignans with platelet activating factor antagonist activity from *Schisandra chinensis* (Turcz.) Baill. *Phytomedicine.* 4(3):229–232.

Ko KM, et al. (1995). Effect of a lignan-enriched fructus schisandrae extract on hepatic glutathione status in rats: protection against carbon tetrachloride toxicity. *Planta Medica.* 61(2):134–137.

Lee IS, et al. (1999). Structure-activity relationships of lignans from *Schisandra chinensis* as platelet activating factor antagonists. *Biologic Pharmacy Bulletin.* 22(3):265–267.

Li PC, et al. (1996). *Schisandra chinensis*-dependent myocardial protective action of sheng mai-san in rats. *American Journal of Chinese Medicine.* 24(3-4):255–262.

Nishiyama N, et al. (1995). Beneficial effects of S-113m, a novel herbal prescription, on learning impairment model in mice. *Biologic Pharmacy Bulletin.* 18(11):1498–1503.

Review of Natural Products. (1997). St. Louis: Facts and Comparisons.

Sun HD, et al. (1996). Nigranoic acid, a triterpenoid from *Schisandra sphaerandra* that inhibits HIV-1 reverse transcriptase. *Journal of Natural Products.* 59(5):525–527.

Upton R. (Ed.). (1999). *American Herbal Pharmacopoeia and Therapeutic Compendium.* Santa Cruz, CA: AHP.

Yamada S, et al. (1993). Preventive effect of gomisin A, a lignan component of schizandra fruits, on acetaminophen-induced hepatotoxicity in rats. *Biochemistry & Pharmacology.* 46(6):1081–1085.

You-Ping Z. (1998). *Chinese Materia Medica.* Amsterdam: Harwood.

 NAME: Scullcap (*Scutellaria laterifolia*)

Common Names: Helmet flower, mad dog, skullcap

Family: *Lamiaceae*

Description of Plant
- A small (1–2 feet) perennial member of the mint family
- Prefers to grow in damp areas

Medicinal Part: Fresh herb

Constituents and Action (if known): Flavonoid glycosides (scutellarein, scutellarin); diterpenoid (scuterivulaetone); bitter iridoid (catapol)

Nutritional Ingredients: None

Traditional Use
- Antispasmodic, nervine, anticonvulsant
- Used for nervous exhaustion with spasms, tics, and palsies
- Mild antispasmodic useful for controlling tremors, stress headaches, back spasms, and facial tics

Current Use
- Useful in nervine formulas with chamomile, lemon balm, fresh oat, and St. John's wort for nervous exhaustion (neurasthenia), insomnia, anxiety with muscle tightness, and mild forms of obsessive-compulsive disorder
- A useful antispasmodic that can be effective for reducing or controlling tremors (Parkinson's disease), restless leg syndrome, Lyme's neuralgias, TMJ pain, mild Tourette's syndrome, and bruxism

Available Forms, Dosage, and Administration Guidelines

Preparations: Fresh plant tincture, freeze-dried capsules. The dried plant has very little activity.

Typical Dosage
- *Fresh plant tincture* (1:2, 30% alcohol): 60 to 120 gtt (3–6 mL) three times a day
- *Freeze-dried capsules:* Two capsules three times per day

Pharmacokinetics—If Available (form or route when known): Not known

Toxicity: Intentional overdoses of the alcoholic tincture from homeopathic provings caused giddiness, stupor, confusion, slowed pulse, and twitching of the limbs.

Contraindications: None

Side Effects: None at normal therapeutic doses

Long-Term Safety: Unknown

Use in Pregnancy/Lactation/Children: Best to avoid due to lack of studies and history of adulteration

Drug/Herb Interactions and Rationale (if known): None known

Special Notes: Be sure of suppliers and botanical identification of all scullcap products. As a result of adulteration with the hepatotoxic herb germander, scullcap has falsely been accused of being hepatotoxic.

BIBLIOGRAPHY

De Smet PAGM, et al. (1993). *Adverse Effects of Herbal Drugs,* Vol. 2. Berlin: Springer-Verlag.

Duke JA. (1985). *Handbook of Medicinal Herbs.* Boca Raton, FL: CRC Press.

Fisher C, Painter G. (1996). *Materia Medica of Western Herbs for the Southern Hemisphere.* Auckland, New Zealand: Authors.

Lawrence Review of Natural Products. (1993). St. Louis: Facts and Comparisons.

McGuffin M, et al. (1997). *American Herbal Products Association's Botanical Safety Handbook.* Boca Raton, FL: CRC Press.

Winston D. (2000). *Herbal Therapeutics: Specific Indications.* (7th ed.). Washington, NJ: Herbal Therapeutics Research Library.

NAME: Shiitake (*Lentinula edodes*)

Common Names: *Hua gu* (Chinese), *Lentinus edodes* (synonym)

Family: *Polyporaceae*

Description of Plant

- A commonly cultivated mushroom, usually grown on oak logs
- Fungus native to Japan, China, and Korea

Medicinal Part: Mushroom, mycelium, mycelium extract (LEM)

Constituents and Action (if known)

- Polysaccharides: lentinin is a highly purified high-molecular-weight polysaccharide used as an injectable medicine: antiviral, immune potentiator, activates NK cells, interleukin 1, interferon, and proliferation of PMNCs
  - LEM (lentinula edodes mycelium extract) contains a heteroglycan protein (a protein-bound polysaccharide), B vitamins, and water-soluble lignans (Hobbs, 1995): antitumor, improves macrophage activity, immune potentiator, antiviral
  - KS-2 is an a-mannan-peptide extract that strongly inhibits cancer cell growth orally and intraperitoneally.
- Water-soluble lignans (EP3, EPS4): antiviral, herpes simplex I and II, polio, measles, mumps, HIV, immunopotentiating
- Eritadenine: lowers cholesterol and lipids
- Tyrosinase: lowers blood pressure
- L-octen-3-ol, ethyl acetate, 2-octenol, and octylalcohol: phytochemicals responsible for the fresh shiitake odor

Nutritional Ingredients: Protein (2%–2.60% fresh, 25.9% dry), minerals (calcium, magnesium, zinc, potassium, phosphorus), vitamins B_2, C, and ergosterol (a vitamin D precursor)

Traditional Use: Long used in the Orient as both a food and medicine. The dry shiitake is known as black mushroom in Chinese cuisine and is considered to be a general tonic for the circulation and immune system and to improve overall health.

Current Use

- Hyperlipidemia: regular use of shiitake can lower cholesterol and blood lipids. In one study of 10 Japanese women, after 1 week of ingesting 9 g dried shiitake per day, serum cholesterol levels fell by 7% (Hobbs, 1995). Another study in a population of 60 years or older saw cholesterol levels drop by 9% (Hobbs, 1995).
- Hepatitis B and C: antiviral and antihepatotoxin effects of LEM have reduced viral load and reduced elevated liver enzyme levels (Jones, 1995).
- LEM strengthens immune response; appropriate for use in patients with cancer, HIV, herpes simplex I and II, frequent colds, and bronchitis.
- May be beneficial for conditions such as CFS, *Candida* overgrowth, and allergies
- Lentinin improved survival times of cancer patients when used concurrently with chemotherapy. It also strengthened the immune function of patients with HIV and tuberculosis.

Available Forms, Dosage, and Administration Guidelines

Preparations: Fresh and dry mushroom, LEM tablets, tincture, lentinin (injectable)

Typical Dosage

- *Fresh mushrooms:* Take as a tonic; medical dosage is unrealistic in this form
- *Dried mushrooms:* 6 to 16 g three times a day
- *LEM tablets:* 2 to 6 g per day for hepatitis or cancer; 0.5 to 1 g per day as a general maintenance dosage
- *Tincture* (1:3, 25% alcohol): 80 to 120 gtt (4–6 mL) three times a day
- *Lentinin (injectable):* 1 to 5 mg intravenously or intramuscularly twice a week. This is an approved medicine in Japan, but has not been approved in the United States.

Pharmacokinetics—If Available (form or route when known): Not known

Toxicity: None known; eaten as a food for thousands of years

Contraindications: None known

Side Effects: LEM occasionally causes mild gastric upset or rashes.

Long-Term Safety: Safe

Use in Pregnancy/Lactation/Children: Safe

Drug/Herb Interactions and Rationale (if known): Thyroxin and hydrocortisone inhibit the antitumor activity of lentinin. Water-soluble extracts may reduce platelet coagulation. Use cautiously with blood thinners.

Special Notes: The most effective oral form of shiitake is the LEM product. Lentinin is widely used in Japan as a prescription medication for cancer, HIV, and hepatitis B and C.

BIBLIOGRAPHY
Hobbs C. (1995). *Medicinal Mushrooms* (2nd ed.). Santa Cruz, CA: Botanica Press.
Jones K. (1995). *Shiitake: The Healing Mushroom.* Rochester, VT: Healing Arts Press.
Jong SC, Birmingham JM. (1993). Medicinal and therapeutic value of the shiitake mushroom. In: *Advances in Applied Microbiology.* New York: Academic Press.
Matsuoka H, et al. (1997). Lentinin potentiates immunity and prolongs the survival time of some patients. *Anticancer Research.* 17:2751–2756.
McCaleb RS, et al. (2000). *Encyclopedia of Popular Herbs.* Roseville, CA: Prima Publishing.
Ying J, Mao X. (1987). *Icones of Medicinal Fungi from China.* Beijing: Science Press.

 NAME: Siberian Ginseng (*Eleutherococcus senticosus*)

Common Names: Eleuthero, ciwujia, *Acanthopanax senticosus*

Family: *Araliaceae*

Description of Plant: A spiny-stemmed shrub native to northeastern China, Siberia, and northern Japan

Medicinal Part: Roots, root bark

Constituents and Action (if known)

- Eleutherosides A to G (0.6%–0.9%) (Bradley, 1992)—adaptogens, hypotensive
- Eleutheroside B is identical to syringin. Syringin in powdered roots decreased by 50% after 12 months and was undetectable after 3 years (Tang & Eisenbrand, 1992).
- Eleutherans A, G (glycans)
- Lignans (sesamin)
- Coumarins (isofraxidin)

Nutritional Ingredients: None known

Traditional Use: Used in TCM as a remedy for "wind damp" arthralgias, muscle spasms, and joint pain and as a *qi* tonic for the Chinese spleen and kidney. Used for low back pain, insomnia, fatigue, and anorexia.

Current Use

- Adaptogen: increases resistance to stress (emotional, occupational, or environmental) and improves performance
- Improves memory and feelings of well-being; reduces fatigue; can be used for mild depression
- Approved in Germany as a tonic for asthenic debility (CFS), impaired concentration, or during convalescence
- Eye problems: in several studies (Blumenthal, 2000), patients taking eleuthero showed significant improvement for primary glaucoma (102 cases), eye burns (58 cases), and myopia (122 cases)
- Normalizes immune and adrenal response; reduces effects of excessive cortisol production
- Supportive therapy for cancer treatment: increases natural killer and T-helper cells and reduces side effects of chemotherapy and radiation
- Ethanol extract of eleuthero dramatically improved the absolute number of immune competent cells, especially T lymphocytes (Wagner, 1999).

Available Forms, Dosage, and Administration Guidelines

Preparations: Dried root, capsules, tablets, tinctures, fluid extract

Typical Dosage

- *Tea:* 1 to 2 tsp powdered root or root bark in 8 oz water, decoct 15 to 20 minutes, steep half-hour; take two or three cups per day
- *Capsules* (dried powdered root): Three to six 500-mg capsules per day
- *Tablets:* One to three 1.25-g tablets (standardized to contain 0.7 mg eleutheroside E) per day
- *Tincture* (1:5, 30% alcohol): 80–120 gtt (4–6 mL) three times a day
- *Fluid extract* (1:1): 1 to 2 mL three times a day

Pharmacokinetics—If Available (form or route when known): None known

Toxicity: None known

Contraindications: Several reports suggest that eleuthero is inappropriate for patients with hypertension (especially blood pressure in excess of 180/90) (Farnsworth, 1985). However, the glycosides contained in this herb have been shown to reduce blood pressure (Blumenthal, 2000).

Side Effects: None

Long-Term Safety: Safe

Use in Pregnancy/Lactation/Children: Safe. One report implicated eleuthero in a report of a "hairy baby," but this problem was due to adulteration with another herb (*Periploca*) (Mills, 1999).

Drug/Herb Interactions and Rationale (if known): Be sure that eleuthero is from a reputable source and has been botanically authenticated. A case of elevated digoxin levels in a 74-year-old man concurrently taking Siberian ginseng has been reported (McRae, 1996). The capsules were analyzed and were found to contain no digoxin or digitoxin. Unfortunately, the herb was not authenticated, so its actual identity is unknown. The possibility of adulteration with *Periploca*, which contains cardiac glycosides, exists. A report of eleuthero being

implicated in causing neonatal androgenization was discovered
to be caused by an adulterant, *Periploca sepium* (Mills, 1999).

BIBLIOGRAPHY

Blumenthal M, et al. (2000). *Herbal Medicine: Expanded Commission E Monographs.* Austin, TX: American Botanical Council.

Bradley P. (Ed.). (1992). *British Herbal Compendium,* Vol. I. Dorset: British Herbal Medicine Association.

Farnsworth NR, et al. (1985). Siberian Ginseng (*Eleutherococcus senticosus*): current status as an adaptogen. In: Wagner H, et al. (Eds.). *Economic and Medicinal Plant Research,* Vol. I. London: Academic Press.

Hson-Mou Chang, Pui-Hay But P. (1986). *Pharmacology and Applications of Chinese Materia Medica.* Singapore: World Scientific.

McRae S. (1996). Elevated serum digoxin levels in a patient taking digoxin and Siberian ginseng. *Canadian Medical Association Journal.* 155(3):293–295.

Mills S, Bone K. (1999). *Principles and Practice of Phytotherapy.* Edinburgh: Churchill Livingstone

Tang W, Eisenbrand G. (1992). *Chinese Drugs of Plant Origin.* Berlin: Springer-Verlag.

Wagner H. (Ed.). (1999). *Immunomodulatory Agents from Plants.* Basel: Birkhauser Verlag.

Waller DP, et al. (1992). Lack of androgenicity of Siberian ginseng. *Journal of the American Medical Association.* 267(17):2329.

NAME: Slippery Elm (*Ulmus rubra*)

Common Names: Red elm, Indian elm, sweet elm, *Ulmus fulva* (synonym)

Family: *Ulmaceae*

Description of Plant
- A deciduous tree native to eastern Canada and eastern and central United States
- Trunk is reddish-brown with gray-white bark on branches
- Can grow 50 to 60 feet high

Medicinal Part: Inner bark (collected in spring or autumn)

Constituents and Action (if known)

- Mucilage (polysaccharides): hexoses, pentoses, menthypentoses, polyuronides, and hexosan
- Tannins (3%–6.5%): responsible for mild astringent properties (Chevallier, 1996; Newall et al., 1996)
- Minerals: calcium

Nutritional Ingredients: Powdered bark has been cooked as a porridge used for feeding babies and weak convalescent patients.

Traditional Use

- Antitussive, demulcent, emollient, nutritive
- Topical use: inner bark mixed with water yields a thick mucilage used as a poultice for styes, boils, carbuncles, sores, and burns.
- Internally, the bark mucilage is used for irritation of the mucous membranes (throat, stomach, bowel). Used for diarrhea (solidifies the stool) and constipation (bulk laxative).

Current Use

- Protects, soothes, and heals irritated tissues such as the esophagus, stomach, and intestinal membranes (colitis, irritable bowel syndrome, diarrhea, leaky gut syndrome, gastric and duodenal ulcers, gastritis, ileitis)
- Local use relieves pain and decreases inflammation of abscesses, varicose ulcers, anal fissures, first-degree burns, styes, and ingrown toenails.
- Soothing demulcent: decreases throat irritation with dry and ticklish coughs, irritation of the vocal cords, and laryngitis

Available Forms, Dosage, and Administration Guidelines

Preparations: Dried bark, cut and sifted, powdered. There are few processors of slippery elm bark because it is highly combustible. Lozenges: powdered bark used to provide demulcent action for throat irritation.

Typical Dosage

- *Capsules:* Up to 12 400-mg capsules a day

- *Tea:* 1 tsp powdered bark in 8 oz cool water, steep for 1 hour; take two or three times a day. This is the most effective dosage form.
- *Tincture:* Ineffective
- *Powdered form:* Mix with boiling water to make a poultice for skin inflammations
- Or follow manufacturer's or practitioner's recommendations

Pharmacokinetics—If Available (form or route when known): Not known

Toxicity: None known

Contraindications: None known

Side Effects: Allergic reaction (rare)

Long-Term Safety: Safe

Use in Pregnancy/Lactation/Children: Safe; long history of use as a food and medicine

Drug/Herb Interactions and Rationale (if known): For all drugs, separate by at least 2 hours when a mucilage preparation is used.

Special Notes: FDA has stated that slippery elm is a safe and effective oral demulcent.

BIBLIOGRAPHY

Bradley PR. (1992). *British Herbal Compendium,* Vol. 1. Bournemouth: British Herbal Medicine Association.

British Herbal Pharmacopoeia. (4th ed.). (1996). Guildford, UK: Biddles Ltd.

Chevallier A. (1996). *Encyclopedia of Medicinal Plants.* New York: DK Publishing.

Integrative Medicine Access: Professional Reference to Conditions, Herbs & Supplements. (2000). Newton, MA: Integrative Medicine Communications.

Morton JF. (1993). Mucilaginous plants and their use in medicine. *Biological & Pharmalogic Bulletin.* 16:735–739.

Newall C, et al. (1996). *Herbal Medicines.* London: Pharmaceutical Press.

Review of Natural Products. (1999). St. Louis: Facts and Comparisons.

NAME: Soy (*Glycine max*)

Common Names: Soya, soybeans

Family: *Fabiaceae*

Description of Plant: Legume that has been cultivated for its edible beans in China for more than 2,000 years

Medicinal Part: Beans and food products made from them, soy protein, soy isoflavones

Constituents and Action (if known)

- Isoflavones (phytoestrogens): genistein, daidzein, glycetein; similar in structure to estradiol, with weak estrogenic and antiestrogenic effects
  - Reduce menopausal symptoms such as hot flashes (Albertazzi et al., 1999; Chiechi, 1999; Duncan et al., 1999; Reinli & Block, 1996; Setchell, 1998; Xu et al., 1998)
  - Increase bone density in some women by up to 6% (Anderson & Garner, 1998)
- Daidzein
  - Boosts immune system function by increasing the phagocytic response of macrophages (Fiedor et al., 1998)
  - Lowers risk of prostatic enlargement and cancer, possibly due to antiestrogen and weak estrogen effect (Geller et al., 1998; Moyad, 1999)
  - Lowers risk of colon and other cancer (Messina & Bennink, 1998)
  - Lowers risk of breast cancer (Messina, 1999; Shao et al., 1998)
  - Antiproliferation effect on breast (Brzezinski & Debi, 1999)
  - Lowers cholesterol and lowers risk of cardiovascular disease (25 g/day is necessary) (Clarkson & Anthony, 1998; Potter, 1998;). Intake of 80 mg/day soy isoflavones improved arterial elasticity by 26% (*Review of Natural Products*, 1998).
  - Antioxidant to protect cells from oxygen free radicals (King & Bursill, 1998)
  - Decreases blood clotting

- Fatty acids (25%): linoleic, palmitic, stearic acids
- Phytates: antinutrients

Nutritional Ingredients: Source of protein, vitamin E, minerals (calcium, iron, potassium), isoflavones, and fatty acids. Generally unaffected by cooking, but extensive processing lowers the medicinal value. Some soy products, such as tamari, contain substantial amounts of added sodium (soy sauce). Traditionally made tofu is high in calcium.

Traditional Use: In the Orient, soy has long been a popular food. Most soy products were traditionally fermented (miso, tempeh, natto) or processed (tofu) to make them more digestible and to remove phytates.

Current Use
- Controls menopausal symptoms such as hot flashes (takes 4 to 6 weeks to notice activity) (Albertazzi et al., 1998)
- Studies show that higher intake of isoflavones prevents cancers of the prostate, breast, endometrium, and bowel.
- Lowers cholesterol
- Reduces prostatic enlargement (BPH)
- Increases bone density; diet must also have adequate calcium, magnesium, boron
- Acts as an antioxidant

Available Forms, Dosage, and Administration Guidelines
Preparations: Foods, soy protein, soy isoflavones
Typical Dosage
- 30 to 100 mg/day isoflavones or 25 to 50 g soy protein lowers cholesterol.

EXCELLENT SOURCES OF SOY	
Fresh soybeans	Tempeh
Miso	Canned/frozen soybeans
Soy flour	Soy nuts (1/2 cup)
Soy protein powders (2–4 tbsp)	Soy milk (2.5–3 cups)
Textured vegetable protein	Tofu (3/4–1 lb)

**POOR SOURCES OF SOY
(TOO PROCESSED TO BE OF MUCH VALUE)**

Soy sauce	Soy cheese
Soy oil	Soy hot dogs
Canned soy drinks	Tofu desserts

- 45 g soy flour increases bone density.
- 25 to 60 g soy protein reduces menopausal signs and changes.
- Revival is a soy meal-replacement drink that tastes good. Both fat and nonfat varieties are available. Research has demonstrated this product's effectiveness. It contains 160 mg isoflavones per serving.

Pharmacokinetics—If Available (form or route when known): The plasma half-life of genistein and daidzein is approximately 8 hours, with peak concentration in 6 to 8 hours. Elimination is by urine.

Toxicity: None

Contraindications: Soy allergies. Large doses are contraindicated if a previous estrogen-positive tumor has been diagnosed, although it is unknown whether soy stimulates estrogen-positive receptor cells. Do not use in patients with

Food	Serving Size	Protein	Isoflavones
Mature soybeans, uncooked	1/2 cup	34.3 g	175.6 mg
Roasted soybeans	1/2 cup	30.2 g	167 mg
Tempeh, uncooked	4 oz	19.4 g	60.5 mg
Soy flour	1/2 cup	8 g	43.8 mg
Tofu, uncooked	4 oz	18 g	38.3 mg
Textured soy protein, dry	1/2 cup	5.4 g	27.8 mg
Soy milk	1 cup	10 g	20 mg

thyroid problems: soy isoflavones may inhibit thyroid synthesis and can induce goiter and thyroid neoplasia in animals.

Side Effects: GI upset: flatulence, diarrhea

Long-Term Safety: Use organic soy products whenever possible. There are concerns about the regular use of large amounts of unfermented soy foods and soy isoflavones because of certain chemicals found in soy. Tripsin inhibitors, hemaglutinin, and phytic acid all may have long-term negative impact on health.

Use in Pregnancy/Lactation/Children: Safe, although there is concern about infants who are fed solely on soy formulas. The phytates (antinutrients) and high levels of isoflavones may have some biological impact. Additional research is needed.

Drug/Herb Interactions and Rationale (if known): None known

Special Notes: Safe for women using birth control pills and hormone replacement therapy concurrently. When buying soy protein powder, make sure the label says "supro," because this means the soy beans have been washed with water and the phytochemicals are intact. Otherwise, the soybeans may have been washed with alcohol, which can change the phytochemical content.

BIBLIOGRAPHY

Albertazzi P, et al. (1998). The effect of dietary soy supplementation on hot flashes. *Obstetrics & Gynecology.* 91:6–11.

Albertazzi P, et al. (1999). Dietary soy supplementation and phytoestrogen levels. *Obstetrics & Gynecology.* 94(2):229–231.

Anderson JJ, Garner SC. (1998). Phytoestrogens and bone. *Bailliere's Clinical Endocrinology & Metabolism.* 12(4):543–557.

Anderson JW, et al. (1995). Meta-analysis of the effects of soy protein intake on serum lipids. *New England Journal of Medicine.* 333(5):276–282.

Brzezinski A, Debi A. (1999). Phytoestrogens: the "natural" selective estrogen receptor modulators? *European Journal of Obstetrics, Gynecology, & Reproductive Biology.* 85(1):47–51.

Chiechi LM. (1999). Dietary phytoestrogens in the prevention of long-term postmenopausal diseases. *International Journal of Gynaecology & Obstetrics.* 67(1):39–40.

Clarkson TB, Anthony MS. (1998). Phytoestrogens and coronary heart disease. *Bailliere's Clinical Endocrinology & Metabolism.* 12(4):589–604.

Duncan AM, et al. (1999). Soy isoflavones exert modest hormonal effects in premenopausal women. *Journal of Clinical Endocrinology & Metabolism.* 84(1):192–197.

Fiedor P, et al. (1998). Immunosuppressive effects of synthetic derivative of genistein on the survival of pancreatic islet allografts. *Transplantation Proceedings.* 30(2):537.

Geller J, et al. (1998). Genistein inhibits the growth of human-patient BPH and prostate cancer in histoculture. *Prostate.* 34(2):75–79.

Greaves KA, et al. (2000). Consumption of soy protein reduces cholesterol absorption compared to casein protein alone or supplemented with an isoflavone extract or conjugated equine estrogen in ovariectomized cynomolgus monkeys. *Journal of Nutrition.* 130(4):820–826.

King RA, Bursill DB. (1998). Plasma and urinary kinetics of the isoflavones daidzein and genistein after a single soy meal in humans. *American Journal of Clinical Nutrition.* 67(5):867–872.

Lindsay SH, Claywell LG. (1999). Considering soy: its estrogenic effects may protect women. *Journal of Obstetrics, Gynecology, & Neonatal Nursing.* 28(6, Suppl. 1):21–24.

Messina M. (1999). Soy, soy phytoestrogens (isoflavones), and breast cancer. *American Journal of Clinical Nutrition.* 70(4):574–575.

Messina M, Bennink M. (1998). Soy foods, isoflavones and risk of colonic cancer: a review of the in vitro and in vivo data. *Bailliere's Clinical Endocrinology & Metabolism* 12(4):707–728.

Moyad MA. (1999). Soy, disease prevention, and prostate cancer. *Seminars in Urology & Oncology.* 17(2):97–102.

Potter SM. (1998). Soy protein and cardiovascular disease: the impact of bioactive components in soy. *Nutrition Review.* 56(8):231–235.

Reinli K, Block G. (1996). Phytoestrogen content of foods—a compendium of literature values. *Nutrition & Cancer.* 26(2):123–128.

Scambia G, et al. (2000). Clinical effects of a standardized soy extract in postmenopausal women: a pilot study. *Menopause.* 7(2):105–111.

Setchell KD. (1998). Phytoestrogens: the biochemistry, physiology, and implications for human health of soy isoflavones. *American Journal of Clinical Nutrition.* 68(6, Suppl.):1333S–1346S.

Shao ZM, et al. (1998). Genistein inhibits proliferation similarly in estrogen receptor-positive and negative human breast carcinoma cell lines characterized by P21WAF1/CIP1 induction, G2/M arrest, and apoptosis. *Journal of Cellular Biochemistry.* 69(1):44–45.

Xu X, et al. (1998). Effects of soy isoflavones on estrogen and phytoestrogen metabolism in premenopausal women. *Cancer Epidemiology, Biomarkers and Prevention.* 7(12):1101–1108.

 NAME: Spirulina (*Spirulina maxima, S. platensis*)

Common Names: None

Family: *Oscillatoriaceae*

Description of Plant

- There are thousands of species of blue-green algae. The species known as spirulina naturally grow in warm alkaline water.
- Most blue-green algaes have cell walls made of cellulose and are difficult to digest. Spirulina's cell walls are made of complex proteins and sugars, and it is easily digestible.
- The blue-green color originates from chlorophyll (green) and phycocyanin (blue) pigments.

Medicinal Part: Dried algae

Constituents and Action (if known)

- Protein, chlorophyll, phycocyanin pigments, carotenoids, sugars
- Sulpholipids (1%)
- Calcium-spirulina (ca-sp): antiviral against HIV-1 and herpes simplex I
- May cause regression of oral tumors in hamsters (Schwartz, 1988)
- Caused tumor regression in oral leukoplakia of tobacco chewers (Mathew et al., 1995)
- May increase TNF production
- Inhibits replication of several viruses—herpes simplex, cytomegalovirus, mumps, influenza, HIV, measles (Hayashi et al., 1996; *Integrative Medicine*, 2000)
- Protects rat livers against hepatotoxicity caused by carbon tetrachloride (Torres-Duran et al., 1999)

Nutritional Ingredients: Source of protein (62%): contains 22 amino acids, B-complex vitamins (all except B_{12}), minerals (zinc, iron, manganese, selenium, potassium, calcium, magnesium), carotenoids. A rich source of GLA (25%–30%); superior to other sources such as evening primrose oil, which contains 10% to 15% GLA.

Traditional Use: Used as a food by the Aztecs and Asian and African peoples

Current Use

- Nutritional supplement with easily absorbed essential fatty acids, trace minerals, protein, and iron
- In a controlled study, spirulina significantly reduced LDL cholesterol in patients with mild hyperlipidemia and hypertension (Belay et al., 1993).
- Rich source of GLA; may be of benefit for skin conditions such as eczema and psoriasis
- Stimulated the growth of healthy intestinal flora, especially lactobacilli and bifidobacteria
- Effective for treating iron-deficiency anemia. The iron in spirulina is absorbed 60% better than iron tablets and also promotes hematopoiesis.
- In animal studies, spirulina exhibited immune-potentiating, anticancer, radiation protective, hepatoprotective, renal protective, and hypotensive activity.

Available Forms, Dosage, and Administration Guidelines

Preparations: Capsules, tablets, powders, supplemental fruit drinks

Typical Dosage: 3 to 5 g per day; four to six 500-mg tablets per day

Pharmacokinetics—If Available (form or route when known): None known

Toxicity: None known for spirulina. Other species of wild-harvested blue-green algae may be contaminated with heavy metals or microcystins.

Contraindications: None known

Side Effects: None known

Long-Term Safety: Safe. Extensive animal studies and a long history of human use as food show no evidence of any acute or chronic toxicity.

Use in Pregnancy/Lactation/Children: Safe: no fetotoxicity or teratogenicity was found with high doses in pregnant animals

Drug/Herb Interactions and Rationale (if known): None known

Special Notes: Promoters of spirulina have claimed that it is a diet product, but an FDA review found no such evidence. One human study found that ingestion of 2.8 g spirulina three times per day for 4 weeks resulted in a significant reduction in body weight (Belay et al., 1993). Blue-green algae is a related product gathered from the Great Klamath Lake in Oregon. It is wild harvested and may contain bacterial toxins (microcystins), which can cause liver damage. It is best to avoid any microalgae products not grown in a controlled environment.

BIBLIOGRAPHY

Belay A, et al. (1993). Current knowledge on potential health benefits of spirulina. *Journal of Applied Phycology.* 5:235–241.

Chamorro G, et al. (1996). Pharmacology and toxicology of Spirulina algae. *Revista de Investigacion Clinica.* 48:389–399.

Hayashi T, et al. (1996). Calcium spirulin, an inhibitor of enveloped virus replication, from a blue-green algae *Spirulina palatensis. Journal of Natural Products.* 59(1):83–87.

Integrative Medicine Access. (2000). *Spirulina.* Newton, MA: Integrative Medicine Communications.

Mathew B, et al. (1995). Evaluation of chemoprevention of oral cancer with *Spirulina fusiformis. Nutrition & Cancer.* 24(2):197–202.

Review of Natural Products. (1998). St. Louis: Facts and Comparisons.

Salazar M, et al. (1998). Subchronic toxicity study in mice fed *Spirulina maxima. Journal of Ethnopharmacology.* 62(3):235–242.

Schwartz J, et al. (1988). Prevention of experimental oral cancer by extracts of *Spirulina-Dunaliella* algae. *Nutrition & Cancer.* 11(2):127–134.

Torres-Duran PV, et al. (1999). Studies on the preventative effect of *Spirulina maxima* on fatty liver development induced by carbon tetrachloride in the rat. *Journal of Ethnopharmacology.* 64(2):141–148.

NAME: St. John's Wort (*Hypericum perforatum*)

Common Names: Klamath weed

Family: *Hypericaceae*

Description of Plant

- Shrubby perennial herb with bright-yellow flowers, grows 1 to 2 feet high
- Native to Europe, but now grows as a weed in many parts of the world in dry gravelly soils with full sun
- The yellow flowers contain small black oil glands that, when crushed, produce a red stain; this was thought to be the blood of St. John the Baptist, hence the name St. John's wort.

Medicinal Part: Flowering tops, especially the flowers and unopened buds. Harvesting at bud stage increases hypericin levels; late harvest increases hyperforin.

Constituents and Action (if known)

- Napthodianthrones (less than 0.1%–0.15%), hypericin, pseudohypericin, isohypericin
  - Increase capillary blood flow
  - Inhibit serotonin uptake at postsynaptic receptors (Muller & Russul, 1994; Perovic, 1995; Upton, 1997)
  - Inhibit reuptake of dopamine and norepinephrine
  - Block presynaptic alpha-2 receptors
  - Antiviral activity against herpes simplex virus I and II, retrovirus (HIV) in vitro and vivo, Epstein-Barr virus, influenza A and B, murine cytomegalovirus, hepatitis C (may work through protein-kinase C-mediated phosphorylation) (Newall et al., 1996; Schempp et al., 1999)
- Phloroglucinols
  - Hyperforin: inhibits uptake of serotonin, GABA, and L-glutamate (Chatterjee et al., 1998; Laakmann et al., 1998), antibacterial (Upton, 1997)
  - Adhyperforin
- Flavonoids and flavonol glycosides (flowers, 11.71%): kaempferol, quercetin, luteolin, amentoflavone: anti-inflammatory and antiulcerogenic activity (Upton, 1997);

inhibition of benzodiazepine binding, rutin, and hyperoside/hyperin

- Essential oils (0.059%–0.35%): monoterpenes (pinenes) and sesquiterpenes: antiviral, antibacterial
- Tannins: astringent activity when applied topically, stimulate wound healing (Newall et al., 1999)
- Other actions:
  - Inhibits catechol-o-methyl-transferase and suppresses interleukin 6 release; may affect mood through neurohormonal pathways
  - Antibacterial activity against gram-positive and gram-negative bacteria
  - Can stimulate and also inhibit cyclic P-450 enzyme metabolism

Nutritional Ingredients: None known

Traditional Use: Antidepressant, antiviral, antibacterial, cholagogue, diuretic, nervine, nervous system trophorestorative, vulnerary. Dioscorides used St. John's wort in the first century for sciatica, burns, and fevers. Gerard noted in 1633 that St. John's wort oil was excellent for wounds, bites, and burns. In Europe, the herb is used for depression, mental exhaustion, liver problems, nerve injuries (internally and topically), bedwetting caused by irritation of the bladder, sciatica, gastric ulcers, and topically for a wide range of skin problems and trauma injuries.

Current Use
Internal

- Mild to moderate depression (not appropriate for severe depression or bipolar disorders) (Linde et al., 1996), seasonal affective disorder (Martinzez et al., 1994); use with lemon balm for greatest activity. Relieves fatigue in depressed persons (Stevinson et al., 1998).
- Most herbalists do not use St. John's wort as monotherapy for depression. The orthodox treatments (selective serotonin reuptake inhibitors [SSRIs] or St. John's wort alone) do not address the full spectrum of this disorder. Effective therapies may require lifestyle changes, counseling, and additional adaptogenic, antidepressant, or nervine herbs such as

Siberian ginseng, schisandra, lemon balm, rosemary, basil, black cohosh, and lavender, which will improve the specificity and effectiveness of the protocol.

- Eases menopausal anxiety, nervousness, and sleep disorders; use with motherwort and blue vervain
- Helps to heal damaged nerve tissue after cerebrovascular accident or neurologic trauma; use with ginkgo, Siberian ginseng, or bacopa
- Oral use concurrent with topical applications for sciatica, neuralgias, diabetic neuropathies, trigeminal neuralgia, and Bell's palsy
- Antiviral activity against herpes type I and II, mononucleosis, influenza. The antiviral effect is mild when taken orally. Use St. John's wort with other antiviral herbs (basil, thyme, oregano, lemon balm, rosemary) as a supportive therapy.

Topical: Topically, *Hypericum* tincture or oil is effective for treating herpetic lesions and shingles. *Hypericum* oil speeds healing of wounds, burns, sunburn, shingles, nerve pain, and nerve damage. It can be useful for neuralgias, hemorrhoids, trauma injuries, gum disease, and painful tooth sockets after dental extractions.

Available Forms, Dosage, and Administration Guidelines

Preparations: Dried herb, capsules, tablets, tinctures. Most products for internal use are standardized to 0.3% hypericin, even though this is no guarantee of efficacy; some products are now standardized to include hyperforin. Well-made tinctures should be dark burgundy red and have a noticeably fragrant aroma.

Typical Dosage

- *Capsules:* For products standardized to 0.3% hypericin, take 300 mg three times a day
- *Tea:* Steep 1 tsp dried herb in 8 oz hot water for 15 to 20 minutes; take two cups per day
- *Tincture* (1:2 or 1:5, 40% alcohol): 40 to 80 gtt (2–4 mL) three times a day
- *Topical:* As an anti-inflammatory or for wound epithelialization, use a tincture or oil and cover wound with gauze or bandage until healing is established

Pharmacokinetics—If Available (form or route when known)

- Onset: absorption 2 to 2.6 hours
- Peak: 5 hours
- Duration: takes 4 to 6 weeks to be effective
- Steady state (with long-term use): 4 days
- Half-life: 24 to 48 hours
- Metabolism and excretion: unknown

Toxicity: Photosensitivity may occur with high doses of hypericin-rich products, so be careful of excessive sun exposure.

Contraindications: Severe depression; use of cyclosporin or other drugs to prevent organ transplant rejection

Side Effects: Headache, pruritus, and GI irritation usually subside with long-term use. If side effects occur, lower dose and then gradually increase again. Photosensitivity may occur (Bowers, 1999; Golsch et al., 1997; Newall et al., 1996). Rash is reversible with withdrawal of herb. If nerve hypersensitivity occurs, discontinue use.

Long-Term Safety: Safe at normal therapeutic dosage

Use in Pregnancy/Lactation/Children: Avoid during pregnancy; safety unknown. May decrease production of milk by inhibiting secretion of prolactin. Avoid in very young children; no research available.

Drug/Herb Interactions and Rationale (if known)

- With concurrent use of theophylline and beta-2 agonists, there is a theoretical possibility of increased anxiety, nervousness, and worsening of panic disorder (Nebel et al., 1999).
- Serotonin syndrome may occur if used with SSRIs (sweating, agitation, tremor) (Gordon, 1998).
- There has been concern about mixing St. John's wort with SSRIs. Most clinicians have not seen interactions, although there is one reported case of a possible serotonin syndrome reaction in a patient taking both medications (Wheatley, 2000). Use cautiously together.

- May increase or decrease cyclic P-450 activity; St. John's wort may affect medications that are metabolized by this pathway (Wheatley, 2000).
  - Protease inhibitors: One poorly done study suggests that St. John's wort may lower blood levels of indinivir in healthy individuals (Henney, 2000). More research is needed to determine whether this herb can reduce the efficacy of this type of drug in HIV-positive patients. Avoid concurrent use until better information is available.
  - Cyclosporin: In two patients taking cyclosporin to prevent heart transplant rejection, therapeutic levels of the drug dropped when they began taking this herb. These preliminary data suggest that patients taking cyclosporin should avoid taking St. John's wort (Henney, 2000).
- Does *not* potentiate alcohol; does *not* interfere with the function of birth control pills or anesthesia

Special Notes: In the past, St. John's wort was believed to have monoamine oxidase inhibitor activity, but recent research has shown little or no such inhibition (Cott, 1997). Concerns associated with the use of monoamine oxidase inhibitors are not germane to St. John's wort (diet, anesthesia, medications). Much of St. John's wort is still picked in the wild, so products are highly variable as a result of proper or improper harvesting, drying, and processing. To date there have been at least 25 well-controlled, placebo trials confirming the efficacy of St. John's wort for depression. Most trials have been short-term (6–8 weeks), so long-term efficacy still needs to be studied fully. A long-term study funded by National Institute of Health in 1998 is ongoing. The FDA has sanctioned hypericin as an investigational new drug; it is in clinical trials under the name VIM RXYN.

BIBLIOGRAPHY

Bennett DA, et al. (1998). Neuropharmacology of St. John's wort. *Annals of Pharmacotherapy.* 5(4):245–252.

Bowers AG. (1999). Phytophotodermatitis. *American Journal of Contact Dermatitis.* 10(2):89–93.

Chatterjee SS, et al. (1998). Hyperforin as a possible antidepressant component of *Hypericum* extracts. *Life Science.* 63(6):499–510.

Cott JM, Fugh-Berman A. (1998). Is St. John's wort (*Hypericum perforatum*) an effective antidepressant? *Journal of Nervous & Mental Disease.* 186(8):500–501.

Cott JM. (1997). In vitro receptor binding and enzyme inhibition by *Hypericum perforatum* extract. *Pharmacopsychiatry.* 30(Suppl.):108–112.

Deltito J, Beyer D. (1998). The scientific, quasi-scientific and popular literature on the use of St. John's wort in the treatment of depression. *Journal of Affective Disorders.* 51(3):345–351.

Golsch S, et al. (1997). Reversible increase in photosensitivity to UV-B caused by St. John's wort extract. *Hautarzt.* 48:249–252.

Gordon JB. (1998). SSRIs and St. John's wort: possible toxicity? *American Family Physician.* 57(5):950.

Henney, J. (2000). Risk of interactions with St. John's wort. *Journal of American Medical Association.* 283(13).

Laakmann G, et al. (1998). St. John's wort in mild to moderate depression: the relevance of hyperforin for the clinical efficacy. *Pharmacopsychiatry.* 31 (Suppl.):54–59.

Lenoir S, et al. (1999). A double-blind randomized trial to investigate three different concentrations of a standardized fresh plant extract obtained from the shoot tips of *Hypericum perforatum* L. *Phytomedicine.* 6(3):141–146.

Linde K, et al. (1996). St. John's wort for depression: an overview and meta-analysis of randomized clinical trials. *British Medical Journal.* 313:253–258.

Martinzez B, et al. (1994). Hypericum in the treatment of seasonal affective disorders. *Journal of Geriatric Psychiatry & Neurology.* 7:S29–S33.

Miller AL. (1998). St. John's Wort (*Hypericum perforatum*): clinical effects on depression and other conditions. *Alternative Medicine Review.* 3(1):18–26.

Mills S, Bone K. (1999). *Principles and Practice of Phytotherapy.* Edinburgh: Churchill Livingstone.

Monograph: hypericum. (1999). *Alternative Medicine Review.* 4(3):190–192.

Muller WEG, Russul R. (1994). Effects of *Hypericum* extract on the expression of serotonin receptors. *Journal of Geriatric Psychiatry and Neurology.* 7:S63–S64.

Mulry M. (1999). First International Conference on St. John's Wort. *HerbalGram.* 45:60–65.

Nathan PJ. (1999). Experimental and clinical pharmacology of St. John's wort (*Hypericum perforatum* L.). *Molecular Psychiatry.* 4:333–338.

Nebel A, et al. (1999). Potential metabolic interaction between St. John's wort and theophylline. *Annals of Pharmacotherapy.* 33(4):502.

Newall C, et al. (1999). *Herbal Medicines.* London: Pharmaceutical Press.

Perovic S. (1995). Pharmacological profile of hypericum extract: effect on serotonin uptake by postsynaptic receptors. *Arzneimittelforschung.* 45(11):1145–1148.

Schempp CM, et al. (1999). Antibacterial activity of hyperforin from St. John's wort, against multiresistant *Staphylococcus aureus* and gram-positive bacteria. *Lancet.* 353(9170):2129.

Schrader E, et al. (2000). Equivalence of St. John's wort extract (Ze 117) and fluoxetine: a randomised, controlled study in mild to moderate depression. *International Clinical Psychopharmacology.* 15:61–68.

Sommer H. (1994). Placebo-controlled double-blind study examining the effectiveness of a hypericum preparation in 105 mildly depressed patients. *Journal of Geriatric Psychiatry and Neurology.* 7:S9–S11.

Stevinson C, et al. (1998). Hypericum for fatigue: a pilot study. *Phytomedicine.* 5(6):443–447.

Upton R. (Ed.). (1997) *American Herbal Pharmacopoeia and Therapeutic Compendium.* Santa Cruz, CA: AHP.

Volz HP. (1997). Controlled clinical trials of *Hypericum* extracts in depressed patients: an overview. *Pharmacopsychiatry.* 30(Suppl.):72–76.

Wheatley D. (1997). LI 160, an extract of St. John's wort, versus amitriptyline in mildly to moderately depressed outpatients: a controlled 6-week clinical trial. *Pharmacopsychiatry.* 30(Suppl.):77–80.

Wheatley D. (2000). St. John's wort: more knowledge needed [letter]. *Pharmacy Journal.* 265(7104):49.

Woelk H. (1994). Benefits and risks of the hypericum extract LI 160: drug monitoring study with 3250 patients. *Journal of Geriatric Psychiatry and Neurology.* 7:S34–S38.

T

 NAME: Tea Tree (*Melaleuca alternifolia*)

Common Names: Australian tea tree oil, Melaleuca oil, tea tree oil

Family: *Myrtaceae*

Description of Plant

- There are many plants known as tea trees, but the species *M. alternifolia* is the source of commercial tea tree oil.
- Small, shrubby evergreen native only to the northeast coastal region of New South Wales, Australia
- It is a member of the myrtle family, grows 8 feet tall, and has sprays of white flowers each summer.

Medicinal Part: EO; leaves are steam-distilled to yield about 2% oil

Constituents and Action (if known)

- Essential oils: terpin-4-ol (40%), alpha-terpenol, alpha-pinene, alpha-terpinene, gamma-terpinene, p-cymene, limonene; more than 100 different compounds have been identified (Bruneton, 1999)
  - Antimicrobial activity against *Candida albicans, Escherichia coli, Pseudomonas aeruginosa, Staphylococcus aureus* (MRSA) (Carson et al., 1995; Chan & Loudon, 1998; Gustafson et al., 1998)
  - Antimicrobial activity against vancomycin-resistant enterococci (Nelson, 1997)
  - Antifungal (Nenoff et al., 1996)
  - Alpha-terpineol and alpha-pinene have antimicrobial activity against *Staphylococcus epidermidis* and *Propionibacterium acnes* (Ramon et al., 1995).

Nutritional Ingredients: None known

Traditional Use

- Analgesic, antibacterial, antifungal, antiviral, anti-inflammatory
- Leaves used by the Aborigines of Australia as a treatment for cuts, abrasions, burns, and insect bites
- Oil used during World War II by soldiers as a disinfectant; used in the 1920s in surgery and dentistry as Australian researchers learned that it was 13 times more active as an antiseptic than carbolic acid, the common disinfectant of that time

Current Use

- Acne (as a 5% solution): in a single-blind randomized study on 124 patients with mild to moderate acne, tea tree was compared with benzoyl peroxide. Both treatments were found to be equally effective; the tea tree patients had no adverse effects (Basset et al., 1990).
- Impetigo: apply EO undiluted two or three times a day to the lesion. May cause mild pain and irritation.
- Boils and topical infections: apply EO undiluted two or three times per day
- Ringworm: apply undiluted to affected area
- First- and second-degree burns: apply freely mixed with lavender EO (1–2 gtt each), in a base of fresh aloe gel
- Mouth ulcers: apply undiluted on a cotton swab two to four times per day
- Gingivitis/pyorrhea: use diluted in water or in commercially made mouthwashes. Swish in mouth two or three times per day.
- Vaginal or oral candidiasis (thrush): use a vaginal suppository once or twice per day for vaginal candidiasis; use mouthwash or EO diluted in water for thrush twice a day
- Bacterial vaginosis: use a vaginal suppository (bolus) once or twice a day
- In shampoos for dandruff: use as needed
- Herpes: apply undiluted to herpetic lesions two or three times per day; may cause irritation and mild pain
- Lung and sinus infections: use 1 to 2 gtt EO in a hot vaporizer or in hot water, once or twice a day. Inhale the steam. Lavender or eucalyptus EO can be added.
- Nail fungus (onychomycosis) and athlete's foot (tinea pedis): helps control infection, but rarely cures it. Apply undiluted to feet and toenails twice a day.

Available Forms, Dosage, and Administration Guidelines

Preparations: EO, vaginal suppositories for vaginal candidiasis, mouthwash, ointments. The Australian quality standard for tea tree oil is 30% terpinene-4-ol and less than 15% cineol.

Typical Dosage
- *For external use:* Follow manufacturer's or practitioner's recommendations.

Pharmacokinetics—If Available (form or route when known): Not known

Toxicity: Ingestion of 0.5 tsp EO has caused symptoms including ataxia, drowsiness, petechial body rash, and neutrophil leukocytosis.

Contraindications: Hypersensitivity

Side Effects: Dermatitis, allergic contact eczema

Long-Term Safety: Safe with topical use; does not cause photosensitization, allergic sensitization, or irritation to the skin or mucous membranes

Use in Pregnancy/Lactation/Children: Safe if used topically

Drug/Herb Interactions and Rationale (if known): None known

Special Notes: Avoid using in or near the eyes. To enhance effectiveness as an antifungal, apply dimethyl sulfoxide (DMSO) immediately afterward to same area (Bucks et al., 1994). Like all EOs, tea tree is a highly concentrated product and should be used internally in very small doses. Overdoses can cause serious health problems.

BIBLIOGRAPHY

Bassett IB, et al. (1990). A comparative study of tea tree benzoyl peroxide oil versus benzoyl peroxide in the treatment of acne. *Medical Journal of Australia.* 153(8):455–458.

Bruneton J. (1999). *Pharmacognosy, Phytochemistry, Medicinal Plants.* Paris: Lavoisier.

Bucks DS, et al. (1994). Comparison of two topical preparations for the treatment of onychomycosis: *Melaleuca alternifolia* (tea tree) oil and clotrimazole. *Journal of Family Practice.* 38:601–605.

Carson CF, et al. (1995). Susceptibility of methicillin-resistant *Staphylococcus aureus* to the essential oil of *Melaleuca alternifolia.* *Journal of Antimicrobial Chemotherapy.* 35:421–424.

Chan CH, Loudon KW. (1998). Activity of tea tree oil on methicillin-resistant *Staphylococcus aureus*. *Journal of Hospital Infection*. 39(3):244–245.

Gustafson JE, et al. (1998). Effects of tea tree oil on *Escherichia coli*. *Letters in Applied Microbiology*. 26:194–198.

Hammer KA, et al. (1996). Susceptibility of transient and commensal skin flora to the essential oil of *Melaleuca alternifolia*. *American Journal of Infection Control*. 24(3):186–189.

Nelson RRS. (1997). In vitro activities of five plant essential oils against methicillin-resistant *Staphylococcus aureus* and vancomycin-resistant *Enterococcus faecium*. *Journal of Antimicrobial Chemotherapy*. 40:305–306.

Nenoff P, et al. (1996). Antifungal activity of the essential Oil of *Melaleuca alternifolia* (tea tree oil) against pathogenic fungi in vivo. *Skin Pharmacology*. 9:388–394.

Ramon A, et al. (1995). Antimicrobial effects of tea-tree oil and its major components on *Staphylococcus aureus, S. epidermidis* and *Propionibacterium acnes*. *Letters in Applied Microbiology*. 21(4):242–245.

Tissarand R, Balacs T. (1995). *Essential Oil Safety*. Edinburgh: Churchill Livingstone.

NAME: Thyme (*Thymus vulgaris*)

Common Names: Creeping thyme, garden thyme, wild thyme (*T. serphyllum*)

Family: *Lamiaceae*

Description of Plant
- Small, highly aromatic member of the mint family with white to pink flowers
- There are hundreds of cultivated species and varieties of thymes.

Medicinal Part: Dried herb, EO

Constituents and Action (if known)
- Volatile oils (1%–2.5%) (monoterpenes)
  - Thymol (30%–70%): antibacterial against *Porphyromonas gingivalis*, *Selenomonas artemidis*, and *Streptococcus sobrinus*, all of which can cause dental caries or gum disease (Mills

& Bone, 1999); antibacterial and antifungal against a wide spectrum of bacteria that cause upper respiratory infections; also active against *Helicobacter pylori* and many fungi

- ○ Carvacrol (3%–15%): antibacterial, antifungal
- Flavonoids: luteolin (antimutagenic), thymonin, cirsilineol, 8-methoxy-cirsilineol (potent spasmolytics), eriodictyol (antioxidant)
- Phenolic acids: rosmarinic acid (antioxidant, inhibits lipid peroxidation, anti-inflammatory, antiallergic), caffeic acid
- Tannins (10%)

Nutritional Ingredients: Fresh and dried herb commonly used as a spice in cooking

Traditional Use

- Antibacterial, antispasmodic, antifungal, antiviral, carminative, diaphoretic, expectorant
- Spasmodic coughs: bronchitis, whooping cough, mild antibacterial/antiviral to the lungs; used for colds, influenza, chest colds, pneumonia, upper respiratory tract congestion
- Expectorant: increases and thins mucus, allowing easier elimination
- Digestive upsets with gas, nausea, vomiting, and abdominal bloating
- Mild urinary antiseptic
- Gargle for sore throats, tonsillitis, gum disease

Current Use

- Effective for spasmodic coughs (bronchospasm) associated with bronchitis, pertussis, asthma, COPD, and emphysema. Use with wild cherry bark and licorice.
- EO (less than 1%) in mouthwashes to prevent cavities and treat gum disease
- EO diluted in a carrier base may be useful for athlete's foot (tinea pedis). Use with tea tree and lavender EOs.
- EO (less than 0.1%) in a cream base was successfully used to treat two cases of vulval lichen sclerosis (Mills & Bone, 1999).
- EO in a vaporizer or in hot water as an inhalation for sinusitis, *Pneumocystis carinii* pneumonia, bronchitis, and bacterial pneumonia

- Herb tea (or tincture), along with eyebright, yerba manza, or osha root, can be effective for allergic rhinitis and otitis media.
- Herb tea useful for GI tract dysbiosis with foul-smelling flatulence, abdominal bloating, and nausea; may also be beneficial for treating gastric ulcers

Available Forms, Dosage, and Administration Guidelines

Preparations: Dried herb, tea, tincture, EO

Typical Dosage

- *Dried herb:* 2 to 6 g per day
- *Tea:* 1 tsp dried herb in 8 oz hot water, steep covered 20 to 30 minutes; take up to three cups per day
- *Tincture* (1:5, 35% alcohol): 40 to 80 gtt (2–4 mL) three times a day
- *EO:* Use dilutions of 1% or less for mouthwashes or vaginal suppositories

Pharmacokinetics—If Available (form or route when known): Not known

Toxicity: Herb is safe in normal therapeutic doses. EO is highly concentrated; do not use internally,

Contraindications: None known

Side Effects: Herb: none known. EO, undiluted or inadequately diluted, can cause irritation of the skin and especially the mucous membranes. Internal use of the EO in mice caused decreased locomotor activity and respiration (ESCOP, 1996).

Long-Term Safety: Safe

Use in Pregnancy/Lactation/Children: Herb: avoid large amounts in pregnancy, but culinary quantities are fine. No adverse effects expected in lactating women or children.

Drug/Herb Interactions and Rationale (if known): None known

Special Notes: Many chemotypes of thyme exist. The chemistry of the herb and EO can be highly variable. Good-quality thyme and thyme extracts should have a strong, aromatic fragrance and taste.

BIBLIOGRAPHY

Bisset NG, Wichtl M. (1994). *Herbal Drugs and Phytopharmaceuticals.* Stuttgart: Medpharm.

ESCOP Monograph on the Medicinal Uses of Plant Drugs. (1996). Exeter: ESCOP.

Fisher C, Painter G. (1996). *Materia Medica of Western Herbs for the Southern Hemisphere.* Oratia, New Zealand: Authors.

Leung A, Foster S. (1996). *Encyclopedia of Common Natural Ingredients* (2nd ed.). New York: John Wiley & Sons.

Mills S. (1991). *Out of the Earth: The Essential Book of Herbal Medicine.* London: Viking Arkana.

Mills S, Bone K. (1999). *Principles and Practice of Phytotherapy.* Edinburgh: Churchill Livingstone.

Tisserand R, Balacs T. (1995). *Essential Oil Safety, A Guide for Health Care Professionals.* Edinburgh: Churchill Livingstone.

Weiss RF. (1988). *Herbal Medicine.* Beaconsfield, UK: Beaconsfield Publishing.

🌿 NAME: Turmeric (*Curcuma longa*)

Common Names: Indian saffron, curcuma

Family: *Zingiberaceae*

Description of Plant
- Perennial member of the ginger family
- Cultivated widely throughout Asia, India, China, and other tropical countries

Medicinal Part: Dried rhizome and curcumin extracts

Constituents and Action (if known)
- Diaryheptanoids (yellow pigments)—curcumin: antioxidant properties
  - Inhibit cancer at initiation, promotion, and progression stages of development, particularly colon cancer (Chen et al., 1999; Chun et al., 1999; Han et al., 1999; Kawamori et al., 1999; Nagabhushan & Bhide, 1992; Plummer et al., 1999; Ranhan et al., 1999; Singhal et al., 1999)

- ○ May be useful in chemoprevention of cancers: tobacco smoke, benzo(alpha)pyrenes, nitrosamines (Li et al., 1998; Mills & Bone, 1999; Polasa et al., 1992)
- ○ Curcumin is as effective as BHA in inhibiting lipid peroxidation; it has anti-inflammatory and antiarthritic activity in rats and mice (Kang et al., 1999; Leung & Foster, 1996; Shah, 1999) and is a dual inhibitor of arachidonic acid metabolism (Mills & Bone, 1999).
- ○ Strong antihepatotoxic properties (Qureshi et al., 1992)
- ○ Prevent doxorubicin (Adriamycin) nephrotoxicity in rats (Venkatesan et al., 2000)
- ○ Increase immune function, including white blood cell counts and macrophage phagocytic activity (Antony et al., 1999)
- ○ Reduce muscle injury after trauma (Thaloor et al., 1999)
- ○ Interfere with replication of viruses, including hepatitis and HIV
- ○ Antithrombotic action while preserving prostacyclin, an anti-inflammatory mediator
- EO (3%–5%): sesquiterpene ketones—ar-turmerone, zingiberene, phellandrene (antifungal, mild antibacterial, anti-inflammatory, antihistamine, choleretic) (Mills & Bone, 1999)
- Tumerin: antioxidant, antimutagen, protects DNA
- Ukonan-A: phagocytic activity (Gonda et al., 1992)
- Ukonan-D: reticuloendothelial system potentiating activity (Gonda et al., 1992); inhibits chemically induced carcinogens, which is probably the basis of anticancer treatment (Azuine et al., 1992)
- Oleo-resins: composed mostly of curcuminoids and essential oils
- Extracts of whole turmeric exhibit antioxidant, antifungal, anticancer, hepatoprotective, and anti-inflammatory activity.

Nutritional Ingredients: Primary component of curry powders and some mustards; vitamin A, carotenoids, and minerals

Traditional Use
- Antihepatotoxin, antioxidant, cholagogue, anti-inflammatory, antiulcerogenic

- Topical use as a poultice with neem leaves in 814 patients resulted in a 97% cure rate in patients with scabies (Mills, 2000). Turmeric is also used for skin infections, bruises, and eczema and to reduce hair growth.
- Liver problems, including hepatitis and jaundice
- Digestive tonic for impaired digestion, gas, and abdominal pain

Current Use

- Cancer prevention and possible treatment, especially bowel, cervical, and liver cancers
- Reduces inflammation of osteoarthritis and rheumatoid arthritis, irritable bowel syndrome, postsurgical inflammation; combines well with sarsaparilla, ginger, and boswellia
- Reduces cholesterol and triglyceride levels; may prevent arteriosclerosis
- An effective hepatoprotective agent: increases glutathione levels and glutathione-S-transferase activity. Use with milk thistle, picrorrhiza, and schisandra to prevent and treat acute and chronic liver disease.

Available Forms, Dosage, and Administration Guidelines

Preparations: Standardized extract, powder, infusion, fresh tincture

Typical Dosage

- Unless otherwise prescribed, 1.5 to 4 g per day of the powdered rhizome as well as other equivalent galenical preparations for internal use
- *Standardized extract* (curcumin 95%): 350 mg twice a day
- *Powder:* 1 to 3 g, 1 to 4 g (Kapoor, 1990), 0.5 to 1 g, several times daily (Wichtl & Biset, 1994). Taking turmeric with lecithin or black pepper increases absorption.
- *Infusion:* 0.5 tsp dried powdered rhizome in 8 oz hot water, steep for 10 to 15 minutes; take twice daily
- *Fresh tincture* (1:2, 60% alcohol): 40 to 80 gtt (2–4 mL) two or three times per day

Pharmacokinetics—If Available (form or route when known): Isolated curcumin is poorly absorbed (in rats) and

mostly excreted by the bowel, with only small amounts found in the bile, liver, kidneys, and adipose tissue.

Toxicity: Long history of human use as a food and medicine. Animal and human studies have revealed no acute or chronic toxicity of turmeric in normal therapeutic doses. Very high doses of curcumin and turmeric oleoresin in rats have led to physiologic and biochemical changes.

Contraindications: Ulcers (isolated curcumin product only); biliary obstruction and gallstones. In women attempting to conceive, high doses of turmeric or curcumin may inhibit fertility.

Side Effects: Allergic contact dermatitis (rare); stomach ulcers: large doses and prolonged use of the curcumin product may irritate the gastric mucosa and reduce mucin production

Long-Term Safety: Safe

Use in Pregnancy/Lactation/Children: Use in small dietary amounts during pregnancy; large amounts may act as an emmenagogue.

Drug/Herb Interactions and Rationale (if known): Avoid using large doses concurrently with anticoagulants and nonsteroidal anti-inflammatories; possible additive effect for bleeding.

Special Notes: Differentiate between turmeric or whole turmeric extracts and standardized curcumin. Both are anti-inflammatory, antihepatotoxic, and antioxidant, but the whole turmeric has a gastroprotective activity, whereas large doses of the curcumin product can irritate the gastric mucosa and suppress mucin production.

BIBLIOGRAPHY

Antony S, et al. (1999). Immunomodulatory activity of curcumin. *Immunologic Investigation.* 28(6-6):291–303.

Azuine MA, et al. (1992). Protective role of aqueous turmeric extract against mutagenicity of direct-acting carcinogens as well as benzo [alpha] pyrene-induced genotoxicity and carcinogenicity. *Journal of Cancer Research & Clinical Oncology.* 118:447.

Chen H, et al. (1999). Curcumin inhibits cell proliferation by interfering with the cell cy and inducing apoptosisin colon carcinoma cells. *Anticancer Research.* 19(5A):3675–3680.

Chun KS, et al. (1999). Antitumor promoting potential of naturally occurring diaryheptanoids structurally related to curcumin. *Mutation Research.* 428(1-2):49–57.

Gonda R, et al. (1992). The core structure of ukonan A, a phagocytosis-activating polysaccharide from the rhizome of *Curcumin longa*, and immunological activities of degradation products. *Chemical and Pharmaceutical Bulletin.* 40:990.

Han SS, et al. (1999). Curcumin causes the growth arrest and apoptosis of B-cell lymphoma by downregulation of egr-1, c-myc, bcl-XL, NF-kappa and p53. *Clinical Immunology.* 93(2):152–161.

Kang BY, et al. (1999). Inhibition of interleukin-12 production in lipopolysaccharide-activated macrophages by curcumin. *European Journal of Pharmacology.* 384(2-3):191–195.

Kapoor LD. (1990). *CRC Handbook of Ayurvedic Medicinal Plants.* Boca Raton, FL: CRC Press.

Kawamori T, et al. (1999). Chemopreventive effect of curcumin, a naturally occurring anti-inflammatory agent, during the promotion/progression stages of colon cancer. *Cancer Research.* 59(3):597–601.

Leung A, Foster S. (1996). *Encyclopedia of Common Natural Ingredients Used in Food, Drugs, and Cosmetics* (2nd ed.). New York: John Wiley & Sons.

Li X, et al. (1998). Study on the antimutagenicity of curcumin. *Wei Sheng Yen Chiu.* 27(4):263–265.

Mills S, Bone K. (1999). *Principles and Practice of Phytotherapy.* Edinburgh: Churchill Livingstone.

Nagabhushan M, Bhide SV. (1992). Curcumin as an inhibitor of cancer. *Journal of the American College of Nutrition.* 11:192.

Plummer SM, et al. (1999). Inhibition of cyclo-oxygenase 2 expression in colon cells by the chemopreventative agent curcumin involves inhibition of NF-kappa activation via the NIK/IKK signalling complex. *Oncogene.* 18(44):6013–6020.

Polasa K, et al. (1992). Effect of turmeric on urinary mutagens in smokers. *Mutagenesis.* 7:107.

Qureshi S, et al. (1992). Toxicity studies on *Alpinia galanga* and *Curcuma longa. Planta Medica.* 58:124.

Ranhan D, et al. (1999). Enhanced apoptosis mediates inhibition of EBV-transformed lymphoblastoid cell line proliferation by curcumin. *Journal of Surgical Research.* 87(1):1–5.

Shah BH, et al. (1999). Inhibitory effect of curcumin, a food spice from turmeric, on platelet-activating factor and arachidonic acid-

mediated platelet aggregation through inhibition of thromboxane
formation and Ca signaling. *Biochemical Pharmacology.*
58(7):1167–1172.

Singhal SS, et al. (1999). The effect of curcumin on glutathione-
linked enzymes in K562 human leukemia cells. *Toxicology Letters.*
109(1-2):87–95.

Thaloor D, et al. (1999). Systemic administration of the NF-kappa B
inhibitor curcumin stimulates muscle regeneration after traumatic
injury. *American Journal of Physiology.* 277 (2 Pt. 1):C320–329.

Venkatesan N, et al. (2000). Curcumin prevents Adriamycin
nephrotoxicity in rats. *British Journal of Pharmacology.*
129(2):231–234.

Wichtl M, Bisset NG. (1994). Herbal drugs and
phytopharmaceuticals. Stuttgart, Germany: Medpharm.

U

 NAME: Uva ursi (*Arctostaphylos uva ursi*)

Common Names: Bearberry, kinnikinnik, beargrape

Family: *Ericaceae*

Description of Plant

- Low-growing evergreen shrub that can form a dark-green
  carpet of leaves and grows up to 20 inches tall.
- Has small, dark-green, leathery leaves and small white or
  pink bell-shaped flowers; blooms April to May. Produces a
  red, edible berry.
- Abundant throughout Northern Hemisphere.

Medicinal Part: Dried leaves

Constituents and Action (if known)

- Phenolic glycosides: arbutin (6%–10%) and methylarbutin
  (up to 4%)
  - Arbutin is hydrolyzed to hydroquinone, which is mildly
    astringent and an effective antimicrobial. Urine must be
    alkaline (pH 8.0) to achieve effect. Most effective against
    *Escherichia coli, Proteus vulgaris, Pseudomonas aeruginosa,
    Staphylococcus aureus.*
  - Anti-immunoinflammatory effects

- Gallotannins (6%–40%): tea can be made by soaking leaves in cold water overnight; this minimizes the extraction of tannins, which contribute to GI discomfort
- Triterpenes (0.4%–0.08%): ursolic acid, uvaole
- Monotropein (iridoid), picein
- Flavone glycosides: hyperin, myricitrin, isoquercitrin, quercitrin
- Saponins: may contribute to disinfective activity (Grases et al., 1994)

Nutritional Ingredients: None known

Traditional Use
- Diuretic, urinary antiseptic, astringent
- Used to treat urinary tract infections,- especially with mucous discharge or blood in the urine
- Decreases inflammation in urinary tract (painful urination and urinary calculi)
- Gout: increases uric acid excretion

Current Use: Urinary antiseptic (cystitis, urethritis). Use with other urinary antiseptic herbs such as corn silk, pipsisscewa, or Oregon grape root.

Available Forms, Dosage, and Administration Guidelines

Preparations: Infusions or cold macerations; tinctures, capsules, and solid forms for oral administration

Typical Dosage
- Unless otherwise prescribed, 10 g per day of crushed leaf or powder corresponding to 400 to 700 mg arbutin. Medication containing arbutin should not be taken for longer than 10 to 14 days or more than five times a year without consulting a physician.
- *Infusion:* 1 tsp dried herb in 8 oz boiling water, steep for 15 minutes; take two or three cups per day
- *Cold maceration:* 1 tsp dried herb in 8 oz cold water, steep for several hours; take up to four times daily
- *Dry extract* (containing 100–210 mg hydroquinone derivatives calculated as water-free arbutin): Take up to four times daily

- *Capsules (ground herb)*: two 500-mg capsules two or three times per day
- *Tincture* (1:5, 30% alcohol): 40 to 60 gtt (2–3 mL) three times a day

Pharmacokinetics—If Available (form or route when known): Maximum urinary antiseptic effect occurs 3 to 4 hours after administration, with 70% to 75% of the dose excreted within 24 hours.

Toxicity: Doses up to 20 g have not caused toxicity in healthy adults.

Contraindications: Kidney disease, pregnancy

Side Effects: GI discomfort (nausea, vomiting); urine may turn greenish

Long-Term Safety: Do not use more than 10 to 14 days.

Use in Pregnancy/Lactation/Children: Large doses are oxytocic. Refrain from use in all.

Drug/Herb Interactions and Rationale (if known): Do not use with cranberry juice; it may acidify the urine and make uva ursi ineffective.

Special Notes: Do not use for more than 10 to 14 days. Urine must be alkaline for herb to be effective. Diet should include dairy products, vegetables (especially tomatoes), fruits, fruit juices, and potatoes. In addition, drink large amounts of water.

BIBLIOGRAPHY

Bradley PR. (1992). *British Herbal Compendium,* Vol. 1. Bournemouth: British Herbal Medicine Association.

Bruneton J. (1999). *Pharmacognosy, Phytochemistry, Medicinal Plants* (2nd ed.). Paris: Lavoisier.

ESCOP Monographs on the Medicinal Uses of Plant Drugs. (1997). Exeter: ESCOP.

Grases F, et al. (1994). Urolithiasis and phytotherapy. *International Urology & Nephrology.* 26(5):507–511.

Review of Natural Products. (1997). St. Louis: Facts and Comparisons.

Weiss R, Fintelmann V. (2000). *Herbal Medicine* (2nd ed.). Stuttgart: Thieme.

NAME: Valerian (*Valeriana officinalis*)

Common Names: All-heal, great wild valerian, setwell, Indian valerian, red valerian

Family: *Valerianaceae*

Description of Plant
- Perennial plant with species native to North America, Europe, and Asia
- White to red flowers bloom June to September

Medicinal Part: Rhizome/root

Constituents and Action (if known)
- Volatile oils (monoterpenes): borneol, bornyl isovalerate, bornyl acetate, camphene—weakly antagonize benzodiazepine receptors (Dressing & Riemann, 1992; Hobbs, 1995; Wagner et al., 1998)
- Sesquiterpenes: valerenal, valerenic acid, valeranone, sedative, spasmolytic—antispasmodic properties, may cause hypotension possibly by influencing serotonin, GABA, and norepinephrine (Schultz et al., 1997)
- Iridoids: valepotriates (insoluble in water)—valtrate, didrovaltrate; bind to barbiturate and peripheral benzodiazepine receptors, resulting in sedation (Leuschner et al., 1993; Lindahl & Lindwall, 1989; Mennini et al., 1993)
- Flavonoids: diosmetin, kaempferol, luteolin
- Amino acids: GABA—calming effect
- Alkaloids (minor amounts)
- Decomposition products (homobaldrinol, valtroxal): sedative activity, well absorbed by the gut (Houghton, 1997)
- Hydroalcoholic extracts: bind to GABA-A receptors (Mennini et al., 1993; Sakamoto et al., 1992; Tatsuya et al., 1992)

Nutritional Ingredients: None

Traditional Use: Used for hundreds of years in Europe as a sedative and antispasmolytic to relieve insomnia, anxiety, muscle spasms, stress-induced palpitations, gastric spasms, hysteria, nervous headaches, and menstrual pain. Northwestern Native Americans boiled the roots into a tea for calming the nerves (*V. stitchensis*).

Current Use
- Anodyne, carminative, antispasmodic, hypotensive, sedative
- Relieves menstrual and intestinal cramps
- Improves sleep quality, with no daytime sedation or impairment of concentration or performance. Those with sleep difficulties such as insomnia benefit the most. Shortens sleep latency and reduces night awakenings. Often mixed with chamomile, lemon balm, or hops.
- Eases muscle pain and spasms: restless leg syndrome, back pain, bruxism; use with kava, black haw, or scullcap
- Acts a sedative; decreases tension headache and anxiety
- Numerous studies have looked at the combination of valerian and St. John's wort for depression and anxiety. This combination was found to be as effective as amitriptyline for depression and more effective than diazepam (Valium) for anxiety. The herb combination also produced dramatically fewer side effects than the pharmaceutical medications (Mills & Bone, 1999).
- Relieves nervous stomach and other stress-induced GI symptoms

Available Forms, Dosage, and Administration Guidelines
Preparations: Dried root, tea, capsules, tablets, tinctures, extracts. Sometimes standardized to contain at least 0.5% EO.

Typical Dosage
- *Dried root:* 3 to 9 g per day
- *Capsules:* For products standardized to 0.5% EO, 300 to 400 mg per day. As a sleep aid, take 1 hour before bedtime. For anxiety, 150 to 500 mg/day divided into several doses.
- *Fresh tincture* (1:2, 70% alcohol): 40 to 90 gtt (2–5 mL) three times a day, or follow manufacturer's or practitioner's recommendations
- *Tea:* 1 tsp root in 8 oz hot water, steep for 20 to 30 minutes covered; take one to three cups daily. Patient compliance may be limited by the unpleasant taste.
- *Fluid extract* (1:1): 0.5 to 1 tsp (1–2 mL)

Pharmacokinetics—If Available (form or route when known): Not known

Toxicity: A patient ingested an overdose of valerian capsules (25 g), and symptoms included fatigue, abdominal cramps, and tremor. All symptoms resolved within 24 hours (Mills & Bone, 1999). Some researchers have noted concerns that some of the valepotriates might be carcinogenic when taken orally; subsequent research showed that these compounds are unstable and are broken down by gastric HCl, forming safe decomposition products (Mills & Bone, 1999).

Contraindications: Theoretical concern that valerian may exacerbate schizophrenia or bipolar disorders (Schellenberg et al., 1993)

Side Effects: Occasionally patients become overstimulated rather than sedated by valerian. Overdose has caused headaches, blurred vision, nausea, stupor.

Long-Term Safety: Safe and approved for food use by the FDA; nontoxic even in large doses

Use in Pregnancy/Lactation/Children: No adverse effects noted or expected

Drug/Herb Interactions and Rationale (if known): May intensify the effects of sedatives; has been shown not to potentiate effects of alcohol

Special Notes: Very unpleasant smell; smells like old sweaty socks. Valerian baths are commonly used in Europe (despite the odor) to relieve stress, muscle tension, anxiety, and insomnia.

BIBLIOGRAPHY

Albrecht M, et al. (1995). Phytopharmaceuticals and safety in traffic: the influence of a plant-based sedative on vehicle operation ability with or without alcohol. *Zeitschrift Allgemeinmedizin.* 71:1215–1221.

Bradley PR. (1992). *British Herbal Compendium*, Vol. 1. Bournemouth: British Herbal Medicine Association.

Donath F, et al. (2000). Critical evaluation of the effect of valerian extract on sleep structure and sleep quality. *Pharmacopsychiatry.* 33(2):47–53.

Dressing H, et al. (1992). Insomnia: are valerian balm combinations of equal value to benzodiazepine? *Therapiewoche.* 42:726–736.

ESCOP Monographs on the Medicinal Uses of Plant Drugs. (1992). Exeter: ESCOP.

Hobbs C. (1995). *Valerian: The Relaxing and Sleep Herb.* Santa Cruz, CA: Botanica.

Houghton PJ. (Ed.). (1997). *Valerian, the Genus Valeriana.* Amsterdam: Harwood.

Leuschner J, et al. (1993). Characterization of the central nervous depressant activity of a commercially valuable valerian root extract. *Arzneimittelforschung.* 43(6):638–643.

Lindahl O, Lindwall L. (1989). Double-blind study of a valerian preparation. *Pharmacology, Biochemistry & Behavior.* 32(4):1065–1066.

Mennini T, et al. (1993). In vitro study on the interaction of extracts and pure compounds from *Valeriana officinalis* roots with GABA, benzodiazepine and barbiturate receptors. *Fitoterapia.* 64:291–300.

Mills S, Bone K. (1999). *Principles and Practice of Phytotherapy.* Edinburgh: Churchill Livingstone.

Sakamoto T, et al. (1992). Psychotropic effects of Japanese valerian root extract. *Pharmaceutical Society of Japan.* 40(3):758–761.

Schellenberg V, et al. (1993). Quantitative EEG monitoring in phyto- and psycho-pharmacological treatment of psychosomatic and affective disorders [abstract]. *Schizophrenia Research.* 9(2,3).

Schultz V, et al. (1997). Clinical trials with phyto-psychopharmacological agents. *Phytomedicine.* 4(4):379–387.

Schulz V, et al. (1998). *Rational Phytotherapy: A Physician's Guide to Herbal Medicine.* (3rd ed.). New York: Springer.

Tatsuya S, et al. (1992). Psychotropic effects of Japanese valerian root extract. *Chemical & Pharmacy Bulletin.* 40(3):758–761.

Vonderheid-Guth B, et al. (2000). Pharmacodynamic effects of valerian and hops extract combination (Ze 91019) on the quantitative-topographical EEG in healthy volunteers. *European Journal of Medical Research.* 5(4):139–144.

Wagner J, et al. (1998). Beyond benzodiazepines: alternative pharmacologic agents for the treatment of insomnia. *American Pharmacotherapy.* 32(6):680–691.

Weiss RF, Fintelmann V. (2000). *Herbal Medicine* (2nd ed.). Stuttgart: Thieme.

Willey LB. (1995). Valerian overdose: a case report. *Veterinary and Human Toxicology.* 37(4):364–365.

NAME: Wild Yam (*Dioscorea villosa*)

Common Names: Wild yam root, colic root, rheumatism root

Family: *Dioscoreaceae*

Description of Plant

- More than 500 species exist worldwide; some are edible, some are medicinal, and some, like the Mexican wild yam, were used as a source of steroidal saponins, which through laboratory synthesis were turned into progesterone.
- Twining vine native to the eastern United States with ovate, heart-shaped leaves
- Inconspicuous white to greenish-yellow female flowers followed by winged seeds.

Medicinal Part: Dried rhizome with rootlets

Constituents and Action (if known)

- Steroidal saponins: dioscin (anti-inflammatory activity), gracilin
- Isoquinuclidine alkaloids: dioscorin
- Tannins

Nutritional Ingredients: None

Traditional Use

- Antispasmodic, anti-inflammatory, cholagogue
- Antispasmodic used for biliary colic, intestinal spasms, gallbladder spasms
- Dysmenorrhea with nausea, and ovarian spasm pain
- Antiemetic used for morning sickness, biliousness, nausea, vomiting
- Used along with fringe tree and celandine to pass small gallstones
- Anti-inflammatory: arthritis, muscular rheumatism

Current Use: An excellent herb for hepatic or intestinal spasms: irritable bowel syndrome, biliary colic, diverticulitis, intestinal colic, painful flatulence, and biliousness. Use with chamomile, kudzu, huang qin, or catnip. Can be useful for dysmenorrhea with nausea along with black haw, ginger, or cyperus.

Available Forms, Dosage, and Administration Guidelines

Preparations: Dried root, tea, capsules, tincture

Typical Dosage

- *Dried root:* 2 to 4 g per day
- *Tea:* 1 tsp dried cut/sifted root to 1 cup water, decoct 15 to 20 minutes, steep half-hour; take up to two cups per day
- *Capsules:* Two 500-mg capsules three times a day
- *Tincture* (1:2, 35% alcohol): 40 to 80 gtt (2–4 mL) three times a day

Pharmacokinetics—If Available (form or route when known): Not known

Toxicity: Overdose may cause nausea, vomiting, diarrhea, and headache.

Contraindications: None known

Side Effects: In overdose, nausea, vomiting, diarrhea, headache

Long-Term Safety: No adverse effects expected with normal therapeutic doses

Use in Pregnancy/Lactation/Children: Small amounts have traditionally been used in formulas for morning sickness. No adverse effects are known. Very little research has been done on this plant. One study suggests that wild yam appeared to suppress progesterone synthesis, but no direct effect on estrogen or progesterone receptors was found (*Review of Natural Products*, 1999). Use with caution.

Drug/Herb Interactions and Rationale (if known): None known

Special Notes: Wild yam has been the subject of numerous myths. Some marketers and publications state that it contains natural progesterone or that natural progesterone can be synthesized in vivo from its steroidal saponin, diosgenin. Other equally inaccurate claims suggest that it contains DHEA or stimulates the body's production of DHEA. The last of these rumors is that wild yam can be used as a "natural" form of birth control. This seems to be based on the fact that progesterone was originally synthesized from diosgenin extracted from the Mexican species. All of these claims are totally wrong and spurred by ignorance and/or avarice (Zava et al., 1998).

Many topical wild yam creams are marketed as natural hormone replacement therapy. There are two types of products on the market: those containing actual pharmaceutical progesterone and those that contain wild yam without added progesterone. Only the creams containing pharmaceutical progesterone (the source of which is unimportant) are clinically useful for relieving hot flashes, formication, and vaginal dryness.

BIBLIOGRAPHY

Bone K. (1997). Progesterogenic herbs? *Modern Phytotherapist.* 3(2):14–16.

Brinker F. (1997). A comparative review of eclectic female regulators. *British Journal of Phytotherapy.* 4(3):123–145.

British Herbal Pharmacopoeia (4th ed.). (1996). Guildford, UK: Biddles Ltd.

Integrative Medicine Access. (2000). *Wild Yam.* Newton, MA: Integrative Medicine Communications.

Review of Natural Products. (1999). St. Louis: Facts and Comparisons.

Zava D, et al. (1998). Estrogen and progestin bioactivity of foods, herbs, and spices. *Proceedings of the Society for Experimental Biology & Medicine.* 217(3):369–378.

NAME: Willow (*Salix* spp.)

Common Names: Bay willow (*S. daphnoides*), crack willow (*S. fragilis*), purple willow (*S. purpurea*), white willow (*S. alba*)

Family: *Salicaceae*

Description of Plant
- Willow trees thrive in moist areas and often grow along river banks.
- Bark is harvested in early spring or autumn from 2- to 3-year-old branches.

Medicinal Part: Dried bark

Constituents and Action (if known)

- Phenolic glycosides (2.5%–11%)
  - Salicin, salicortin, tremulacin, populin (Wichtl & Bisset, 1994): anti-inflammatory activity (ESCOP, 1997; Mills et al., 1996)
- Tannins (8%–20%): catechins, procyanidins, gallotannins (Newall et al., 1996)
- Flavonoids (isoquercitrin, naringenin) (Wichtl & Bisset, 1994)
- Other actions: has no effect on platelet function (Bradley, 1992)

Nutritional Ingredients: None known

Traditional Use

- Anti-inflammatory, analgesic, antipyretic, antirheumatic, astringent
- Internally: to reduce fevers, muscle aches, arthritic pains, headaches, and inflammation
- Externally: as a wash for wounds, a poultice or bath for sore joints and muscle pain

Current Use

- Mild pain reliever (anodyne); can be used for arthritic pain, mild headaches, gout, fevers, and aches associated with influenza and colds
- Anti-inflammatory activity for arthralgias, lumbago, tendinitis, bursitis, and sprains. According to the *British Herbal Pharmacopoeia* (1996), willow combines well with guaiac, black cohosh, and celery seed for rheumatoid arthritis.
- Can be useful for mild diarrhea with cramps

Available Forms, Dosage, and Administration Guidelines

Preparations: Dried bark, capsules, tea, tincture. European products are standardized to 1% salicin.

Typical Dosage

- Unless otherwise prescribed: Liquid and solid preparations for internal use with an average daily dosage corresponding

to 60 to 120 mg total salicin (Blumenthal, 2000), which is
equivalent to 6 to 12 g dried bark (Schilcher, 1997)

- *Dried bark:* 1 to 3 g, three times daily (Newall et al., 1996)
- *Decoction:* 1 to 2 tsp finely chopped or coarsely powdered
  bark in 8 oz cold water, bring to a boil and simmer for 10
  minutes, steep half-hour; take 8 oz three times per day
  (Meyer-Buchtela, 1999; Wichtl & Bisset, 1994)
- *Tincture* (1:5, 30% alcohol): 80–120 gtt (4–6 mL) three
  times daily
- *Spray-dried extract:* Standardized to contain 20 to 40 mg
  total salicin, three times daily

**Pharmacokinetics—If Available (form or route when
known):** In a human study, 86% of orally administered
salacin was excreted in the urine as metabolites (mainly
salicyluric acid) over several hours, showing a more prolonged
effect than acetylsalicylic acid (Upton, 1999). The half-life is
2.5 hours.

Toxicity: None known

Contraindications: There is a theoretical concern that salicin
may cause a response in patients with allergies to ASA.
Although they have similar activity, salicin is metabolized
differently and does not provoke many of the adverse responses
associated with ASA (reduced clotting, Reye's syndrome, gastric
irritation, and allergic reaction).

Side Effects: Mild GI irritation from tannins

Long-Term Safety: No adverse effects expected with
appropriate dosage

Use in Pregnancy/Lactation/Children: No restriction
known; use with caution

Drug/Herb Interactions and Rationale (if known): Use
cautiously with nonsteroidal anti-inflammatories: may increase
likelihood of GI irritation and bleeding from tannins

Special Notes: There are few clinical trials, but extensive
empirical and ethnobotanical use clearly shows the benefits of
willow bark. More research would be useful to clarify the

differences between willow bark and pure acetylsalicylic acid and to put to rest fears concerning adverse reactions.

BIBLIOGRAPHY

Bartram T. (1995). *Encyclopedia of Herbal Medicine.* Dorset: Grace Publishing.

Blumenthal M, et al. (2000). *Herbal Medicine, Expanded Commission E Monographs.* Austin, TX: American Botanical Council.

Bradley PR. (Ed.). (1992). *British Herbal Compendium,* Vol. I. Bournemouth: British Herbal Medicine Association.

British Herbal Pharmacopoeia. (1996). Exeter: British Herbal Medicine Association.

Bruneton J. (1999). *Pharmacognosy, Phytochemistry, Medicinal Plants* (2d ed.). Paris: Lavoisier.

ESCOP Monographs on the Medicinal Uses of Plant Drugs. (1997). Exeter: ESCOP.

Kudriashov BA, et al. (1986). Hemostatic system function as affected by thromboplastic agents from higher plants. *Nauchnye Doki Vyss Shkoly Biol Nauki.* (4):58–61.

Meyer-Buchtela E. (1999). *Tee-Rezepturen- Ein Handbuch fur Apotheker und Arzte.* Stuttgart: Deutscher Apotheker Verlag.

Mills SY, et al. (1996). Effect of a proprietary herbal medicine on the relief of chronic arthritic pain: a double-blind study. *British Journal of Rheumatology.* 35(9):874–878.

Newall CA, et al. (1996). *Herbal Medicines: A Guide for Healthcare Professionals.* London: Pharmaceutical Press.

Schilcher H. (1997). *Phytotherapy in Paediatrics: Handbook for Physicians and Pharmacists.* Stuttgart: Medpharm.

Upton R. (Ed.). (1999). *American Herbal Pharmacopoeia and Therapeutic Compendium.* Santa Cruz, CA: AHP.

Wichtl M, Bisset NG. (1994). *Herbal Drugs and Phytopharmaceuticals.* Stuttgart: Medpharm.

Y

 NAME: Yarrow (*Achillea millefolium*)

Common Names: Thousand-leaf, milfoil, woundwort

Family: *Asteraceae*

Description of Plant

- Hardy aromatic perennial, growing 2 to 3 feet tall; blooms June to October
- Native to Europe, Asia, and North America; common in fields and waste places
- Adapts to environment; plant can change its morphology and chemical composition depending on growing conditions.

Medicinal Part: Dried leaves and flowers

Constituents and Action (if known)

- EO (0.2%–1%): monoterpenes—linalool, camphor, borneol (antimicrobial)
  - Sesquiterpenes (chamazulene): anti-inflammatory and antiallergenic properties (rat models) (Newall et al., 1996), beta-caryophyllene, sabinene, alpha- and beta-pinenes
- Flavonoids: apigenin, artemetin, casticin, luteolin, rutin (Wichtl, 1994)
  - Antispasmodic activity (Newall et al., 1996)
  - Effective against diarrhea, flatulence, and cramping
- Sesquiterpene lactones: achillicin, achillin, leucodin, achillifolin, millefin—anti-inflammatory, digestive bitters
- Alkaloids: stachydrine, achilleine—hemostatic (Newall et al., 1996), digestive bitters
- Tannins (3%–4%)
- Coumarins (Newall et al., 1996; Wichtl & Bisset, 1994)

Other actions

- Improves circulation and tones varicose veins (Chevallier, 1996)

Nutritional Ingredients: None

Traditional Use

- Antibacterial, antispasmodic, anti-inflammatory, bitter tonic, diuretic, diaphoretic, styptic, vulnerary, menstrual amphoteric, peripheral vasodilator
- Fresh leaf or flower can be applied topically as a poultice to stop bleeding from wounds (styptic).
- A bitter digestive tonic used for gas, nausea, poor fat digestion, and biliousness

- Reduces pain of toothache (fresh leaves, flowers, or roots, chewed)
- Helps regulate menstrual cycle (menorrhagia or amenorrhea)
- Used as a diaphoretic to increase sweating and lower fevers

Current Use
- Anti-inflammatory and antispasmodic activity, especially to GI tract; used for irritable bowel syndrome, gastric ulcers with bleeding, mucous colitis, intestinal colic, enteritis, and diarrhea
- Styptic: used topically for cuts and scratches and hemorrhoids and episiotomy incisions (sitz bath; add 1–2 gtt lavender EO)
- Internally for menorrhagia, hematuria, nosebleeds, and hemoptysis
- Effective remedy for the early stages of influenza and fever management. Take as a hot tea with boneset or elderflower.
- A digestive tonic, useful for biliary dyskinesia, nervous dyspepsia, impaired fat digestion, and flatulence

Available Forms, Dosage, and Administration Guidelines
Preparations: Dried herb, tea, tincture, succus (pressed juice from fresh herb); sitz baths

Typical Dosage
- *Infusion:* 1 tsp dried herb/flowers in 8 oz hot water, steep covered 20–30 minutes; take up to three cups per day
- *Succus:* 1 tsp (5 mL) three times daily between meals
- *Tincture* (1:5, 40% alcohol): 40 to 100 gtt (2–5 mL) three times a day
- *Sitz bath:* 4 oz dried yarrow in 1 gallon hot water, steep covered 40 minutes, add to just enough water to cover the hips with the knees up. Wrap upper body in towels, soak 10 to 20 minutes, rinse.

Pharmacokinetics—If Available (form or route when known): Not known

Toxicity: No acute or chronic toxicity known

Contraindications: Serious allergy to the aster family (ragweed, chamomile, chrysanthemum, and so forth)

Side Effects: Contact dermatitis (rare)

Long-Term Safety: No adverse effects expected with normal therapeutic doses

Use in Pregnancy/Lactation/Children: Use cautiously during pregnancy; may have mild emmenagogue qualities. No adverse effects expected in lactating mothers or in children.

Drug/Herb Interactions and Rationale (if known): None known

Special Notes: Although there is little current research on yarrow, it has a long history of clinical use by herbalists and naturopathic and eclectic physicians. It also has extensive ethnobotanical use, and we have detailed knowledge of the herb's phytochemistry. This accumulated information gives adequate support for use of this herb.

BIBLIOGRAPHY

Bradley PR. (1992). *British Herbal Compendium,* Vol. 1. Bournemouth: British Herbal Medicine Association.

Chevallier A. (1996). *Encyclopedia of Medicinal Plants*. New York: DK Publishing.

Hedley C. (1996). Yarrow: a monograph. *European Journal of Herbal Medicine*. 2(3):14–18.

Mills S. (1991). *Out of the Earth: The Essential Book of Herbal Medicine*. London: Viking Arkana.

Montanari T, et al. (1998). Antispermatogenic effect of *Achillea millefolium* L in mice. *Contraception*. 58(5):309–313.

Newall C, et al. (1996). *Herbal Medicines*. London: Pharmaceutical Press.

Review of Natural Products. (1998). St. Louis: Facts and Comparisons.

Wichtl M, Bisset NG. (1994). *Herbal Drugs and Phytopharmaceuticals*. Stuttgart: Medpharm.

 NAME: Yohimbe (*Pausinystalia yohimbe*)

Common Names: None

Family: *Rubiaceae*

Description of Plant: A tall evergreen tree native to West Africa (Nigeria, Cameroon, Gabon, and the Congo).

Medicinal Part: Dried bark

Constituents and Action (if known)
- Indole alkaloids (1%–6% total): yohimbine (10%–15%), coryanthine, pseudo-yohimbine, allo-yohimbine
- Yohimbine is a monoamine oxidase inhibitor (Leung & Foster, 1996) and a selective inhibitor of presynaptic alpha-2-adrenergic receptors, increasing sympathetic nervous system activity, norepinephrine release, and lipolysis.
- Low doses are hypertensive and higher doses are hypotensive; it is a peripheral vasodilator (Bruneton, 1999).

Nutritional Ingredients: None

Traditional Use: Aphrodisiac, CNS stimulant, antidiuretic; used by tribal peoples in West Africa as an aphrodisiac for men with erectile dysfunction, as a stimulant, and for anginal pain and hypertension

Current Use: The prescription drug yohimbine HCl is used for erectile dysfunction in diabetic patients. Yohimbine HCl has also been used for orthostatic hypotension, chronic constipation, narcolepsy, diabetic patients with incapacitating paresthesia of the lower limbs, and obesity, especially in the thighs and buttocks. Stimulates alpha-2-adrenergic receptors, which increases lipolysis of fat cells. Inhibits hunger pangs (Mitchell, 2000).

Available Forms, Dosage, and Administration Guidelines
Preparations: Crude herb, tincture
Typical Dosage
- *Tincture* (1:5, 50% alcohol): 5 to 10 gtt (0.25–0.5 mL) twice a day
- *Yohimbine HCl* (prescription only): 5.4 to 6 mg three times a day; increased risk of adverse effects with doses of more than 10 mg

Pharmacokinetics—If Available (form or route when known): Most bioavailable if patient is fasting. Oral doses of

10 mg yohimbine HCl resulted in rapid absorption (absorption half-life of 0.17 ± 0.11 hours) and elimination (elimination half-life 0.60 ± 0.26 hours) (de Smet, 1997).

Toxicity: Associated with a lupus-like syndrome, nausea, vomiting, tachycardia, hypertension, tremor, acute renal failure, psychiatric disorders (de Smet, 1997; Reichert, 1997; Sandler & Aronson, 1993). Long-term use of yohimbine HCl (more than 5 years at 5.4 mg three times a day) has been linked to agranulocytosis.

Contraindications: Hepatic insufficiency and liver disease, renal insufficiency and kidney disease, hypotension, hypertension (oral doses of 15–20 mg yohimbine HCl can increase blood pressure), depression, prostatitis, bipolar disorders (a dose of yohimbine HCl as low as 10 mg can trigger a manic episode in bipolar patients), schizophrenia, asthma, cardiac disease

Side Effects: Priapism, hypertension or hypotension depending on dosage, irritability, migraines, dizziness, tremors, bronchospasm, insomnia, tachycardia, nausea and vomiting

Long-Term Safety: Inappropriate for long-term use

Use in Pregnancy/Lactation/Children: Avoid in all.

Drug/Herb Interactions and Rationale (if known):
Phenothiazines such as chlorpromazine increase yohimbe's toxicity; monoamine oxidase inhibitors; tricyclic antidepressants (12 mg yohimbine HCl elicited hypertensive crisis in patients taking these medications [de Smet, 1997]); antihypertensive medications (antagonizes effects of drugs such as clonidine)

Special Notes
- This herb's use should be restricted to trained clinicians.
- It has been suggested that yohimbe is effective for erectile dysfunction. There are no studies of the crude drug for this claim. Only yohimbine HCl has been tested, and results of studies on this alkaloid are contradictory.

- Yohimbine is also an active stimulant of the alpha-2-adrenergic receptors of adipocytes. This process is believed to increase lipolysis, but most trials using yohimbine HCl for weight loss have had negative results.

- Body builders tout yohimbe as a natural way to build muscle. Not only is this unproven, but it is potentially dangerous.

- Studies of commercial yohimbe products (crude herb) have often shown little or no yohimbe in the product. Yohimbine concentrations have ranged from less than 0.1 to 489 parts per million, compared with 7,089 parts per million in authentic material. Some of these products showed only yohimbine HCl and none of the other indole alkaloids that should be present in the crude herb, suggesting the product was "spiked" with minute amounts of the isolated alkaloid. With the problems of adulteration, possible drug/herb interactions, and toxicity, it is unwise for patients to self-medicate with this herb.

BIBLIOGRAPHY

Betz JM, et al. (1995). Gas chromatographic determination of yohimbine in commercial yohimbe products. *Journal of AOAC International.* 78(5):1189–1194.

Blumenthal M, et al. (2000). *Herbal Medicine: Expanded Commission E Monographs.* Austin, TX: American Botanical Council.

Brinker F. (1997). *Herb Contraindications and Drug Interactions.* Sandy, OR: Eclectic Institute, Inc.

Bruneton J. (1999). *Pharmacognosy, Phytochemistry, Medicinal Plants* (2nd ed.). Paris: Lavoisier.

de Smet PA. (1997). Yohimbe alkaloids. In: *Adverse Effects of Herbal Drugs,* Vol. 3. New York: Springer-Verlag.

de Smet PA, Oscar S. (1994). Potential risks of health food products containing yohimbe extracts. *British Medical Journal.* 309:958.

Ernst E, Pittler MH. (1998). Yohimbe for erectile dysfunction: a systematic review and meta-analysis of randomized clinical trials. *Journal of Urology.* 159(2):433–436.

Leung A, Foster S. (1996). *Encyclopedia of Common Natural Ingredients* (2nd ed.). New York: John Wiley & Sons.

Miller WW. (1968). Afrodex in the treatment of male impotence: a double-blind cross-over study. *Current Therapeutic Research.* 10:354.

Mitchell W. (2000). *Plant Medicine: Applications of the Botanical Remedies in the Practice of Naturopathic Medicine.* Seattle: Author.

Reichert R. (Spring 1997). Yohimbine pharmacokinetics. *Quarterly Review of Natural Medicine*, pp. 17–18.

Riley AJ. (1994). Yohimbine in the treatment of erectile disorder. *British Journal of Clinical Practice.* 48(3):133–136.

Sandler B, Aronson P. (1993). Yohimbine-induced cutaneous drug eruption, progressive renal failure, and lupus-like syndrome. *Urology.* 41(4):343–345.

Susset JG, et al. (1989). Effect of yohimbine hydrochloride on erectile impotence: a double-blind study. *Journal of Urology.* 141:1360–1363.

PART III

Nutritional Supplements

NAME: L-**arginine**

Common Names: Argenine

Description and Source: Essential amino acid

Biologic Activity
- Substrate necessary for nitric oxide synthesis and maintenance of activity
- Nitric oxide acts as a vasodilator, reduces platelet aggregation, reduces monocyte/vessel wall interactions, and reduces smooth muscle cell proliferation (Cooke & Tsao, 1994)
- Improves endothelium-dependent dilation with significant hypercholesterolemia (7 g three times a day) (Clarkson et al., 1996)
- Improves blood flow and reduces total and very-low-density lipoproteins (Maxwell & Anderson, 1999)
- Improves blood flow and reduces chest pain in patients with nonobstructive coronary artery disease (Lerman et al., 1998)
- Improves blood flow and walking ability in patients with intermittent claudication (Maxwell et al., 1999)

Nutritional Sources: Peanuts and peanut butter, brown rice, cashews, pecans, almonds, chocolate, sunflower seeds

Current Use
- Improves coronary blood flow in persons with atherosclerosis
- Improves walking distance in persons with intermittent claudication
- May reduce cholesterol (very-low-density lipoproteins)
- May enhance penile engorgement

Available Forms, Dosage, and Administration Guidelines: Dosages found to be effective for the treatment of cardiovascular disease range from 6 to 9 g/day. Heart Bar (Cooke Pharmaceuticals, Belmont, CA) contains 2 to 3 g arginine.

Pharmacokinetics—If Available (form or route when known): Not known

Toxicity: None known

Contraindications: Persons susceptible to herpes: arginine activates herpesvirus replication

Side Effects: GI intolerance

Long-Term Safety: Not known

Use in Pregnancy/Lactation/Children: Not known

Drug/Herb Interactions and Rationale (if known): Not known

Special Notes: Current studies are very short (6 months or less); long-term studies are necessary.

BIBLIOGRAPHY

Chaitow L. (1985). *Amino Acids in Therapy.* Wellingborough, England: Thorsons.

Clarkson P, et al. (1996). Oral L-arginine improves endothelium-dependent dilation in hypercholesterolemic young adults. *Journal of Clinical Investigation.* 97(8):1989–1994.

Cooke JP, Tsao PS. (1994). Is NO an endogenous antiatherogenic molecule? *Arteriosclerosis & Thrombosis.* 14(5):653–655.

Lerman A, et al. (1998). Long-term L-arginine supplementation improves small-vessel coronary endothelial function in humans. *Circulation.* 97(21):2123–2128.

Maxwell AJ, Anderson BA. (1999). A nutritional product designed to enhance nitric oxide activity restores endothelium-dependent function in hypercholesterolemia. *Journal of the American College of Cardiology.* 33:282A.

Maxwell AJ, et al. (1999). Improvement in walking distance and quality of life in peripheral arterial disease by a nutritional product designed to enhance nitric oxide activity. *Journal of the American College of Cardiology.* 33:277A.

 NAME: L-carnitine

Common Names: L-carnitine (LC), acetyl-L-carnitine (ALC), L-propionylcarnitine (LPC)

Description and Source

- LC is an essential amino acid that is necessary for the conversion of fatty acids into energy for muscle activity. It is primarily stored in the muscles, including the heart.

- Three forms of LC are available
  - LC: the most common form, it has the most research and costs less than the other forms
  - ALC (or L-acetyl-carnitine): effects are primarily directed toward cerebral function and memory
  - LPC: may have the most profound effect on the heart and its function

Biologic Activity

- ALC stimulates message transmission in brain cells, retards loss of receptors in brain cells (rats) (Castorina & Ferraros, 1994), and increases cerebral blood flow and enzyme activity in the brain.
- LC is therapeutically active in hyperlipidemia, lowering LDL and very-low-density lipoprotein cholesterol and triglyceride levels and elevating HDL. It is also indicated for preventing and treating atherosclerosis. LC has shown benefits for ischemic heart disease, CHF, angina pectoris, and mild arrhythmias (Pepine, 1991).
- Levels of L-carnitine may be low in patients with CFS; more research is necessary (Werbach, 2000).
- LC may play a role in reversing insulin resistance (Kelly, 2000).
- When low, LC may play a role in complications of diabetes mellitus; supplementation may also improve glucose tolerance (Tamamogullari et al., 1999).

Nutritional Sources: Red meats and to a lesser degree poultry, fish, and dairy products

Current Use

- ALC may improve mental functioning in patients with Alzheimer's disease, senile dementia, and Down syndrome (more research is necessary) (Pettegrew, 1995; Sano et al, 1992).
- ALC enhances behavioral performance and results on memory tests (Cucinotta et al., 1988; Salvioli & Neri, 1994).
- LC or LPC can be used to prevent and treat ischemic heart disease (Singh et al., 1996).

- LC is being given to AIDS patients (6 g/day) to reduce the toxicity of AZT on the muscle cells, thus reducing muscle fatigue and pain (Integrative Medicine Access, 2000).
- LC should be considered in treating hyperlipidemia and atherosclerosis.
- LC has shown benefits in reducing muscle pain and fatigue associated with CFS/fibromyalgia (Plioplys & Plioplys, 1997).

Available Forms, Dosage, and Administration Guidelines: 1 to 3 g/day, divided into two or three doses

Pharmacokinetics—If Available (form or route when known): Not known

Toxicity: None known. Avoid the D- or DL-carnitine, which has caused adverse effects.

Contraindications: Seizure activity, bipolar disorders, liver or kidney disease

Side Effects: Diarrhea, nausea, vomiting with 4 g or more per day; fishy body odor

Long-Term Safety: Unknown; additional research needed

Drug/Herb Interactions and Rationale (if known): Co-Q10 seems to enhance LC's effects.

BIBLIOGRAPHY

Castorina M, Ferraros L. (1994). Acetyl-L-carnitine affects aged brain receptorial system in rodents. *Life Science.* 54:1205–1214.

Cucinotta D, et al. (1988). Multicenter clinical placebo-controlled study with acetyl-L-carnitine (LAC) in the treatment of mildly demented elderly patients. *Drug Development Research.* 14:213–216.

Integrative Medicine Access. (2000). *L*-carnitine. Newton, MA: Integrative Medicine Communications.

Kelly GS. (1998). L-carnitine: therapeutic applications of a conditionally essential amino acid. *Alternative Medicine Review.* 3(5):345–360.

Kelly GS. (2000). Insulin resistance: lifestyle and nutritional interventions. *Alternative Medicine Review.* 5(2):109–132.

Pepine CJ. (1991). The therapeutic potential of L-carnitine in cardiovascular disorders. *Clinical Therapeutics.* 13(1):2–21.

Pettegrew JW, et al. (1995). Clinical and neurochemical effects of acetyl-L-carnitine in Alzheimer's disease. *Neurobiology of Aging.* 16:1–4.

Plioplys AV, Plioplys S. (1997). Amantadine and L-carnitine treatment of chronic fatigue syndrome. *Neuropsychology.* 35(1):16–23.

Salvioli G, Neri M. (1994). L-acetyl-carnitine treatment of mental decline in the elderly. *Drugs: Experimental & Clinical Research.* 20:169–176.

Sano M, et al. (1992). Double-blind parallel design pilot study of acetyl levo-carnitine in patients with Alzheimer's disease. *Archives of Neurology.* 49:1137–1141.

Singh RB, et al. (1996). A randomized, double-blind, placebo-controlled trial of L-carnitine in suspected acute myocardial infarction. *Postgraduate Medicine.* 72:45–50.

Tamamogullari N, et al. (1999). L-carnitine deficiency in diabetes mellitus complications. *Journal of Diabetes Complications.* 13(5-6):251–253.

Werbach MR. (2000). Nutritional strategies for treating chronic fatigue syndrome. *Alternative Medicine Review.* 5(2):93–108.

NAME: Chondroitin

Common Names: Chondroitin sulfate

Description and Source

- A high-viscosity mucopolysaccharide (glycosaminoglycan)
- Can be extracted from natural sources or synthesized in the laboratory
- Is a flexible connecting matrix between proteins and filaments in cartilage
- May replace proteoglycans, a substance that forms cartilage (Morreale et al., 1996)

Biologic Activity

- Helps and attracts essential fluid into proteoglycan molecules, "water magnets" that act as shock absorbers, and moves nutrients into cartilage
- Stimulates chondrocyte activity. Chondrocytes must get their nutrition from the synovial fluid because there is no vasculature to nourish them. During inflammation, chondrocyte activity is disturbed.

- May inhibit human leukocyte elastase and hyaluronidase, which are found in high concentrations in persons with rheumatoid disease

Nutritional Sources: Bovine or shark cartilage

Current Use: Osteoarthritis (Theodosakis, 1997); chondroitin sulfate B inhibits venous thrombosis; antithrombolytic and may decrease heparin requirements

Available Forms, Dosage, and Administration Guidelines: Follow manufacturer's directions. Usually combined with glucosamine sulfate. Dosage is based on weight.
    <120 lb: 800 mg
    120 to 200 lb: 1,200 mg
    >200 lb: 1,600 mg
    Divide into two to four smaller doses and take with food (Theodosakis, 1997).

Pharmacokinetics—If Available (form or route when known): Absorption, 0% to 13%; very large molecule size

Toxicity: None known; long-term clinical trials needed

Contraindications: Bleeding disorders

Side Effects: GI upset (dyspepsia, nausea), headache

Long-Term Safety: Unknown

Use in Pregnancy/Lactation/Children: Unknown; do not use

Drug/Herb Interactions and Rationale (if known): Do not take with anticoagulants: may potentiate bleeding.

Special Notes: Mixed research on effectiveness is found in the literature. Those arguing against its use suggest that chondroitin may be too large to be delivered to cartilage cells. In clinical practice, the effects of chondroitin seem marginal, especially compared with those of glycosamine sulfate. The American College of Rheumatology suggests that more definitive studies be performed to determine its efficacy. In

2000, the National Institute of Health funded research in nine centers.

BIBLIOGRAPHY

McAlindon TE, et al. (2000). Glucosamine and chondroitin for treatment of osteoarthritis: a systematic quality assessment and meta-analysis. *Journal of the American Medical Association.* 283(11):1469–1475.

McCarty MF, et al. (2000). Sulfated glycosaminoglycans and glucosamine may synergize in promoting synovial hyaluronic acid synthesis. *Medical Hypotheses.* 54(5):798–802.

Morreale P, et al. (1996). Comparison of the anti-inflammatory efficacy of chondroitin sulfate and diclofenac sodium in patients with knee osteoarthritis. *Journal of Rheumatology.* 23:1385–1391.

Review of Natural Products. (1998). St. Louis: Facts and Comparisons.

Theodosakis J. (1997). *The Arthritis Cure.* New York: St. Martin's Press.

 NAME: Chromium

Common Names: None

Description and Source
- Naturally occurring trace element
- The organic form found in natural foods appears to be absorbed better than the inorganic form.

Biologic Activity
- Required for normal glucose metabolism (Ducros, 1992; Kimura, 1996)
- Glucose tolerance factor chromium increases HDL after 2 months in patients taking beta-blockers (Roeback et al., 1991)
- May exert anabolic effect by enhancing the effect of insulin and increasing the uptake of amino acids into muscle cells

Nutritional Sources: Brewer's yeast, liver, lean meats, whole grains, and cheese. Cooking with stainless-steel cookware increases the chromium content of foods (Integrative Medicine Access, 2000).

Current Use
- Low chromium levels may contribute to hypoglycemia, cardiovascular disease, glaucoma, and osteoporosis.
- Chromium promotes a normal insulin activity in persons with diabetes (enhances insulin use) (McCarty, 1980, 1981).
- May benefit insulin resistance (Syndrome X)

Available Forms, Dosage, and Administration Guidelines
Preparations: Capsules, tablets. Several forms of chromium are available in the marketplace, including chromium polynicotinate and chromium picolinate (the best forms to use), chromium-enriched yeast, and chromium chloride.
Typical Dosage: 50 to 200 mcg per day

Pharmacokinetics—If Available (form or route when known): Eliminated through the kidney

Toxicity: Irritation of GI tract (nausea, vomiting, ulcers) at high doses. Hexavalent (industrial) chromium is a heavy metal and causes kidney, liver, and lung damage.

Contraindications: Not known

Side Effects: Not known

Long-Term Safety: Safe

Use in Pregnancy/Lactation/Children: Safe

Drug/Herb Interactions and Rationale (if known):
Calcium carbonate and antacids reduce chromium absorption.

Special Notes
- Glucose tolerance factor (GTF) chromium, which is combined with niacin, improves carbohydrate use and may improve binding of insulin to insulin receptors.
- Although rare, chromium deficiency (eg, peripheral neuropathy or encephalopathy, increased glucose use during pregnancy) may play a role in the development of adult diabetes.

- Chromium deficiency leads to impaired lipid and glucose metabolism and may put the person at risk for cardiovascular disease (Simonoff, 1984).

BIBLIOGRAPHY

Cerulli J, et al. (1998). Chromium picolinate toxicity. *Annals of Pharmacotherapy.* 32:428–431.

Ducros V. (1992). Chromium metabolism, a literature review. *Biological Trace Element Research.* 32:65–77.

Kimura K. (1996). Role of essential trace elements in the disturbance of carbohydrate metabolism. *Nippon Rinsho.* 54(1):79–84.

Integrative Medicine Access. (2000). *Chromium.* Newton, MA: Integrative Medicine Communications.

Lawrence Review of Natural Products. (1992). St. Louis: Facts and Comparisons.

McCarty MF. (1980). Therapeutic potential of glucose tolerance factor. *Medical Hypotheses.* 6(11):1177–1189.

McCarty MF. (1981). Maturity-onset diabetes mellitus: toward a physiologically appropriate management. *Medical Hypotheses.* 7(10):1265–1285.

Roeback JR Jr., et al. (1991). Effects of chromium supplementation on serum high-density lipoprotein cholesterol levels in men taking beta-blockers. A randomized, controlled trial. *Annals of Internal Medicine.* 115(12):917–924.

Simonoff M. (1984). Chromium deficiency and cardiovascular risk. *Cardiovascular Research.* 18(10):591–596.

 NAME: Coenzyme Q10

Common Names: Vitamin Q, ubiquinone, Co-Q10

Description and Source: Lipid-soluble benzoquinones, similar in structure to vitamin K. They are found in almost all aerobic organisms in the mitochondria. The Q10 structure is unique to humans.

Biologic Activity

- Powerful lipophilic antioxidant present in all tissue (Kontush et al., 1997)
- Membrane-stabilizing properties

- Improves stroke volume and cardiac output in patients with CHF (Soja & Mortensen, 1997)
- Improves ejection fraction (Sinatra et al., 1997)
- Inhibits platelet vitronectin receptor to reduce thrombotic complications (Serebruany et al., 1997)
- Works with other enzymes to bring about its effects (Langsjoem, 1994)
- Precursor to energy production in mitochondria (adenosine triphosphate)
- Oxygen free radical scavenger
- Regenerates vitamin E from its oxidized form (Ernster et al., 1995)
- Improves immune function

Nutritional Sources: Small amounts in meat and seafood

Current Use
- Improves CHF. Research suggests that patients with New York Hospital Association class III and IV disease with Co-Q10 deficiencies can become class I and II with treatment (Morisco et al., 1993).
- Benefits cardiomyopathies caused by ischemia and toxins: angina, cardiotoxicity caused by doxorubicin (Adriamycin)
- Slows progression of breast cancer (Langsjoem et al., 1994; Lockwood et al., 1994) and enhances immune response
- Improves tissue health and healing in gingivitis (Hansen et al., 1976; Integrative Medicine Access, 2000)
- Prevents gastric ulcers
- May improve survival after MI if administered within 3 days (120 mg/day) (Singh et al., 1998; Singh & Niaz, 1999)
- Decreases blood pressure (Singh et al., 1999): 39% of patients with hypertension have a Co-Q10 deficiency. Four to 12 weeks of supplementation showed benefit (Integrative Medicine Access, 2000).
- Improves tissue reperfusion after cross-clamping during cardiac bypass surgery (Chillo et al., 1996; Nibori et al., 1998)
- May improve mitral valve prolapse (use with hawthorn), arrhythmias, and diabetes

Available Forms, Dosage, and Administration Guidelines: Varies with condition; take 50 mg/day as baseline. Use oil-based soft gel for better absorption. Take with food. Take with piperine (Bioperine) (black pepper) for increased absorption (by 30%).

Pharmacokinetics—If Available (form or route when known): Not known

Toxicity: None known

Contraindications: None known

Side Effects: loss of appetite (rare), nausea, diarrhea (rare)

Long-Term Safety: Not known

Use in Pregnancy/Lactation/Children: Unknown; do not use

Drug/Herb Interactions and Rationale (if known)

- Warfarin is less effective; monitor INR carefully (Landbo & Almdal, 1998).
- HMG-CoA reductase or statin drugs (lovastatin [Mevacor], simvastatin [Zocor]) decrease absorption of Co-Q10. Supplement with 60 to 90 mg/day as a replacement dose (Folkers et al., 1990; Mortensen et al., 1997; Palomaki et al., 1998).

Special Notes: Mixed research exists. There are more positive results than negative (Watson et al., 1999), but further research is needed. The number in Co-Q10 refers to the number of isoprene units of the terpenoid side chain.

BIBLIOGRAPHY

Chillo M, et al. (1996). Protection by coenzyme Q10 of tissue reperfusion injury during abdominal aortic cross-clamping. *Journal of Cardiovascular Surgery (Torino).* 37(3):229–235.

Ernster L, et al. (1995). Co-enzyme Q10. *Biochemica Biophysica Acta.* 1271(1):195–204.

Folkers K, et al. (1990). Lovastatin decreases coenzyme Q levels in human. *Proceedings of the National Academy of Science USA.* 87(22):8931–8934.

Hansen J, et al. (1976). Bioenergetics in clinical medicine. *Research Communications in Chemical Pathology and Pharmacology.* 14(4):729–738.

Integrative Medicine Access. (2000). *Co-enzyme Q10*. Newton, MA: Integrative Medicine Communications.

Kontush A, et al. (1997). Plasma ubiquinol-10 is decreased in patients with hyperlipidaemia. *Atherosclerosis*. 28;129(1):119–126.

Landbo C, Almdal TP. (1998). Interaction between warfarin and coenzyme Q10. *Ugeskrift for Laeger*. 160(22):3226–3227.

Langsjoem PH. (1994). *Introduction to Coenzyme Q10*. Tyler, TX: Research Reports.

Langsjoem P, et al. (1994). Treatment of essential hypertension with coenzyme Q10. *Molecular Aspects of Medicine*. 15(Suppl.):S265–272.

Lockwood K, et al. (1994). Apparent partial remission of breast cancer in high risk patients supplemented with nutritional antioxidants, essential fatty acids and coenzyme Q10. *Molecular Aspects of Medicine*. 15(Suppl.):S231–240.

Morisco C, et al. (1993). Effect of coenzyme Q10 therapy in patients with congestive heart failure: a long-term multicenter randomized study. *Clinical Investigations*. 71(8 Suppl.):S134–136.

Mortensen SA, et al. (1997). Dose-related decrease of serum coenzyme Q10 during treatment with HMG-CoA reductase inhibitors. *Molecular Aspects of Medicine*. 18(Suppl.):S137–144.

Nibori K, et al. (1998). Acute administration of liposomal coenzyme Q10 increases myocardial tissue levels and improves tolerance to ischemia reperfusion injury. *Journal of Surgical Research*. 79(2):141.

Palomaki A, et al. (1998). Ubiquinone supplementation during lovastatin treatment: effect on LDL oxidation ex vivo. *Journal of Lipid Research*. 39(7):1430–1437.

Review of Natural Products. (1997). St. Louis: Facts and Comparisons.

Serebruany UL, et al. (1997). Could coenzyme Q10 affect hemostasis by inhibiting platelet vitronectin (CD51/CD61) receptor? *Molecular Aspects of Medicine*. 18(Suppl.):S189–194.

Sinatra ST, et al. (1997). Coenzyme Q10: a vital therapeutic nutrient for the heart with special application in congestive heart failure. *Connecticut Medicine*. 65:707–711.

Singh RB, et al. (1998). Randomized, double-blind placebo-controlled trial of coenzyme Q10 in patients with acute myocardial infarction. *Cardiovascular Drugs & Therapy*. 12(4):347–353.

Singh RB, et al. (1999). Effect of hydrosoluble coenzyme Q10 on blood pressures and insulin resistance in hypertensive patients with coronary artery disease. *Journal of Human Hypertension*. 13(3):203–208.

Singh RB, Niaz MA. (1999). Serum concentration of lipoprotein(a) decreases on treatment with hydrosoluble coenzyme Q10 in patients with coronary artery disease: discovery of a new role. *International Journal of Cardiology.* 68(1):23–29.

Soja AM, Mortensen SA. (1997). Treatment of congestive heart failure with coenzyme Q10 illuminated by meta-analyses of clinical trials. *Molecular Aspects of Medicine.* 18(Suppl.):S159–168.

Watson PS, et al. (1999). Lack of effect of coenzyme Q on left ventricular function in patients with congestive heart failure. *Journal of the American College of Cardiology.* 33(6):1549–1552.

 NAME: Glucosamine Sulfate (2-amino 2-deoxyglucose)

Common Names: GS, chitosamine

Description and Source: A simple molecule composed of glucose, an amine (nitrogen and hydrogen), and sulfur. Glucosamine is a fundamental building block of cartilage glycosaminoglycan (GAG) and is a natural substance found in mucopolysaccharides, mucoproteins, and chiten. Glucosamine sulfate is manufactured. Sulfate is the preferred form. Sulfur is an essential nutrient for joint tissue that stabilizes the connective tissue matrix of cartilage.

Biologic Activity

- Glucosamine is formed from the glycolytic intermediate fructose-6-phosphate via amination, with glutamine acting as the donor, yielding glucosamine-6-phosphate, which is acetylated and/or converted to galactosamine for incorporation into the growing GAG (Noack, 1994).
- Stimulates the manufacture of cartilage components and promotes the incorporation of sulfur into cartilage (Kelly, 1998)
- Stimulates joint repair; some people lose the ability to manufacture glucosamine and therefore cannot repair joints (Barclay et al., 1998; Da Camara & Dowless, 1998).
- Allows cartilage to act as a shock absorber (Setnikar, 1992)
- Reduces tenderness and improves mobility (Qiu et al., 1998)

Nutritional Sources: None known

Current Use: Antiarthritic for osteoarthritis; prevents joint space narrowing. May stimulate hyaluronic acid, which is anti-inflammatory and an anodyne. Glucosamine is as effective as nonsteroidal anti-inflammatories in improving mobility and decreasing the pain of osteoarthritis without irritating the gastric mucosa.

Available Forms, Dosage, and Administration Guidelines

Preparations: Capsules, tablets
Typical Dosage

Pounds	Glucosamine (mg)
<120	1,000
120–200	1,500
>200	2,000

Divide the total dosage into three or four doses per day and take with food. As improvement occurs, reduce the dose to the lowest effective dose. European studies suggest that people who are very obese or are taking diuretics may need higher doses (McCarty, 1994; Qiu et al., 1998).

Pharmacokinetics—If Available (form or route when known): Ninety percent is absorbed with oral administration, but substantial amounts are metabolized by the liver, and only 26% reaches the blood.

Toxicity: None known

Contraindications: Patients with type 2 diabetes should monitor blood sugar levels. Patients with Syndrome X (insulin resistance) may find that glucosamine worsens their symptoms (elevated triglycerides, obesity, carbohydrate cravings).

Side Effects: Mild GI upset and irritation, diarrhea, and flatulence; may increase insulin resistance and elevate blood sugar levels; drowsiness, skin reactions, headaches

Long-Term Safety: Short-term studies suggest safety, but no long-term studies are available.

Use in Pregnancy/Lactation/Children: Not known; do not use

Drug/Herb Interactions and Rationale (if known): None known

Special Notes: The Arthritis Foundation does not recommend the use of glucosamine for the treatment of any form of arthritis because of the lack of well-designed studies. Most studies are short-term and have serious design flaws. In 2000, the National Institutes of Health funded nine centers to study glucosamine. Chronic use of nonsteroidal anti-inflammatories has been shown to prevent joint repair. Glucosamine sulfate has been shown to reduce pain and inflammation and allows the joint to heal.

BIBLIOGRAPHY

Barclay TS, et al. (1998). Glucosamine. *Annals of Pharmacotherapy.* 32(4):574–579.

Da Camara CC, Dowless GV. (1998). Glucosamine sulfate for osteoarthritis. *Annals of Pharmacotherapy.* 32(5):580–587.

Integrative Medicine Access. (2000). *Glucosamine.* Newton, MA: Integrative Medicine Communications.

Kelly GS. (1998). The role of glucosamine sulfate and chondroitin sulfates in the treatment of degenerative joint disease. *Alternative Medicine Review.* 3(1):27–39.

McAlindon TE, et al. (2000). Glucosamine and chondroitin for treatment of osteoarthritis: a systematic quality assessment and meta-analysis. *Journal of the American Medical Association.* 283(11):1469–1475.

McCarty M. (1994). The neglect of glucosamine as treatment for osteoarthritis. *Medical Hypotheses.* 42:3223–3227.

Murray MT. (1996). *Encyclopedia of Nutritional Supplements.* Rocklin, CA: Prima Publishing.

Noack W. (1994). Glucosamine sulfate in osteoarthritis of the knee. *Osteoarthritis and Cartilage.* 2:51–59.

Qiu GX, et al. (1998). Efficacy and safety of glucosamine sulfate versus ibuprofen in patients with knee osteoarthritis. *Arzneimittelforschung.* 48(5):469–474.

Rindone JP, et al. (2000). Randomized, controlled trial of glucosamine for treating osteoarthritis of the knee. *Western Journal of Medicine.* 172(2):91–94.

Rovati LC. (1994). A large randomized, placebo-controlled, double-blind study of glucosamine sulfate vs. piroxicam and vs. their association, on the kinetics of the symptomatic effect in knee osteoarthritis. *Osteoarthritis and Cartilage.* 2(Suppl. 1): 56.

Setnikar I. (1992). Antireactive properties of "chondroprotective" drugs. *International Journal of Tissue Reactions.* 14(5):253–261.

Vaz AL. (1982). Double-blind clinical evaluation of the relative efficacy of ibuprofen and glucosamine sulfate in the management of osteoarthritis of the knee in out-patients. *Current Medical Research and Opinion.* 8:145–149.

 NAME: 5-hydroxytryptophan

Common Names: 5-HTP

Description and Source
- An amino acid that occurs in the human body and is the precursor of serotonin
- Extracted from natural source

Biologic Activity: Natural precursor to serotonin; enhances mood and lifts depression

Nutritional Sources: *Griffonia simplicifolia* seed

Current Use
- Relieves mild to moderate depression and related symptoms such as anxiety, insomnia, and fatigue
- For bipolar (manic) depression (200 mg three times a day), along with lithium
- Relieves migraine headaches: a dosage of 200 to 600 mg/day for 2 to 6 months has been shown to decrease the severity and frequency of migraines (Integrative Medicine Access, 2000)
- Fibromyalgia: studies of fibromyalgia sufferers taking 300 mg three times a day for 1 to 3 months showed improved sleep quality and improvements in depression, insomnia, and somatic pain
- Insomnia: reduced sleep latency and improved sleep quality in double-blind clinical trials

Available Forms, Dosage, and Administration
Guidelines: Take 150 mg at bedtime on an empty stomach

(can cause sleepiness); dosage can be increased after several weeks to as much as 300 mg three times a day.

Pharmacokinetics—If Available (form or route when known): Well absorbed; approximately 70% of an oral dose

Toxicity: Serotonin syndrome is possible when combined with many drugs. See notes on drug interactions.

Contraindications: Cardiac disease

Side Effects: Mild nausea, heartburn, borborygmus, flatulence

Long-Term Safety: Unknown

Use in Pregnancy/Lactation/Children: Unknown; do not use

Drug/Herb Interactions and Rationale (if known)
- Do not take with antidepressants, antiparkinsonian drugs, barbiturates, tranquilizers, weight loss products, antihistamines, cold medications, alcohol, chemotherapy, or antibiotics: all may be potentiated, particularly side effects.
- Do not take with selective serotonin reuptake inhibitors: increased likelihood of serotonin syndrome.
- May potentiate effects of St. John's wort

Special Notes
- Vitamin B_6, niacin, and magnesium should be taken on the same day as 5-HTP, preferably 6 hours before 5-HTP because these substances are cofactors for the conversion of 5-HTP into serotonin.
- There have been recent reports that the Peak X contaminants, originally found in L-tryptophan, have been found in 5-HTP. This is a serious issue because the Peak X contaminants are responsible for eosinophilia-myalgia syndrome. More studies are needed to clarify this concern.

BIBLIOGRAPHY
Birdsall TC. (1998). 5-Hydroxytryptophan: a clinically-effective serotonin precursor. *Alternative Medicine Review.* 3:271–280.
Cangiano C, et al. (1998). Effects of oral 5-hydroxy-tryptophan on energy intake and macronutrient selection in non-insulin-

dependent diabetic patients. *International Journal of Obesity & Related Metabolic Disorders.* 22:648–654.

Integrative Medicine Access. (2000). *5-Hydroxytryptophan (5-HTP).* Newton, MA: Integrative Medicine Communications.

Juhl JH. (1998). Primary fibromyalgia syndrome and 5-hydroxy-L-tryptophan: a 90-day open study. *Alternative Medicine Review.* 3:367–375.

Klarskov K, et al. (1999). Eosinophilia-myalgia syndrome case-associated contaminants in commercially available 5-hydroxytryptophan. *Advances in Experimental Medicine & Biology.* 467:461–468.

Puttini PS, Caruso I. (1992). Primary fibromyalgia and 5-hydroxy-L-tryptophan: a 90-day open study. *Journal of International Medical Research.* 20:182–189.

Review of Natural Products. (1998). St. Louis: Facts and Comparisons.

Van Praag HM. (1982). Serotonin precursors in the treatment of depression. *Advances in Biochemistry & Psychopharmacology.* 34:259–286.

 NAME: Lipoic Acid

Common Names: Alpha lipoic acid, thioctic acid, lipoicin, thioctacid, acetate replacing factor

Description and Source: Fat- and water-soluble, sulfur-containing antioxidant that can be synthesized in the body

Biologic Activity
- May be the most powerful antioxidant made by the body (Ley, 1996; Packer & Coleman, 1999)
- Boosts levels and can recycle glutathione by 30%
- Recycles other antioxidants, vitamins A and C
- Turns off "bad" genes (aging, cancer)
- Enhances immune function
- Protects neurotransmitters
- Functions as a coenzyme with pyrophosphatase in carbohydrate metabolism (Ensminger et al., 1994)
- Oxygen free radical scavenger inside and outside cell (Packer & Coleman, 1999)

Nutritional Sources: Yeast, liver, and spinach are fairly good sources; broccoli, kidney, heart, and potatoes contain small amounts of lipoic acid.

Current Use
- May benefit patients with HIV and prevent cancer
- Prevents cataracts and other degenerative eye diseases
- Decreases stroke-related injuries
- Treats hepatotoxicity caused by poisonous mushroom ingestion, so initial evidence suggests it may protect the liver in cirrhosis and hepatitis B and C (Budavari et al., 1989; Berkson, 1999)
- Decreases complications in diabetes (diabetic retinopathy, cataracts, neuropathy) (Ziegler et al., 1997); prescribed in Germany for diabetic neuropathy (Murray, 1996); improves blood sugar metabolism

Available Forms, Dosage, and Administration Guidelines: 100 mg/day divided into two doses

Pharmacokinetics—If Available (form or route when known): Not known

Toxicity: None known

Contraindications: None known

Side Effects: None known

Long-Term Safety: Unknown

Use in Pregnancy/Lactation/Children: No data suggests toxicity. Pregnant and lactating women should consult with their physician.

Drug/Herb Interactions and Rationale (if known): If taken with insulin and antidiabetic drugs, dosage may need to be reduced. Monitor blood sugar levels closely (Murray, 1996).

Special Notes: Recent research suggests that lipoic acid does not change current symptoms but may decrease overall complications associated with diabetic neuropathy. More research is needed (Ziegler et al., 1999a, 1999b).

BIBLIOGRAPHY

Berkson BM. (1999). A conservative triple antioxidant approach to the treatment of hepatitis C. Combination of alpha-lipoic acid (thioctic acid), silymarin, and selenium: three case histories. *Medizinische Klinikum.* 94(Suppl. 3), 84–89.

Budavari S, et al. (Eds.). (1989). *The Merck Index* (11th ed.). Rahway, NJ: Merck & Co.

Ensminger A, et al. (1994). *Foods and Nutrition Encyclopedia.* (2nd ed.). Boca Raton, FL: CRC Press.

Gleiter CH, et al. (1999). Lack of interaction between thioctic acid, glibenclamide and acarbose. *British Journal of Clinical Pharmacology.* 48(6):819–825.

Ley B. (1996). *The Potato Antioxidant, Alpha Lipoic Acid.* Colorado Springs, CO: BL Publications.

Marangon K, Devaraj S. (1999). Comparison of the effect of alpha-lipoic acid and alpha-tocopherol supplementation on measures of oxidative stress. *Free Radicals Biology in Medicine.* 27(9-10): 1114–1121.

Murray M. (1996). *Encyclopedia of Nutritional Supplements.* Rocklin, CA: Prima Publishing.

Packer L, Coleman C. (1999). *The Antioxidant Miracle.* Philadelphia: John Wiley & Sons.

Review of Natural Products. (1998). St. Louis: Facts and Comparisons.

Ruhnau KJ, et al. (1999). Effects of 3-week oral treatment with the antioxidant thioctic acid (alpha-lipoic acid) in symptomatic diabetic polyneuropathy. *Diabetes Medicine.* 16(12):1050–1053.

Ziegler D, et al. (1997). Effects of treatment with the antioxidant alpha-lipoic acid on cardiac autonomic neuropathy in NIDDM patients. A 4-month randomized controlled multicenter trial. *Diabetes Care.* 20:369–373.

Ziegler D, et al. (1999a). Alpha-lipoic acid in the treatment of diabetic polyneuropathy in Germany: current evidence from clinical trials. *Experimental & Clinical Endocrinology & Diabetes.* 107(7):421–430.

Ziegler D, et al. (1999b). Treatment of symptomatic diabetic polyneuropathy with the antioxidant alpha-lipoic acid: a 7-month multicenter randomized controlled trial. *Diabetes Care.* 22(8):1296–1301.

 NAME: Lycopene

Common Names: None

Description and Source: A carotenoid that occurs in ripe fruits

Biologic Activity

- Antioxidant: twice as effective as beta-carotene (Agarwal & Roa, 1998)
- Lowers activity of oxygen free radicals (Klebanov et al., 1998)
- Inhibits serum lipid peroxidation, decreases LDL cholesterol, and reduces risk of MI (Kohlmeier et al., 1997)
- Lowers risk of prostate enlargement and prostate cancer, especially when combined with tocopherols (Amir et al., 1999; Gann et al., 1999)
- Enhances immune function and cell-to-cell communication and inhibits tumor cell growth
- Prevents macular degeneration, a leading cause of blindness in the elderly (Seddon et al., 1994); use with lutein, blueberry, and ginkgo for best results
- Lowers incidence of many cancers (stomach, pancreatic, prostate, colon, rectum, cervix) (Kantesky et al., 1998; Sengupta & Das, 1999)

Nutritional Sources: Red and pink fruits. Tomatoes are the best source, especially if cooked (increases the available lycopene; tomato paste, sauce, juice). Also watermelon, guava, pink grapefruit, strawberries.

Available Forms, Dosage, and Administration Guidelines: To enhance intestinal absorption of lycopene, consume oils or fats at the same time (Porrini et al., 1998). Intake goal is 10 half-cup servings of lycopene-rich food a week, or one 10- to 15-mg gel cap per day.

Pharmacokinetics—If Available (form or route when known): Not known

Toxicity: None known

Contraindications: None known

Side Effects: None known

Long-Term Safety: Safe in dietary quantities

Use in Pregnancy/Lactation/Children: Safe in dietary quantities; large amounts as an isolate, safety unknown

Drug/Herb Interactions and Rationale (if known): None known

Special Notes: Carotenoid mixtures, especially with lycopene and lutein, have a synergistic antioxidant and anticancer activity.

BIBLIOGRAPHY

Agarwal S, Rao AV. (1998). Tomato lycopene and low-density lipoprotein oxidation: a human dietary intervention study. *Lipids.* 33(10):981–984.

Amir H, et al. (1999). Lycopene and 1,25-dihydroxyvitamin D3 cooperate in the inhibition of cell cycle progression and induction of differentiation in HL-60 leukemic cells. *Nutrition & Cancer.* 33(1):105–12.

Clinton S. (1998). Lycopene: chemistry, biology, and implications for human health and disease. *Nutrition Review.* 56(2 pt. 1):35–51.

Gann PH, et al. (1999). Lower prostate cancer risk in men with elevated plasma lycopene levels: results of a prospective analysis. *Cancer Research.* 59(6):1225–1230.

Kantesky P, et al. (1998). Dietary intake and blood levels of lycopene: association with cervical dysplasia among non-Hispanic, black women. *Nutrition & Cancer.* 31(1):31–40.

Klebanov Gi, et al. (1998). The antioxidant properties of lycopene. *Membranes & Cell Biology.* 12(2):287–300.

Kohlmeier I, et al. (1997). Lycopene and myocardial infarction risk in the EURAMIC Study. *American Journal of Epidemiology.* 146(8):618–626.

Krinsky N. (1998). Overview of lycopene, carotenoids, and disease prevention. *Proceedings of the Society for Experimental Biology & Medicine.* 218(2):95–97.

Porrini M, et al. (1998). Absorption of lycopene from single or daily portions of raw and processed tomato. *British Journal of Nutrition.* 80(4):353–361.

Review of Natural Products. (1999). St. Louis: Facts and Comparisons.

Seddon NJ, et al. (1994). Dietary carotenoids, vitamins A, C, and E, and advanced age-related macular degeneration. *Journal of the American Medical Association.* 272:1413–1420.

Sengupta A, Das S. (1999). The anti-carcinogenic role of lycopene, abundantly present in tomato. *European Journal of Cancer Prevention.* 8(4):325–330.

Weisburger J. (1998). International symposium on the role of lycopene and tomato products in disease prevention. *Proceedings of the Society for Experimental Biology & Medicine.* 218(2):93–94.

NAME: Melatonin (*N*-acetyl-5-methoxytryptamine)

Common Names: Mel

Description and Source

- Melatonin is a hormone produced by the pineal gland during sleep. For melatonin to be produced, the pineal gland must perceive darkness; thus, people who work swing shifts and must sleep during the day make less melatonin and therefore have difficulty obtaining restful sleep and multiple REM cycles. Melatonin enhances REM cycles.
- Melatonin production is highest in children and decreases with age.
- Natural or synthetically produced hormone
- Melatonin is produced from tryptophan → serotonin → melatonin.

Biologic Activity

- Enhances sleep (Zhdanova & Wurtman, 1997)
- Modulates circadian rhythm (Petrie et al., 1993; Reiter et al., 1995; Zawilska & Nowak, 1999)
- Enhances immune system function (Morrey et al., 1994)
- May decrease incidence of hormone-dependent cancers (eg, breast, prostate cancers) (Erren & Piekarski, 1999)
- May reduce stress (Kirby, 1999)
- Reduces core temperature, which decreases arousal (Dawson & Encel, 1993)
- Acts as oxygen (hydroxyl) free radical scavenger

Nutritional Sources

FOODS HIGH IN MELATONIN	
Food	**Melatonin (picograms per gram)**
Oats	1.796
Sweet corn	1.366
Rice	1.006
Japanese radish	687
Ginger	583

(continued)

FOODS HIGH IN MELATONIN *(Continued)*	
Tomatoes ("Sweet 100s")	500
Bananas	460
Barley	378

FOODS HIGH IN TRYPTOPHAN	
Food	**mg**
Seaweed (2 oz)	580
Soy nuts (1/2 cup)	495
Turkey (3.5 oz)	332
Tofu (1/2 cup)	310
Milk (1 cup)	100

Current Use

- May be useful for sleep disorders in children associated with autism, Down's syndrome, epilepsy, and cerebral palsy
- Used to enhance sleep (blind persons, jet lag, insomnia, and the elderly) (Kendler, 1997; Zhdanova et al., 1995)
- May be useful for seasonal affective disorder
- Stimulates the immune system: monocytes and NK cells
- Acts as an antioxidant, oxygen free radical scavenger
- Nightly supplement (10 mg) may improve cancer survival rates in persons with metastatic non-small cell lung cancer, especially if combined with interferon or interleukin 2 therapy. It enhances their activity and reduces adverse effects.
- Prevents pregnancy in large doses

Available Forms, Dosage, and Administration Guidelines

- For sleep only: 0.1 to 0.3 mg (up to 1 mg), 1 hour before sleep
- For jet lag: Start a day before travel. Traveling west, take it on waking; traveling east, take it mid-afternoon. When you arrive, continue on the same pill-taking schedule according to your hometown clock.
- Slow-release melatonin, in 2-mg doses, may enhance sleep (Garfinkel et al., 1995; Samuel, 1999).
- For blind persons with sleep problems: 5 mg orally at bedtime

- For elderly persons with insomnia: 1 to 2 mg (Haimov et al., 1995)
- Does not alter endogenous melatonin production

Pharmacokinetics—If Available (form or route when known): Half-life, 20 to 50 minutes; metabolized in liver

Toxicity: No acute toxicity, but long-term potential for health problems unknown

Contraindications: Pregnancy and lactation; trying to get pregnant; severe mental illness; autoimmune disease; cancers of the blood or bones; hepatic insufficiency from reduced clearance

Side Effects: Headache; vivid dreams, nightmares (Guardiola-Lemaitre, 1997); transient depression; morning lethargy; drowsiness (use caution driving for 30 minutes after taking melatonin); unfavorable shifts in circadian rhythm

Long-Term Safety: No acute toxicity, but long-term safety issues are yet to be researched. In rats, long-term use inhibits uptake of T_4 and T_3.

Use in Pregnancy/Lactation/Children: Avoid in pregnant and lactating women; use in children under professional supervision only.

Drug/Herb Interactions and Rationale (if known)
- Do not use with Ca++ channel blockers: enhances effects of light on retina and interferes with melatonin (Benloucif et al., 1999).
- Do not use with benzodiazepines: enhances anxiolytic action.
- Do not use with methamphetamine: may exacerbate insomnia.
- The following drugs may deplete melatonin: alcohol, antidepressants, anxiolytics, beta-blockers, Ca++ channel blockers, caffeine, nonsteroidal anti-inflammatories, steroids, tobacco, vitamin B_{12} in large doses.

Special Notes
- There is no standardization for quality, purity, and hormone among OTC products.

- OTC products may contain cellulose, lactose, cornstarch, magnesium stearate, and isopropyl alcohol.
- May have some potential for use as contraceptive, but more research is needed
- Patient should be told that sleep disorders need a comprehensive program of behavior modification and counseling, as well as pharmacologic agents.
- According to the FDA, there are no assurances of long-term safety with melatonin.
- More research is necessary to establish dose–response relations and drug interactions (Chase & Gidal, 1997).

BIBLIOGRAPHY

Benloucif S, et al. (1999). Nimodipine potentiates the light-induced suppression of melatonin. *Neuroscience Letters.* 272(1):67–71.

Blaicher W, et al. (2000). Melatonin in postmenopausal females. *Archives of Gynecology & Obstetrics.* 263(3):116–118.

Chase JE, Gidal BE. (1997). Melatonin: therapeutic use in sleep disorders. *Annals of Pharmacotherapy.* 31(10):1218–1226.

Citera G, et al. (2000). The effect of melatonin in patients with fibromyalgia: a pilot study. *Clinical Rheumatology.* 19(1):9–13.

Dawson D, Encel N. (1993). Melatonin and sleep in humans. *Journal of Pineal Research.* 15(1):1–12.

Erren TC, Piekarski C. (1999). Does winter darkness in the Arctic protect against cancer? The melatonin hypothesis revisited. *Medical Hypotheses.* 53(1):1–5.

Garfinkel D, et al. (1995). Improvement of sleep quality in elderly people by controlled-release melatonin. *Lancet.* 346:541–544.

Guardiola-Lemaitre B. (1997). Toxicology of melatonin. *Journal of Biologic Rhythms.* 12(6):697–706.

Haimov I, et al. (1995). Melatonin replacement therapy of elderly insomniacs. *Sleep.* 18:598–603.

Integrative Medicine Access. (2000). *Melatonin.* Newton, MA: Integrative Medicine Communications.

Kendler B. (1997). Melatonin: media hype or therapeutic breakthrough? *Nurse Practitioner.* 22(2):66–72.

Kirby AW, et al. (1999). Melatonin and the reduction or alleviation of stress. *Journal of Pineal Research.* 27(2):78–85.

Lissoni P, et al. (1991). Clinical results with the pineal hormone melatonin in advanced cancer resistant to standard antitumor therapies. *Oncology.* 48:448–450.

Lissoni P, et al. (1996). Is there a role for melatonin in the treatment of neoplastic cachexia? *European Journal of Cancer.* 32A:1340–1343.

Morrey KM, et al. (1994). Activation of human monocytes by the pineal hormone melatonin. *Journal of Immunology.* 153(6):2671.

Nagtegaal JE, et al. (2000). Effects of melatonin on the quality of life in patients with delayed sleep phase syndrome. *Journal of Psychosomatic Research.* 48(1):45–50.

Ozbek E, et al. (2000). Melatonin administration prevents the nephrotoxicity induced by gentamicin. *BJU International* 85(6):742–746.

Petrie K, et al. (1993). A double-blind trial of melatonin as a treatment for jet lag in international cabin crew. *Biological Psychiatry.* 33:526.

Reiter RJ, et al. (1995). A review of the evidence supporting melatonin's role as an antioxidant. *Journal of Pineal Research.* 18(1):1.

Samuel A. (1999). Melatonin and jet-lag. *European Journal of Medical Research.* 4(9):385–388.

Zawilska JB, Nowak JZ. (1999). Melatonin: from biochemistry to therapeutic applications. *Polish Journal of Pharmacology.* 51(1):3–23.

Zhdanova IV, Wurtman RJ. (1997). Efficacy of melatonin as a sleep-promoting agent. *Journal of Biologic Rhythms.* 12(6):644–650.

Zhdanova IV, et al. (1995). Sleep-inducing effects of low doses of melatonin ingested in the evening. *Clinical Pharmacy & Therapeutics.* 57:552–558.

NAME: Methylsulfonylmethane (DMSO₂)

Common Names: MSM, crystalline DMSO

Description and Source

- MSM is a natural chemical found in green plants such as algae, fruit, vegetables, and grains.
- It occurs naturally in fresh food but is destroyed by heat, dehydration, and processing.

Biologic Activity

- MSM is the normal oxidation product of DMSO (dimethyl sulfoxide). It is odor-free and provides sulfur for methionine (Richmond, 1986).
- May bind to surface receptors, preventing binding of parasite and host; therefore may prevent fungal and amebic infections (*Giardia lamblia, Trichomonas vaginalis*).

- May have chemopreventive action (in rats) (McCabe et al., 1986; O'Dwyer et al., 1988)
- Anti-inflammatory; may reduce fibroblast production

Nutritional Sources: Common in raw milk, uncooked grains, fruits, and vegetables

Current Use
- Clinical use to control GI upset and GRD
- Relieves arthritis and musculoskeletal pain (bursitis, carpal tunnel syndrome, fibromyalgia, low back pain, tendinitis)
- May boost the immune system; it has delayed tumor growth in animals
- May benefit allergies and allergic asthma
- Local application (intraurethral) has shown some effectiveness for reducing the inflammation and pain of interstitial cystitis.

Available Forms, Dosage, and Administration Guidelines
Preparations: Crystals, capsules
Typical Dosage: Take 2 to 4 g/day with meals. Clinicians may recommend much higher doses. Follow manufacturer's directions.

Pharmacokinetics—If Available (form or route when known): Not known

Toxicity: None known

Contraindications: None known

Side Effects: Occasional GI upset, diarrhea

Long-Term Safety: Unknown

Use in Pregnancy/Lactation/Children: Unknown; do not use

Drug/Herb Interactions and Rationale (if known): Use cautiously with ASA, heparin, or dicumarol: possible potentiation.

Special Notes: Additional research on this promising sulfur compound is needed to confirm its activity.

BIBLIOGRAPHY

Childs SJ. (1994). Dimethyl sulfone (DMSO$_2$) in the treatment of interstitial cystitis. *Urological Clinics of North America.* 21(1):85–88.

Jacob SW, et al. (1999). *The Miracle of MSM: The Natural Solution for Pain.* New York: GP Putnam's Sons.

Lawrence RM. (1998). Methylsulfonylmethane (MSM): a double-blind study of its use in degenerative arthritis. *International Journal of Antiaging Medicine.* 1(1):50.

McCabe D, et al. (1986). Polar solvents in the chemoprevention of dimethylbenzanthracene-induced rat mammary cancer. *Archives of Surgery.* 121(12):1455–1459.

O'Dwyer P, et al. (1988). Use of polar solvents in chemoprevention of 1,2-dimethylhydrazine-induced colon cancer. *Cancer.* 62(5):944–948.

Review of Natural Products. (1999). St. Louis: Facts and Comparisons.

Richmond V. (1986). Incorporation of methylsulfonylmethane sulfur into guinea pig serum proteins. *Life Science.* 39(3):263–268.

 NAME: Phosphatidylserine

Common Names: PS

Description and Source

- Fatty nutrient present in all cell membranes but is most concentrated in brain cells
- Derived from soybeans (most research was originally performed on cow brain-derived PS)
- Similar to acetylcholine

Biologic Activity

- Memory rejuvenator, particularly in elderly
- Improves cognitive function and may reduce decline in as few as 3 months (Crook, 1992)
- Decreases apathy and withdrawal in elderly (Maggioni et al., 1990)
- Increases brain activity
- Protects cell membranes from oxygen free radical damage
- May increase T-cell activity (Guarcello et al., 1990)

Nutritional Sources: Animal brains (not recommended) and soy

Current Use: Protects brain cells from oxygen free radical damage. May be useful to prevent ischemic damage after strokes. Boosts memory and cognitive function; may benefit patients with Alzheimer's and senile dementia. Can be useful for geriatric depression and menopausal cloudy thinking.

Available Forms, Dosage, and Administration Guidelines: Take 100 to 300 mg three times a day with meals. Action may persist for several months after stopping PS.

Pharmacokinetics—If Available (form or route when known): Not known

Toxicity: Not known

Contraindications: Not known

Side Effects: Nausea with large doses (more than 200 mg)

Long-Term Safety: Probably safe

Use in Pregnancy/Lactation/Children: Not known

Drug/Herb Interactions and Rationale (if known): Not known

Special Notes: Ninety-five percent of all PS is produced by Lucas Meyer in Decatur, Florida, under the trademark Leci-PS. It is packaged for many other companies.

BIBLIOGRAPHY

Abood LG, Host WP. (1975). Stereospecific binding of morphine to phosphatidyl serine. *Psychopharmacology Communications.* 1(1):29–35.

Crook, T, et al. (1992). Effects of phosphatidylserine in Alzheimer's disease. *Psychopharmacology Bulletin.* 28(1):61–66.

Guarcello V, et al. (1990). Phosphatidylserine counteracts physiological and pharmacological suppression of humoral immune response. *Immunopharmacology.* 19(3):185–195.

Maggioni M, et al. (1990). Effects of phosphatidylserine therapy in geriatric patients with depressive disorders. *Acta Psychiatrica Scandinavica.* 81(3):265–270.

NAME: Red-Yeast Rice (*Monascus purpureus*)

Common Names: Cholestin (product name), *xue zhi kang* (Chinese)

Description and Source
- Red yeast fermented in cooked rice
- Red yeast is a natural source of at least 10 cholesterol-lowering chemicals known as HMG-CoA reductase inhibitors (the "statin" drugs).

Biologic Activity
- Mevinolin (chemically similar to but a different compound from lovastatin): lowers cholesterol (Heber et al., 1999)
- Inhibits HMG-CoA reductase, thus limiting cholesterol biosynthesis. Decreases LDL and very-low-density cholesterol and triglycerides, elevates HDL (*Review of Natural Products*, 1997).
- Unsaturated fatty acids, which help lower triglycerides (Heber et al., 1999)
- Inhibits atherosclerotic plaque formation

Nutritional Sources: Used for centuries in China for making rice wine and Peking duck

Current Use: To lower cholesterol

Available Forms, Dosage, and Administration Guidelines
A dosage of 600 mg twice a day with meals delivers 10 mg HMG-CoA reductase inhibitors daily. Do not take more than four capsules in 24 hours. Available from Pharmanex (1-800-800-0255; *www.pharmanex.com*).

Pharmacokinetics—If Available (form or route when known): Not known

Toxicity: None found

Contraindications: Liver disease; intake of more than two alcoholic drinks per day; serious infection; recent surgery; yeast allergies

Side Effects: Mild and similar to those of HMG-CoA drugs: muscle pain, tenderness, weakness, gastric upset

Long-Term Safety: Probably safe

Use in Pregnancy/Lactation/Children
- Pregnancy: do not take—cholesterol is needed for fetal development.
- Lactation/children: do not take

Drug/Herb Interactions and Rationale (if known): Do not take with any cholesterol-lowering drug (Heber et al., 1999).

BIBLIOGRAPHY

Bliznakov EG. (2000). More on the Chinese red-yeast rice supplement and its cholesterol-lowering effect. *American Journal of Clinical Nutrition.* 71(1):152–154.

Heber D. (1999). Dietary supplement or drug? The case for cholestin. *American Journal of Clinical Nutrition.* 70(1):106–108.

Heber D, et al. (1999). Cholesterol-lowering effects of a proprietary Chinese red-yeast-rice dietary supplement. *American Journal of Clinical Nutrition.* 69(2):231–236.

Review of Natural Products. (1997). St. Louis: Facts and Comparisons.

Wigger-Alberti W, et al. (1999). Anaphylaxis due to *Monascus purpureus*-fermented rice (red-yeast rice). *Allergy.* 54(12):1330–1331.

 NAME: SAMe (S-adenosylmethionine)

Common Names: Sammy, SAM

Description and Source
- Synthesized naturally in the body from the amino acid methionine and adenosine triphosphate
- Necessary for mood-building neurotransmitters such as serotonin and dopamine (which it increases) by supplementing carbon where it is needed; folic acid, vitamin B_{12} (cobalamin), and vitamin B_6 (pyridoxine) are also required. Norepinephrine is stabilized.
- SAMe is grown in yeast before conversion to tablets

Biologic Activity
- Contributes to production of glutathione, a major antioxidant (Kaplowitz, 1981)

- Generates taurine and cysteine in the body, essential amino acids (Murray, 1996; Proceedings, 1987)
- Lowers homocysteine, an amino acid associated with heart disease
- Improves nerve function and transmission time by increasing fat found in nerve cell membrane (Cestaro, 1994; Scott et al., 1994)
- Regenerates cartilage (Harmand et al., 1987)
- Enhances liver health (Barak et al., 1993)
- Enhances methylation, the process necessary for making neurotransmitters. SAMe is a methy-group donor (donates one carbon atom and three hydrogen atoms). When there is a shortage of methy-donors, the risk of heart attack and stroke increases, and depression and memory loss occur. SAMe also promotes methylation of phospholipids, which is crucial to maintain the fluidity and responsiveness of nerve cell membranes. Vitamins B_6 and B_{12} and folic acid are also important for methylation (Bressa, 1994; Proceedings, 1987).

Nutritional Sources: Small quantities are found in foods, but not enough for therapeutic benefits.

Current Use
- Discovered in 1952; available in Europe since 1975 by prescription
- Numerous clinical studies have shown SAMe to be as effective or more effective than conventional antidepressants for mild to moderate depression (Bell et al, 1994; Bressa, 1994).
- Arthritis has responded very well to SAMe. SAMe is as effective as nonsteroidal anti-inflammatories without the side effects, such as gastric irritation (Brandt, 1987; Caruso et al., 1987; Harmand et al., 1987).
- Protects against dementia
- Reduces symptoms of Alzheimer's disease, spinal cord degeneration, HIV-type neuropathies (Bottigueri et al., 1994; Lesley et al., 1999)
- Reduces progression of Parkinson's disease
- Improves fatigue, depression, muscle pain, and morning stiffness in fibromyalgia (Murray, 1996)

- Benefits liver disease with depletion of hepatic glutathione (alcohol-induced cirrhosis) and intrahepatic cholestasis

Available Forms, Dosage, and Administration Guidelines: SAMe is very unstable and easily absorbs moisture. Use only enteric-coated tablets in blister packs. Keep SAMe in its packaging until used. Do not take at night; may cause restlessness.

Typical Dosage
- Arthritis: 200 mg three times a day. Begins to reduce inflammation in 3 weeks; begins to build cartilage in about 3 months. Maintenance dose: 200 mg twice a day.
- Mild depression: 400 mg in the morning on an empty stomach and 400 mg before lunch. After 1 week, if depression is not improving, add another 400-mg dose 1 hour before dinner. Most European studies used 800 to 1,600 mg/day.

Pharmacokinetics—If Available (form or route when known): None known

Toxicity: None known

Contraindications: Should not be used in bipolar conditions

Side Effects: Rare: heartburn, nausea, dry mouth, restlessness, diarrhea, headaches, change from depression to mania

Long-Term Safety: Very safe; no reports of toxicity in Europe

Use in Pregnancy/Lactation/Children: Unknown

Drug/Herb Interactions and Rationale (if known): Use cautiously with antidepressants, including supplements such as 5-HTP. Adjust dosages if necessary.

Special Notes: Short-term clinical use (3–4 weeks) in Europe suggests both efficacy and safety of SAMe. Most European studies have used intramuscular SAMe, which is unavailable in the United States. Most studies have been relatively short-term; longer human trials are needed. Most studies of depression used a dosage of 1,600 mg/day. At that dose, it would cost about $230 per month. Product can be obtained from *www.immunesupport.com* (Health Resources, 1-800-366-6056).

BIBLIOGRAPHY

Barak A, et al. (1993). Dietary betaine promotes generation of hepatic S-adenosylmethionine and protects the liver from ethanol-induced fatty infiltration. *Alcohol: Clinical & Experimental Research.* 17(3):552–555.

Bell K, et al. (1994). S-adenosylmethionine blood levels in major depression: changes with drug treatment. *Acta Neurologica Scandinavica.* (Suppl. 154):15–18.

Bottigueri T, et al. (1994). S-adenosylmethionine levels in psychiatric and neurological disorders: a review. *Acta Neurologica Scandinavica* (Suppl. 154):19–26.

Brandt K. (1987). Effects of nonsteroidal anti-inflammatory drugs on chonodrocyte metabolism in vitro and in vivo. *American Journal of Medicine.* 83(5A):29–34.

Bressa GM. (1994). SAMe (S-adenosyl-methionine) as antidepressant: meta-analysis and clinical studies. *Acta Neurologica Scandinavica.* 89(154):7–14.

Brown R, Bottigueri T. (1999). *Stop Depression Now.* New York: Putnam.

Caruso I, et al. (1987). Italian double-blind multicenter study comparing S-adenosylmethionine, naproxen, and placebo in the treatment of degenerative joint disease. *American Journal of Medicine.* 83(5A):66–71.

Cestaro B. (1994). Effects of arginine, S-adenosylmethionine and polyamines on nerve regeneration. *Acta Neurologica Scandinavica.* (Suppl. 154):32–41.

Harmand L, et al. (1987). Effects of S-adenosylmethionine on human articular chondrocyte differentiation and in vitro study. *American Journal of Medicine.* 83(5A):48–54.

Integrative Medicine Access. (2000). *S-adenosylmethionine (SAMe).* Newton, MA: Integrative Medicine Communications.

Kaplowitz N. (1981). The importance and regulation of hepatic glutathione. *Yale Journal of Biology & Medicine.* 54:407–502.

Lesley D, et al. (1999). Brain S-adenosylmethionine levels are severely decreased in Alzheimer's disease. *Journal of Neurochemistry.* 67(3):1328.

Murray M. (1996). *Encyclopedia of Nutritional Supplements.* Rocklin, CA: Prima Publishing.

Proceedings of a Symposium on SAMe. (1987). Osteoarthritis: the clinical picture, pathogenesis, and management with studies on a new therapeutic agent, S-adenosylmethionine. *American Journal of Medicine.* 83(5A):1–110.

The Review of Natural Products. Facts and Comparisons. Wolters Kluwer Company, St Louis, MO, Oct. 1999.

SAMe for depression. (1999). *Medical Letter.* 41(1065):107–108.

Scott J, et al. (1994). Effects of the disruption of transmethylation in the central nervous system: an animal model. *Acta Neurologica Scandinavica.* (Suppl. 154):27–31.

 NAME: Shark Cartilage

Common Names: Spiny dogfish shark (*Squalus acanthias*), hammerhead shark (*Sphyrna lewini*), blue shark (*Prionace glauca*), and other shark species

Description and Source
- Prepared from freshly caught sharks in both the Atlantic and Pacific oceans
- Cartilage is cleaned, shredded, and dried

Biologic Activity
- Tetranectin-like protein: enhances plasminogen and may reduce cancer metastases (Moore et al., 1993); no human studies have confirmed this (Miller et al., 1998)
- Potent angiogenesis inhibitor: U-995 has been isolated from blue shark cartilage. Animal studies have shown potent inhibition of collagenolysis, angiogenesis, and tumor cell growth.
- Squalamine: may have antibacterial activity against gram-positive and gram-negative bacteria (Moore et al., 1993)

Nutritional Sources: In the Orient, shark fin soup has long been a prized delicacy and restorative tonic.

Current Use
- Cancer cure: the rationale is that sharks rarely get cancer. Sharks are cartilaginous fish. Cartilage is avascular and contains agents that inhibit vascularization (angiogenesis). Inhibited vascularization inhibits cancer development, and this is why shark cartilage is theorized to be a treatment for cancer (Masslo Anderson, 1993). Although animal studies have shown some promise, recent research has found no benefit in treating human cancers (Miller et al., 1998).

- Psoriasis: may have anti-inflammatory activity (Dupont et al., 1998; Fontenele et al., 1997)
- Prevention of macular degeneration (Integrative Medicine Access, 2000)

Available Forms, Dosage, and Administration Guidelines

Preparations: Gelatin capsules containing 750 mg shark cartilage without additives or fillers

Typical Dosage
- *Powdered concentrate:* 1 to 2 tbsp daily
- *Ampules:* One per day
- *Capsules:* 750 mg, 3 to 4 capsules per day

Pharmacokinetics—If Available (form or route when known): Not known

Toxicity: No data available

Contraindications: None known

Side Effects: Nausea; one report of hepatitis (Ashar & Vorgo, 1996)

Long-Term Safety: Not known

Use in Pregnancy/Lactation/Children: Unknown; do not use

Drug/Herb Interactions and Rationale (if known): Not known

Special Notes: Studies have found no beneficial effects (Hunt & Connelly, 1995; Miller et al., 1998), so this product cannot be recommended for cancer (Oneschuk et al., 1998). Additional research is ongoing on shark cartilage's anti-inflammatory activity. Overfishing of many types of sharks has depleted their populations. Lack of evidence of the effectiveness of this product and the threatened status of any shark species strongly suggest against using shark cartilage products.

BIBLIOGRAPHY

Ashar B, Vargo E. (1996). Shark cartilage-induced hepatitis. *Annals of Internal Medicine.* 125:780–781.

Berbari P, et al. (1999). Antiangiogenic effects of the oral administration of liquid cartilage extract in humans. *Journal of Surgical Research.* 87(1):108–113.

Dupont E, et al. (1998). Antiangiogenic properties of a novel shark cartilage extract: potential role in the treatment of psoriasis. *Journal of Cutaneous Medicine & Surgery.* 2(3):146–152.

Fontenele JB, et al. (1997). The analgesic and anti-inflammatory effects of shark cartilage are due to a peptide molecule and are nitric oxide (NO) system dependent. *Biology & Pharmacy Bulletin.* 20(11):1151–1154.

Horsman MR, et al. (1998). The effect of shark cartilage extracts on the growth and metastatic spread of the SCCVII carcinoma. *Acta Oncologica.* 37(5):441–445.

Hunt TJ, Connelly JF. (1995). Shark cartilage for cancer treatment. *American Journal of Health-System Pharmacy.* 52:1756–1760.

Integrative Medicine Access. (2000). *Cartilage.* Newton, MA: Integrative Medicine Communications.

Lawrence Review of Natural Products. (1995). St. Louis: Facts and Comparisons.

Masslo Anderson J. (1993). Biotech discovers the shark. *MD Magazine.* 37:43.

Miller DR, et al. (1998). Phase I/II trial of the safety and efficacy of shark cartilage in the treatment of advanced cancer. *Journal of Clinical Oncology.* 16:3649–3655.

Moore KS, et al. (1993). Squalamine: an aminosterol antibiotic from the shark. *Proceedings of the National Academy of Science USA.* 90(4):1354.

Oneschuk D, et al. (1998). The use of complementary medications by cancer patients attending an outpatient pain and symptom clinic. *Journal of Palliative Care.* 14(4):21–26.

Sheu JR, et al. (1998). Effect of U-995, a potent shark cartilage-derived angiogenesis inhibitor, on anti-angiogenesis and anti-tumor activities. *Anticancer Research.* 18(6A):4435–4441.

APPENDICES

Herbs Contraindicated During Pregnancy and Breast-Feeding

HERBS CONTRAINDICATED DURING PREGNANCY

Herb	Latin Name	Action
Andrographis herb	*Andrographis paniculata*	E
Angelica root	*Angelica archangelica*	E
Arnica flowers	*Arnica montana*	AT
Barberry root bark	*Berberis vulgaris*	US
Bethroot	*Trillium erectum*	E
Bitter melon	*Momordica charantia*	E
Black cohosh root	*Cimicifuga racemosa*	E, US
Blessed thistle herb	*Cnicus benedictus*	E
Bloodroot	*Sanguinaria canadensis*	AT, US
Blue cohosh	*Caulophyllum thalictroides*	E, US, T
Blue vervain	*Verbena hastata*	E
Borage herb	*Borago officinalis*	FH
Buchu herb	*Agathosma betulina*	E
Calamus root	*Acorus calamus*	E
Celandine herb	*Chelidonium majus*	US
Celery seed*	*Apium graveolens*	E
Chamomile (Roman)	*Anthemis nobilis*	E
Chaparral herb	*Larrea divaricata*	Possible FH
Chinese coptis	*Coptis teeta*	US
Chinese ligusticum	*Ligusticum chuanxiong*	E
Cinchona bark	*Cinchona* spp.	T, E
Coltsfoot leaves	*Tussilago farfara*	FH
Comfrey root or leaf	*Symphytum officinale*	FH
Cotton root	*Gossypium herbaceum*	E, US
Dan shen root	*Salvia miltiorrhiza*	US

(continued)

HERBS CONTRAINDICATED DURING PREGNANCY—cont'd

Herb	Latin Name	Action
Devil's claw root	*Harpagophytum procumbens*	US
Fenugreek seed*	*Trigonella foenum-graecum*	US, E
Feverfew herb	*Tanacetum parthenium*	E
Goldenseal root	*Hydrastis canadensis*	US
Guarana seed	*Paullinia cupana*	S
Guggal gum resin	*Commiphora mukul*	E
Hyssop herb	*Hyssopus officinalis*	E
Ipecac root	*Cephalis ipecacuanha*	US
Jamaica dogwood bark	*Piscidia erythrina*	AT
Juniper berries	*Juniperus communis*	E, US
Khella seed	*Amni visnaga*	E
Life root	*Senecio aureus*	FH
Lomatium root	*Lomatium disecctum*	E
Ma huang herb	*Ephedra sinica*	CNS stimulant, US
Male fern root	*Dryopteris filix-mas*	AT, E
Mayapple root/ rhizome	*Podophyllum peltatum*	AT, T
Mistletoe herb	*Viscum album*	US
Motherwort herb	*Leonurus cardiaca*	E
Mugwort herb	*Artemisia vulgaris*	E
Mustard seed*	*Brassica nigra*	E
Myrrh gum	*Commiphora* spp.	E
Nutmeg seed*	*Myristica fragrans*	E
Oregon grape root	*Mahonia* spp.	US
Osha root	*Ligusticum porterii*	E
Parsley seed*	*Petroselinum crispus*	E
Pennyroyal herb/ essential oil	*Hedeoma pulegioides*	E, US, AT
Periwinkle herb	*Vinca rosea*	T, E
Petasites rhizome	*Petasites frigida*	H
Picrorrhiza root	*Picrorrhiza kurroa*	E

(continued)

HERBS CONTRAINDICATED DURING PREGNANCY—cont'd

Herb	Latin Name	Action
Pink root	*Spigelia marilandica*	AT
Pleurisy root	*Asclepias tuberosa*	E
Pokeweed root	*Phytolacca americana*	AT, SL, T
Pulsatilla herb	*Anemone pulsatilla*	AT
Pygeum bark	*Prunus africanum*	US
Quassia	*Picrasma excelsa*	US
Rauwolfia root	*Rauwolfia serpentaria*	AT
Rue herb	*Ruta graveolens*	E, US
Sandalwood	*Santalum album*	E
Shepherd's purse herb	*Capsella bursa-pastoris*	US
Tansy herb	*Tanacetum vulgare*	E, US
Thuja	*Thuja occidentalis*	E
Thyme herb*	*Thymus vulgaris*	E
Tienchi ginseng	*Panax pseudo-ginseng*	E
Tobacco leaves	*Nicotiana tabacum*	AT, US, T
Una de gato	*Uncaria tomentosa*	T
Uva-ursi herb/bark	*Arctostyphylos uva-ursi*	US
Wild carrot seed	*Daucus carota*	E
Wild cherry bark	*Prunus serotina*	T
Wild ginger rhizome	*Asarum canadense*	E
Wild indigo	*Baptisia tinctoria*	AT
Wormseed	*Chenopodium ambrosioides*	AT, E
Wormwood	*Artemesia absinthium*	E
Yellow jasmine herb	*Gelsemium sempervirens*	AT
Yellow root	*Xanthorrhiza simplicissema*	US
Yohimbe bark	*Pausinystalia yohimbe*	AT

*Small amounts for culinary use are safe; E, emmenagogue, abortifacient; US, uterine stimulant; FH, fetal hepatotoxin; T, teratogenic; AT, acute toxin; SL, stimulant laxative.

HERBS TO USE ONLY UNDER PROFESSIONAL GUIDANCE DURING PREGNANCY

Black horehound	Kava
Chaste tree	Lobelia
Dong quai	Prickly ash

STIMULANT LAXATIVES (CONTRAINDICATED DURING PREGNANCY BECAUSE THEY CAN STIMULATE CONTRACTIONS)

Herb	Latin Name
Aloe latex	*Aloe* spp.
Blue flag rhizome	*Iris versicolor*
Buckthorn bark	*Rhamnus cathartica*
Cascara sagrada bark	*Rhamnus purshiana*
Castor oil	*Ricinus communus*
Culvers root	*Veronicastrum virginiana*
Rhubarb root	*Rheum palmatum*
Senna herb	*Cassia senna*

HERBS CONTRAINDICATED DURING BREAST-FEEDING

Herb	Latin Name	Action
Aloe latex	*Aloe* spp.	SL
Borage herb	*Borago officinalis*	H
Buckthorn bark	*Rhamnus cathartica*	SL
Cascara sagrada	*Rhamnus purshiana*	SL
Comfrey root and leaf	*Symphytum officinalis*	H
Life root	*Senecio aureus*	H
Ma huang (ephedra) herb	*Ephedra sinica*	S
Mayapple root	*Podophyllum peltatum*	SL, AT
Petasites root	*Petasites frigida*	H
Poke root	*Phytolacca americana*	SL, AT
Pulsatilla herb	*Amemone* spp.	AT
Rhubarb root	*Rheum palmatum*	SL
Rue herb	*Ruta gravelens*	E, US
Sage herb*	*Salvia officinalis*	*
Senna herb	*Cassia senna*	SL
Wild ginger root	*Asarum canadenis*	E, AT

SL, stimulant laxative; H, hepatotoxic; S, CNS stimulant; AT, acute toxin;
*decreases milk flow.

REFERENCES

Brinker F. (1999). *Herb Contraindications and Drug Interactions.* 2nd ed. Sandy, OR: Eclectic Institute, Inc.

De Smet PAGM, et al. (Eds.). (1993). *Adverse Effects of Herbal Drugs,* Vol. 2. Berlin: Springer-Verlag.

De Smet PAGM, et al. (Eds.). (1997). *Adverse Effects of Herbal Drugs,* Vol. 3. Berlin: Springer-Verlag.

Hobbs C, Keville K. (1998). *Women's Herbs, Women's Health.* Loveland, CO: Interweave Press, Inc.

McGuffin M, et al. (eds.). (1997). *Botanical Safety Handbook.* Boca Raton, FL: CRC Press.

Winston D. (2000). *Herbal Therapeutics, Specific Indications for Herbs and Herbal Formulas.* 7th ed. Washington, NJ: Herbal Therapeutics Research Library.

Condition/Disease and Possible Herbal/Supplemental Therapy

Condition/Disease	Possible Herbal/Supplemental Therapy
Achlorhydria	Angelica root, cayenne, ginger, orange peel (Citris)*
Adrenal exhaustion	American ginseng, Asian ginseng, licorice, reishi, schisandra, Siberian ginseng
AIDS	
Immune support	American ginseng, ashwagandha, Asian ginseng, astragalus, cat's claw, reishi, schisandra, shiitake, spirulina, carnitine, lipoic acid, SAMe
Antivirals	Aloe (50:1) extract (oral), bitter melon, garlic, hyssop, rosemary, shiitake, St. John's wort, turmeric
Alcoholism	Kudzu, fresh oat glycerite (Avena)*
Allergies	
Allergic rhinitis	Bilberry/blueberry, eyebright, huang qin, kudzu, licorice, ma huang, nettle leaf, reishi, thyme
Allergic dermatitis	Borage seed oil, calendula (topical), evening primrose seed oil, flaxseed oil/omega-3 fatty acids, gotu kola, huang qin, sarsaparilla, turmeric

(continued)

Possible Herbal/Supplemental Therapy (Continued)

Condition/Disease	Possible Herbal/Supplemental Therapy
Alzheimer's disease	Ashwagandha, basil, ginkgo, lemon balm, rosemary, Siberian ginseng, acetyl-L-carnitine, phosphatidylserine, Bacopa monniera*
Anemia	Ashwagandha, dong quai, nettles, spirulina, parsley (Petroselinum)*
Angina pectoris	Astragalus, dan shen, dong quai, hawthorn, kudzu, carnitine, Co-Q10, cactus (Selenicereus)*
Ankylosing spondylitis	Ashwagandha, gotu kola, hawthorn, licorice, picrorrhiza, reishi, maitake (Grifola)*
Anorexia nervosa	Angelica root, artichoke leaf, dandelion root, fenugreek seed, saw palmetto, Siberian ginseng
Anxiety disorder	Ashwagandha, gotu kola, kava, lavender, lemon balm, motherwort, passion flower, reishi, scullcap, valerian, 5-HTP, blue vervain (Verbena hastata)*
Arrhythmias (mild)	Hawthorn, motherwort, reishi extract, carnitine, Co-Q10
Arteriosclerosis/ atherosclerosis	Cayenne, dan shen, flaxseed, garlic, gingko, grape seed extract, gum guggul, hawthorn, reishi, turmeric, carnitine
Asthma	Angelica root, evening primrose oil, ginkgo, green tea, huang qin (allergic asthma), licorice, lobelia, ma huang, picrorrhiza, reishi, schisandra, thyme, MSM, khella (Amni visnaga)*
Athlete's foot	Lavender essential oil, myrrh, tea tree essential oil, thyme essential oil
Attention deficit disorder	Lemon balm, hawthorn, rosemary, Siberian ginseng, basil (Ocimum sanctum),* linden flower (Tilea),* Bacopa monniera*
Autoimmune disorders	Dan shen, flaxseed oil/omega-3 fatty acids, huang qin, licorice, picrorrhiza, reishi, maitake (Grifola)*
Bacterial vaginosis	Garlic, goldenseal, usnea*

Bedwetting	Ma huang, raspberry, St. John's wort
Benign prostatic hyperplasia	Nettle root, pygeum bark, saw palmetto, soy, agrimony (Agrimonia),* pumpkin seed oil,* rye pollen,* zinc*
Biliary dyskinesia	Angelica, artichoke leaf, barberry, blessed thistle, dandelion root, gentian, lavender, yarrow, wild yam
Blepharitis	Calendula, flaxseed, goldenseal
Bronchitis	Black cohosh, Boswellia, echinacea, fenugreek, garlic, huang qin, hyssop, licorice, plantain, red clover, saw palmetto, thyme
Buerger's disease	Dong quai, dan shen, hawthorn, Co-Q10
Burns (topical application)	Aloe gel, calendula, echinacea, gotu kola, lavender essential oil, plantain, St. John's wort
Bursitis	Black cohosh, Boswellia, grape seed extract, meadowsweet, sarsaparilla, turmeric, willow, MSM
Cancer	
General preventive/ immune stimulation	Aloe (50:1) extract (oral), ashwagandha, Asian ginseng, astragalus, bilberry/blueberry, burdock root, cat's claw, flaxseed, garlic, grape seed extract, green tea, kudzu, reishi, Siberian ginseng, turmeric, Co-Q10, lipoic acid, lycopene, maitake (Grifola),* violet leaf (Viola),* green tea
Breast cancer	American ginseng, flaxseed, green tea, melatonin, red clover, soy
Colon cancer	Cat's claw, flaxseed, turmeric
Prostate cancer	Flaxseed, green tea, nettle root, saw palmetto, soy
Candidiasis	Barberry, echinacea, goldenseal, Oregon grape root, pau d'arco, tea tree essential oil, Chinese coptis (Coptis teeta)*

(continued)

Possible Herbal/Supplemental Therapy (Continued)

Condition/Disease	Possible Herbal/Supplemental Therapy (Continued)
Carpal tunnel syndrome	Ginger, sarsaparilla, St. John's wort, turmeric
Chronic fatigue syndrome	American ginseng, ashwagandha, Asian ginseng, astragalus, gotu kola, licorice, reishi, schisandra, shiitake, Siberian ginseng, carnitine
Cirrhosis of the liver	Artichoke leaf, dong quai, licorice, milk thistle, picrorrhiza, schisandra, turmeric, lipoic acid, SAMe
Cold sores	Calendula, chamomile, goldenseal, lavender essential oil, lemon balm, myrrh
Colitis	Chamomile, flaxseed, kudzu, slippery elm, yarrow
Common cold	Andrographis, echinacea, ginger, hyssop, meadowsweet, thyme, yarrow, catnip (Nepeta), elderberry (Sambucus)*
Congestive heart failure (mild)	Astragalus, dan shen, dandelion leaf (edema), dong quai, hawthorn, kudzu, carnitine, Co-Q10, cactus (Selenicereus)*
Conjunctivitis (eyewash)	Barberry, calendula, goldenseal, Oregon grape root
Constipation	Aloe gel (mild), artichoke, dandelion root, fenugreek, flaxseed, psyllium seed, slippery elm, butternut bark (Juglans cineraria)*
Coughs	
Dry coughs	Coltsfoot, fenugreek, flaxseed, licorice, psyllium seed, saw palmetto, slippery elm, ginger, thyme, horehound (Marrubium),* yerba santa (Eriodictyon),* thyme, black cohosh, licorice, lobelia
Wet coughs	
Spastic coughs	
Crohn's disease	Cat's claw, dan shen, kudzu, licorice, reishi, slippery elm

Condition/Disease	Possible Herbal/Supplemental Therapy
Cystitis	Barberry root, cranberry, echinacea, Oregon grape root, meadowsweet, uva ursi, MSM
Depression (mild/moderate)	American ginseng, ashwagandha, black cohosh (menopausal), ginkgo, gotu kola, lavender, lemon balm, rosemary, schisandra, Siberian ginseng, St. John's wort, 5-HTP, melatonin, phosphatidyserine, SAMe, basil (Ocimum sanctum)*
Diabetes (type II)	Asian ginseng, astragalus, bitter melon, cinnamon, evening primrose seed oil, fenugreek, grape seed extract, guggul, gymnema, chromium, Co-Q10, lipoic acid
Diabetic retinopathy	Bilberry/blueberry, ginkgo, grape seed extract, lipoic acid, lutein*
Diarrhea	Barberry, bilberry/blueberry, cat's claw, chamomile, cinnamon, flaxseed, garlic, ginger, goldenseal, huang, kudzu, meadowsweet, plantain, psyllium seed, raspberry leaf, schisandra, slippery elm, yarrow
Diverticulitis	Cat's claw, kudzu, plantain, sarsaparilla, slippery elm, turmeric, wild yam, yarrow
Dry skin	Evening primrose seed oil, flaxseed oil/omega-3 fatty acids
Eczema	Borage seed oil, burdock seed, calendula (topical), chamomile (topical), echinacea (topical), evening primrose seed oil, flaxseed oil/omega-3 fatty acids, gotu kola
Edema	Dandelion leaf, gotu kola, green tea, hawthorn, nettle leaf
Emphysema	Astragalus, thyme, prince seng (Pseudostellaria)*
Endometriosis	Black cohosh, blue cohosh (pain), chaste tree
Fatigue	Ashwuganda, American ginseng, Asian ginseng, gotu kola, guarana (stimulant), reishi, schisandra, Siberian ginseng, St. John's wort, L-carnitine
Fibrocystic disease	Burdock root, chaste tree, red clover, red root (Ceanothus),* violet leaf (Viola)*of the breast

(continued)

Condition/Disease	Possible Herbal/Supplemental Therapy (Continued)
Fibroids, uterine	Chaste tree, cinnamon, dong quai, white ash bark (Fraxinus),* white peony (Peonia)
Fibromyalgia syndrome	American ginseng, ashwagandha, black cohosh, kava, carnitine, 5-HTP, MSM, SAMe
Flatulence	Angelica, artichoke, blessed thistle, chamomile, cinnamon, dandelion root, lavender, lemon balm, peppermint, rosemary, thyme, yarrow, catnip (Nepeta),* fennel (Foeniculum)
Gastric ulcers	Aloe gel, bilberry/blueberry, calendula, cinnamon, garlic, goldenseal, grape seed extract, licorice, meadowsweet, pau d'arco, plantain, thyme, yarrow, Co-Q10
Gastroenteritis	Chamomile, licorice, marshmallow, meadowsweet, plantain, yarrow
Gastroesophageal reflux disorder (GERD)	Chamomile, devil's claw, meadowsweet, slippery elm, wild yam, MSM
Gingivitis/pyorrhea	Calendula, echinacea, goldenseal, myrrh, tea tree essential oil, Co-Q10
Headache	
Migraine	Black cohosh, chaste tree (PMS migraine), evening primrose seed oil, feverfew, ginger (nausea), guarana, 5-HTP
Stress-induced	Chamomile, hops, kava, lemon balm, meadowsweet, motherwort, passion flower, rosemary, scullcap, valerian, willow
Hemorrhoids	Aloe gel (topical), bilberry/blueberry, horse chestnut, plantain (topical), yarrow, collinsonia (C. canadensis),* Figwort (Scrophularia)*
Hepatitis B and C	Andrographis, artichoke leaf, bitter melon, dan shen, huang qin, licorice, milk thistle, picrorrhiza, reishi, schisandra, shiitake, St. John's wort, turmeric, lipoic acid

Herpes	
Simplex I & II	Bitter melon, hyssop, lemon balm, licorice, pau d'arco, reishi, shiitake, St. John's wort
Zoster	Lemon balm, licorice, St. John's wort, capsaicin cream (topical pain relief)
Hyperacidity (gastric)	Meadowsweet, slippery elm
Hyperinsulinemia (syndrome X)	Artichoke leaf, Asian ginseng, cinnamon, dandelion root, carnitine, chromium
Hyperlipidemia	Artichoke leaf, cayenne, fenugreek, flaxseed, gum guggul, hawthorn, psyllium seed, reishi, shiitake, spirulina
Hypertension (mild/moderate)	Black haw, dandelion leaf, dan shen, evening primrose seed oil, garlic, grape seed extract, hawthorn, huang qin, kava, linden flower, motherwort, olive leaf, reishi, spirulina, red yeast rice
Hyperthyroidism	Lemon balm, motherwort, brassicas,* bugleweed (Lycopus)*
Hypoglycemia	American ginseng, dandelion root
Hypothyroidism	Gum guggul, schisandra
Immune deficiency	American ginseng, Asian ginseng, astragalus, licorice, reishi, saw palmetto, schisandra, shiitake, Siberian ginseng
Impotence	Ashwagandha, ginkgo, yohimbe, muira-puama (Liriosma)*
Indigestion	Artichoke leaf, chamomile, dandelion root, devil's claw, gentian root, ginger, lavender, meadowsweet, peppermint, thyme
Influenza	Andrographis, echinacea, ginger, hyssop, pau d'arco, St. John's wort, willow, yarrow, elderberry (Sambucus)*

(continued)

Condition/Disease	Possible Herbal/Supplemental Therapy *(Continued)*
Insomnia	Ashwagandha, black cohosh (menopausal), chamomile, dan shen, hops, kava, lavender, passion flower, reishi, scullcap, valerian, 5-HTP, melatonin
Interstitial cystitis	Kava (for pain), plantain, saw palmetto, MSM, couch grass *(Elymus repens)**
Irritable bowel syndrome	Cat's claw, chamomile, evening primrose seed oil, hops, kudzu, licorice, meadowsweet, peppermint essential oil, sarsaparilla, slippery elm, wild yam, yarrow
Jaundice	Artichoke leaf, dan shen, huang qin, milk thistle, picrorrhiza, turmeric
Kidney disease	Dan shen, nettle leaf, nettle seed, Corydyceps*
Macular degeneration	Bilberry/blueberry, grape seed extract, ginkgo, lycopene, lutein*
Memory problems	Ashwagandha, Asian ginseng, ginkgo, gotu kola, lavender, reishi, rosemary, schisandra, acetyl-L-carnitine, phosphatidyserine, SAMe, *Bacopa monniera*,* basil *(Ocimum sanctum)**
Meniere's disease	Ginger, ginkgo
Menopausal problems	
Hot flashes, night sweats	Black cohosh, chaste tree, dong quai, flaxseed, motherwort, red clover, soy
Anxiety, insomnia	Chamomile, kava, lavender, motherwort, passion flower, blue vervain *(Verbena hastata)**
Menstrual cramps	Angelica, black cohosh, black haw, chamomile, chaste tree, dong quai, feverfew, motherwort
Morning sickness	Chamomile, ginger, raspberry leaf, wild yam
Muscle spasm	Ashwagandha, black cohosh root, black haw, kava, lobelia, Roman chamomile, scullcap, valerian

Nausea/vomiting	Angelica, cinnamon, chamomile, blessed thistle, ginger, hyssop, lavender, lemon balm, peppermint, rosemary, thyme
Obesity	Ephedra, gum guggul (used with *Triphila*), *Gymnema*, yohimbe
Osteoarthritis	Ashwagandha, black cohosh, *Boswellia*, cayenne (capsaicin cream topically), dandelion root, devil's claw, feverfew, ginger, grape seed extract, gum guggul, meadowsweet, nettle leaf, turmeric, chondroitin, glucosamine sulfate, SAMe
Osteoporosis	Black cohosh, kudzu, red clover, soy, boron,* calcium*
Otitis media	Echinacea, eyebright, garlic, goldenseal, kudzu, plantain, thyme
Pancreatitis	Milk thistle, fringe tree (*Chionanthus*),* red root (*Ceanothus*)*
Peripheral vascular disease	Blueberry, cayenne, cinnamon, ginger, ginkgo, hawthorn, horse chestnut, alpha-lipoic acid, L-carnitine, prickly ash (*Zanthoxylum*)*
Pneumonia	Andrographis, echinacea, garlic, huang qin, hyssop, elecampane *(Inula)**
Premenstrual syndrome	Barberry, black cohosh, black haw, blue cohosh, borage seed oil, chaste tree, dong quai, evening primrose seed oil, flaxseed oil/omega-3 fatty acids, ginkgo, lavender, motherwort
Prostatitis	Echinacea, pygeum bark
Psoriasis	Barberry, borage seed oil, burdock seed, evening primrose oil, flaxseed oil/omega-3 fatty acids, gotu kola, guggal, Oregon grape root, picrorrhiza, sarsaparilla
Pyelonephritis	Cranberry juice, huang qin, uva ursi
Raynaud's disease	Bilberry/blueberry, cayenne, dong quai, ginger, ginkgo, horse chestnut

(continued)

Condition/Disease	Possible Herbal/Supplemental Therapy (Continued)
Rheumatoid arthritis	Ashwagandha, borage seed oil, Boswellia, flaxseed oil/omega-3 fatty acids, ginger, picrorrhiza, reishi, sarsaparilla, turmeric, willow, chondroitin, maitake (Grifola)*
Seasonal affective disorder	Lavender, lemon balm, St. John's wort
Sore throat	Burdock seed, cinnamon, echinacea, hyssop, licorice, myrrh, thyme, sage (Salvia)*
Systemic lupus erythematosus	Ashwagandha, flaxseed oil/omega-3 fatty acids, gotu kola, huang qin, licorice, reishi, maitake (Grifola)*
Tendinitis	Devil's claw, grape seed extract, hawthorn, St. John's wort, sarsaparilla
Tinnitus	Ginkgo, kudzu
Ulcerative colitis	Boswellia, calendula, chamomile, flaxseed, kudzu, plantain, slippery elm, yarrow
Uterine prolapse	Raspberry leaf
Vertigo	Ginger, ginkgo, kudzu
Vitiligo	Picrorrhiza, psorela seed (Psoralea)*
Warts	
Common (topical)	Dandelion latex, garlic, celandine latex (Chelidonium)*
Venereal (topical)	Calendula, goldenseal, thuja (T. occidentalis)*

*Not covered in this text; see Appendix C.

An Annotated Guide to Recommended References

HERBAL MEDICINE

Eldin S, Dunford A. (1999). *Herbal Medicine in Primary Care.* Oxford: Butterworth-Heinemann. A handbook for practitioners who want to integrate good herbal medicine into a primary care practice. Written by a British herbalist and a physician, it offers useful insights into the benefits of phytotherapy.

ESCOP Monographs on the Medicinal Uses of Plant Drugs. (1999). Exeter, UK: Author. Detailed monographs on plant drugs commonly used in European phytotherapy.

Hobbs C. (1995). *Medicinal Mushrooms.* (2nd ed.). Santa Cruz, CA: Botanica Press. The most comprehensive guide to medicinal fungi, complete with research and clinical information.

Hoffmann D. (1992). *Therapeutic Herbalism.* Santa Rosa, CA: Author. A notebook of practical clinical herbal medicine that includes therapeutics, phytochemistry, and materia medica.

McGuffin M, et al. (1997). *American Herbal Products Association's Botanical Safety Handbook.* Boca Raton, FL: CRC Press. Guide to the safety, toxicity, and contraindications of botanical medicines.

Mills S. (1991). *The Essential Book of Herbal Medicine.* This title is currently out of print, but finding a used copy will be worth your efforts. Mills is a prominent English herbalist who in this book creates a synthesis of Eastern and Western herbal practices. He combines Eastern energetics with Western physiology to explain herbal therapies in a an easy-to-understand manner.

Mills S, Bone K. (1999). *Principles and Practice of Phytotherapy.* Edinburgh: Churchill Livingstone. An exceptional work combining the knowledge of English herbal medicine and modern scientific research. The materia medica is small (only 40 herbs), but each plant is covered in a wonderfully

detailed and accurate monograph. The section on
therapeutics is one of the best in all of herbal literature.

Mitchell W. (1999). *Plant Medicine: Applications of the
Botanical Remedies in the Practice of Naturopathic Medicine.*
Seattle: Author. Dr. Bill Mitchell (*wmitchell@seanet.com*) is
one of the most respected naturopathic physicians in the
United States. This preparatory manuscript is an
accumulation of his and his teachers' more than 60 years of
clinical practice and experience.

Moore M. (1993). *Medicinal Plants of the Pacific West.* Santa
Fe, NM: Red Crane Books. Michael Moore is one of the
most respected and talented American herbalists in the
past 30 years. This title, as well as his study guide series,
offers clear, insightful, humorous, and effective
information on the use of herbs in clinical practice.
His SWSBM study guides can be ordered from eherbs at
www.eherbsplus.com.

Moore M. (1990). *Herbal Repertory in Clinical Practice.* (3rd
ed.). A manual of differential therapeutics in 23 sections,
with a cross-index of symptoms. Dose and media are found
in the herbal materia medica.

Moore M. (1995). *Herbal Energetics in Clinical Practice.* A
concise approach to defining constitutional imbalances by
evaluating organ systems, patterns of stress, and imbalances
in fluid transport; discussing the herbs that will strengthen
any deficient functions; and explaining their physiologic
effects. A sample patient questionnaire, formula worksheet,
and record form are included. Thirteen pages of graphs
provide a metabolic profile for more than 400 widely used
herbs, showing their primary and secondary effects on organ
systems and on neuroendocrine functions. Evaluating these
overt and covert effects can both prevent unwanted synergies
and define the iatrogenic potential for professional or OTC
herb formulas.

Moore M. (1995). *Herbal Formulas for Clinic and Home.*
Herbal formulas, compounds, and recipes for the clinician
and the adventurous. A diverse collection of formulations,
ranging from constitutional tonics to cough syrups,
suppositories to garam masala, tea blends to tooth powders,
and ointments to guarana fudge.

Moore M. (1995). *Herbal Materia Medica* (5th ed.). A brief outline of more than 400 botanical medicines, giving preparation methods, strengths, media, and common adult dosages.

Moore M. (1995). *Herbal/Medical Dictionary.* A glossary of terms used in herbalism, medicine, and physiology, giving descriptions, explanations, and implications for involved holistic and vitalist therapy and a dictionary for terms used in the other manuals.

Moore M. (1995). *Herbal Tinctures in Clinical Practice.* (3rd ed.). A concise manual for the health care professional, giving symptom pictures, dosages, side effects, and contraindications for 166 botanicals best used as tinctures. Preparations follow herbal materia medica.

Moore M. (1997). *Specific Indications.* (2nd ed.). More than 400 herbs, formulas, and essential oils, with their specific clinical indications in botanical medicine.

Trickey R. (1998). *Women, Hormones, and the Menstrual Cycle.* St. Leonards, Australia: Allen & Unwin. An exceptional work by an Australian medical herbalist; combines detailed knowledge of female physiology, gynecology, and the use of herbs to treat female reproductive problems.

Upton R. (Ed.). *The American Herbal Pharmacopoeia and Therapeutic Compendium.* Santa Cruz, CA: AHP. An important scholarly project that brings together the most accurate information on each herb covered in this ongoing series. So far, monographs include astragalus, black haw, cramp bark, hawthorn berry, hawthorn flower and leaf, schisandra, St. John's wort, and willow bark. Each monograph includes the botany, history, pharmacognosy, clinical uses, and relevant research on the herb.

Weiss RF. (1988). *Herbal Medicine.* Beaconsfield, UK: Beaconsfield Publishing. Weiss's text is a testament to 50 years of practice as an herbal physician (MD) in Germany. His book is full of clinical pearls left out of most texts. An exceptional guide for the physician wanting to include good herbal medicine into his or her practice. Now out of print; finding a used copy would be worthwhile.

Weiss RF, Fintelmann V. (2000). *Herbal Medicine.* Stuttgart: Thieme. The new edition of this text is not as useful as the

book it replaces. Although it still offers valuable information
for the physician, nurse, or herbalist, it is less experiential
and based more on the very flawed German Commission E
monographs.

Yance D. (1999). *Herbal Medicine, Healing and Cancer.* The
author of this book specializes in the treatment of cancer. He
is an herbalist who works closely with prominent oncologists
and has won their respect and admiration for his knowledge,
compassion, and clinical skills. This book shares many
insights from his 20 years of clinical practice.

ECLECTIC TEXTS

All of the following texts contain outdated terminology and
medical concepts, but despite these limitations, they provide
superb insights into the use of botanical medicine in daily clinical practice.

Ellingwood F. (1919). *The American Materia Medica,
Therapeutics, and Pharmacognosy.* [Reprint of the 1919 2nd
ed.]. Sandy, OR: Eclectic Medical Publishers. Dr.
Ellingwood was an excellent clinician and his book provides
a remarkable view into the use of botanical remedies. He
includes specific indications for each medicine to help the
clinician develop a clear understanding of the benefits of
each herb.

Felter HW, Lloyd JU. (1919). *Kings American Dispensatory.*
[Reprint of 1919 19th ed.]. Sandy, OR: Eclectic Medical
Publishers. This huge two-volume reference contains the
accumulated knowledge on the eclectic materia medica from
thousands of physicians over a period of 90 years.

Felter HW. (1922). *The Eclectic Materia Medica, Pharmacology,
and Therapeutics.* [Reprint of 1922 ed.]. Sandy, OR: Eclectic
Medical Publishers. Another excellent reference to the use of
the (mostly botanical) eclectic remedies. Felter clearly notes
the uses as well as the limitations of each herbal medicine.

Jones E. (1911). *Cancer, Its Causes, Symptoms and Treatment.*
[Reprint of 1911 ed.]. India: Jain Publishing; available from
Homeopathic Education Resources, Berkeley, CA. Dr. Eli
Jones was the pre-eminent cancer specialist of his day. His

therapies are not only of historical interest but also provide many valuable clinical insights for the botanical treatment of cancer today.

Jones E. (1919). *Definite Medication.* [Reprint of 1919 ed.]. Pomeroy, WA: Health Research (*publish@pomeroy-wa.com*). Dr. Jones was perhaps the most eclectic of all eclectic physicians. He was trained as an allopathic physician, an eclectic, a homeopath, and a physiomedicalist. He practiced each of these unique forms of medicine for more than 50 years and combined the best of each into a system he called definite medication.

CHINESE MEDICINE

Bensky D, Barolet R. (1990). *Chinese Herbal Medicine— Formulas and Strategies.* Seattle: Eastland Press. Rarely are Chinese herbs used as single herbs. This complete text reviews the major TCM formulas, how they are applied to illness, and how they can be altered to fit the patient.

Bensky D, Gamble A. (1993). *Chinese Herbal Medicine: Materia Medica.* Seattle: Eastland Press. A Bencao or Chinese materia medica that is comprehensive and nicely put together. The individual medicines (herbs, minerals, animal parts) are discussed from a TCM perspective.

Bone K. (1996). *Clinical Applications of Ayurvedic and Chinese Herbs.* Queensland, Australia: Phytotherapy Press. A succinct materia medica of the best-known Chinese and Ayurvedic herbs. The focus is on Western medical uses of these Asian plants.

Maccioca G. (1993). *Foundations of Chinese Medicine.* Edinburgh: Churchill Livingstone. If you don't understand the philosophy and theories of TCM, this book is the best place to learn an entirely new way of perceiving health and disease.

You-Ping Z. (1998). *Chinese Materia Medica: Chemistry, Pharmacology, and Applications.* Amsterdam: Harwood Academic Publishers. Very useful clinical guide to Chinese materia medica, including TCM uses as well as clinical studies and recent research data.

NUTRITION/COMPLIMENTARY ALTERNATIVE MEDICINE

Erasmus U. (1995). *Fats That Heal, Fats That Kill: The Complete Guide to Fats, Oils, Cholesterol and Human Health.* Vancouver, Canada: Alive Books. Despite this book's alarmist title, it is the best introduction to the topic of dietary fats and fatty acid metabolism.

Heber D, et al. (1999). *Nutritional Oncology.* San Diego: Academic Press. An excellent clinical reference to diet and nutrition as they relate to cancer.

Integrative Medicine Access. (2000). *Integrative Medicine Communications.* Newton, MA: Author. Ongoing botanical and nutritional reference compiled by medical doctors, pharmacognosists, herbalists, and naturopathic physicians. Sections include herbal medicines, supplements, and medical conditions.

Pizzorno J, Murray M. (1999). *Textbook of Natural Medicine.* (2nd ed.). Edinburgh: Churchill Livingstone. Detailed text on the practice of naturopathic medicine and naturopathic therapies (nutritional, botanical, hydrotherapy, homeopathy, and so forth).

Werbach M, Moss J. (1999). *Textbook of Nutritional Medicine.* Tarzana, CA: Third Line Press. Two experienced clinicians combined their knowledge and experience to create an encyclopedia of nutritional therapies for treating disease.

RECOMMENDED JOURNALS FOR CLINICIANS

European Journal of Herbal Medicine: National Institute of Medical Herbalists, 56 Longbrook St., Exeter, Devon, EX4 6AH, UK; e-mail: *herbmed@dialopipex.com*

HerbalGram: P.O. Box 144345, Austin, TX, 78714-4345; Website: *www.herbalgram.org*

Journal of the American Herbalists Association: AHG, 1931 Gaddis Rd., Canton, GA, 30015; Website: *www.healthy.net/herbalists/*

Medical Herbalism: P.O. Box 20512, Boulder, CO, 80308; Website: *www.medherb.com*

Modern Phytotherapist: Mediherb, Ltd., P.O. Box 713, Warwick, Queensland, 4370 Australia; e-mail: *reception@mediherb.com.au*

WEBSITES

American Botanical Counsel (*www.herbalgram.org*): A great assortment of information about herbs with an especially nice introduction for beginners and excellent links to other herbal sites.

Henriette's Herbal Homepage (*megalab.unc.edu/herbmed*): An eclectic assortment of good herb information with many good links.

Herb Research Foundation (*www.herbs.org*): Good reviews of the most recent research in herbal medicine. Offers many good links.

Soaring Bear (*www.dkotacom.net/~bear/*): Researcher Soaring Bear has put together an impressive compilation of biochemistry, herbal, medical, and pharmacy sites.

Southwest School of Herbal Medicine (*chili.rt66.com/hrbmoore/HOMEPAGE*): Michael Moore's homepage. Includes great information on herbs and education, plus plant images and research reviews.

PROFESSIONAL ORGANIZATIONS

Herbalists

American Herbalists Guild (AHG), 1931 Gaddis Rd., Canton, GA, 30115; phone: 770-751-6021; Website: *www.healthy.net/herbalists/*

Nutritionists

International American Association of Clinical Nutritionists (IAACN), 16775 Addison Rd., Suite 102, Addison, TX, 75001; phone: 972-407-9089

Explanation of Abbreviations

ACH	acetylcholine
ADD	attention deficit disorder
ADHD	attention deficit hyperactivity disorder
ADP	adenosine diphosphate
AIDS	acquired immunodeficiency syndrome
ALA	alpha-linolenic acid
ASA	aspirin
BPH	benign prostatic hypertrophy
Ca++	calcium
CFS	chronic fatigue syndrome
CHF	congestive heart failure
CNS	central nervous system
COPD	chronic obstructive pulmonary disease
EFAs	essential fatty acids
EO	essential oil
ERT	estrogen replacement therapy
ETOH	ethanol, alcohol
FDA	Food and Drug Administration
FOS	fructo-oligo-saccharides
GABA	gamma-amino-butyric acid
GLA	gamma-linolenic acid
GH	growth hormone
GI	gastrointestinal
GRAS	generally recognized as safe
GRD	gastric reflux disease
HDL	high-density lipoprotein
HIV	human immunodeficiency virus
HPA	hypothalamus-pituitary-adrenal axis
INR	International Normalized Ratio
LDL	low-density lipoprotein
LH	luteinizing hormone
MI	myocardial infarction
MRSA	methicillin-resistant *Staphylococcus aureus*
MS	multiple sclerosis

NK	natural killer (cells)
OPC	oligomeric procyanidins
OTC	over the counter
PAF	platelet activating factor
PMNC	polymorphonuclear cells
PMNNC	polymorphonuclear neutrophil cells
PO	by mouth
PVCs	premature ventricular contractions
REM	rapid eye movement
SGPT	serum glutamatic-pyruvatic transaminase
SLE	systemic lupus erythematosus
SOD	superoxide dismutase
TCM	traditional Chinese medicine
TMJ	temporomandibular joint
TNF	tumor necrosis factor
UTIs	urinary tract infections
WHO	World Health Organization

Glossary

Glossary of Herbal/Medical Terms That May Not be in Current Medical Dictionaries

Adaptogen: A substance that helps a living organism adapt to stress (environmental, physical, or psychological). According to the Soviet researcher I. I. Brekhman, who did most of the early research on adaptogens, these substances have very low toxicity, have little physiologic effect in healthy organisms, and improve endocrine, immune, and nervous system function in stressed subjects. Examples: Asian ginseng, Siberian ginseng.

Alterative: A substance that, by increasing elimination, helps to alter an unhealthy state into a healthier one; also known as a "blood purifier." Examples: burdock root, sarsaparilla.

Amphoteric: An herb that normalizes the function or activity of an organ. It can either potentiate a deficient immune response or reduce excessive immune activity in conditions such as autoimmune diseases. Example: reishi.

Antihepatotoxin: A hepatoprotective; a substance that prevents liver damage and helps to improve liver function in hepatic disease caused by alcohol, solvents, and viruses. Examples: milk thistle, picrorrhiza.

Biliary dyskinesia: Improper bile flow associated with regulatory failure of the biliary system, pancreas, duodenum, and jejunum

Bitter tonic: A bitter-tasting herb that stimulates digestive, absorptive, and eliminatory functions. Bitters before or with meals increase gastric HCl production, bile secretion, pancreatic and small intestine juices, and bowel function. Examples: artichoke, gentian.

Borborygmus: Intestinal rumbling or gurgling, usually associated with flatulence and abdominal bloating

Carminative: An herb that relaxes the intestinal sphincters, relieving gas pain, and, as a result of high levels of volatile oils, reduces gas formation. Examples: chamomile, fennel.

Cholagogue: An herb that stimulates bile production. Examples: artichoke, dandelion root.

Choleretic: An herb that stimulates bile flow; usually considered interchangeable with the term cholagogue

Decoction: A method of making tea in which the plant material (usually bark or root) is gently simmered to increase the extraction of its constituents

Diaphoretic: A substance that gently increases body temperature and stimulates sweating to lower fevers. Examples: elderflower, yarrow.

Dysbiosis: Abnormal digestion and bowel flora causing flatulence, borborygmus, belching

Emmenagogue: An herb that stimulates menstrual flow. If taken during pregnancy, emmenagogues can cause abortion. Examples: blue cohosh, pennyroyal.

Galactogogue: An herb that stimulates milk flow in breast-feeding mothers. Examples: fennel seed, milk thistle leaf.

Hyperinsulinemia (syndrome X): A cell-level insulin resistance with compensatory elevated insulin levels. Clinical manifestations include elevated triglyceride levels, decreased HDL cholesterol, elevated cortisol levels, abdominal obesity, and a host of cardiovascular and systemic illnesses (atherosclerosis, hypertension, type 2 diabetes, PCOD). The causes of Syndrome X include excessive intake of calories, carbohydrates, and omega-6 fatty acids (relative to omega-3 fatty acids), mineral deficiencies (magnesium, chromium), and lack of exercise.

Infusion: A method of making tea in which the plant material (usually leaf or flower) is steeped. Heat-sensitive materials are best prepared by this method.

Nervine: An herb that tonifies the nervous system, producing a mild sense of relaxation. Examples: chamomile, lemon balm.

Rubefacient: A substance that acts as a counterirritant, causing increased localized blood flow and irritation. Examples: cayenne, ginger.

Solid extract: Also known as a native extract, this is a highly concentrated extract, usually in a glycerin or honey base. A good way to take blueberry or hawthorn fruit.

Tincture: A hydroalcoholic extract of an herb. Tinctures made with dry herbs are usually prepared in a ratio of 1 part herb to 5 parts menstruum (1:5). Fresh plant (green) tinctures are usually prepared in a ratio of 1 part fresh herb to 2 parts menstruum (1:2).

Trophorestorative: An herb that nourishes, strengthens, and tonifies a specific organ or function. Considered "food for the organ." Hawthorn, with its specificity for the heart and circulatory system, is a cardiovascular trophorestorative. Examples: fresh oat (nervous system), nettle seed (kidney).

Vulnerary: An old term for wound-healing plants. Vulneraries tend to have antibacterial, anti-inflammatory, and pro-cuticularization activities. They reduce healing time, prevent infection, increase granulation of tissue, and prevent scarring. Examples: calendula, plantain.

INDEX